Using Nutrigenomics within Personalized Nutrition

Personalized Nutrition and Lifestyle Medicine for Healthcare Practitioners
Edited by Lorraine Nicolle, this series of accessible, evidence-based, practical guides is essential reading for practitioners and students of clinical nutrition, and all other primary and complementary healthcare professionals interested in an approach that responds to the unique health needs of every individual. Each book in the series is a powerful new tool to help practitioners achieve significant clinical improvements for their clients/patients through the cutting-edge paradigm of personalized nutrition and lifestyle medicine.

Lorraine Nicolle MSc is a Registered Nutritionist (MBANT) and an educator and author in personalized nutrition. www.lorrainenicollenutrition.co.uk

in the same series

Case Studies in Personalized Nutrition
Edited by Angela Walker
ISBN 978 1 84819 394 9
eISBN 978 0 85701 351 4

Mitochondria in Health and Disease
Ray Griffiths
Foreword by Lorraine Nicolle
ISBN 978 1 84819 332 1
eISBN 978 0 85701 288 3

of related interest

Oral Health and Systemic Disease
A Clinical Guide for Nutritional Therapists and Functional Medicine Practitioners
Rose Holmes
ISBN 978 1 84819 411 3
eISBN 978 0 85701 366 8

Biochemical Imbalances in Disease
A Practitioner's Handbook
Edited by Lorraine Nicolle and Ann Woodriff Beirne
ISBN 978 1 84819 033 7
eISBN 978 0 85701 028 5

Using Nutrigenomics within Personalized Nutrition

Part of

Personalized Nutrition and Lifestyle
Medicine for Healthcare Practitioners *series*

Anne Pemberton

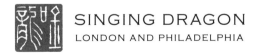

SINGING DRAGON
LONDON AND PHILADELPHIA

First published in Great Britain in 2022 by Singing Dragon
An imprint of Jessica Kingsley Publishers
An imprint of Hodder & Stoughton Ltd
An Hachette Company

1

A CIP catalogue record for this title is available from the
British Library and the Library of Congress

ISBN 978 1 84819 413 7
eISBN 978 0 85701 368 2

Printed and bound in Great Britain by TJ Books Limited

Jessica Kingsley Publishers' policy is to use papers that are natural, renewable and recyclable
products and made from wood grown in sustainable forests. The logging and manufacturing
processes are expected to conform to the environmental regulations of the country of origin.

Jessica Kingsley Publishers
Carmelite House
50 Victoria Embankment
London EC4Y 0DZ

www.singingdragon.com

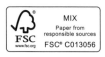

Contents

Acknowledgements

I send my immense gratitude to those who have supported the production of this book in many ways. First and foremost, I would like to thank my sons who helped change my career pathway.

I would like to thank Dr Damien Downing and Dr Patricia Kane for the wonderful opportunity of working with and learning from both of them. Dr Kane first introduced me to consumer genetic testing before the UK had a glimpse of it, which sparked my interest in nutrigenomics. Both doctors taught me the importance of cell membrane integrity on all levels.

I would like to show gratitude to Dr Ben Lynch for that pat on the shoulder in 2011 when I was the supporting act at the CAM nutrigenomic conference. I am really appreciative that Ben gave permission to reproduce his pathway planners. Thanks also go to Dr Donald Epstein and Dr Dietrich Klinghardt for permission to reproduce and incorporate their models of wellness into Chapter 8 to make this a truly integrative approach. I was heartened by their overt interest in reading the book on completion and by Donny editing the section on reorganizational healing.

My appreciation also goes to my dear friend Dr Jess Armine. Dr Jess is a wizard with neurotransmitters, and we have shared many a conversation and the occasional stage. My knowledge on neurotransmitters increased significantly due to our mutual interest.

Niki Gratrix – thank you also, my friend and colleague, for many exchanges since we both left the Institute for Optimum Nutrition (ION) many moons ago. The pooling of ideas and the sharing of the latest evidence on all things energy has helped us both to grow exponentially.

I would like to thank my dear long-time friend and colleague Angela Bailey. From that first day of SNP (single nucleotide polymorphism) comparing back in 2010, Angela helped me to grow as a person. Angela was instrumental in helping me put together the Genesnippers nutrigenomic course for practitioners and to gain NTEC (National Therapy Education Commission) short course certification.

Finally, I would like to thank one my graduates from NCA (Northern College of Acupuncture), now a successful NT (nutrition therapist) colleague – Wendy Urwin. Wendy critiqued the first section on gut health to ensure it was readable at recent graduate level.

There are so many more practitioners who have followed and supported Genesnippers and me. You all know who you are and I thank you from the bottom of my heart. You gave me the strength and courage to be me. This book would not exist if it were not for you guys.

Introduction

This book teaches the reader how to approach nutrigenomics from an integrative framework. It is not a book that teaches practitioners how to find and treat a gene in isolation or to treat genes per se. The book moves as far away from this methodology as is humanly possible.

Although the book does teach the reader how to follow the biochemical pathways and understand the single nucleotide polymorphisms within the pathways, it also makes it very clear that successful outcomes can only be achieved when the epigenetics have also been addressed.

Clients now have access to direct-to-consumer genetic testing (DTC-GT), which can be both a great bonus or a curse to them. Sensitive and often fearful data being presented by DTC-GT may be the reason they contact the practitioner. It is crucial that practitioners act responsibly and have an established referral network, especially when dealing with nutrigenomics and those with mental health profiles. It is really important to have a full understanding of the metabolic pathways and how they affect that individual. Without this level of understanding, it can become custom and practice to treat a gene with a vitamin or herb – in effect, produce a protocol. These are outdated methods of practice in the field of integrative or lifestyle medicine. Nutrigenomics research is still very much in its infancy and practitioners need to respect this. Allopathic medicine and natural medicine have very different understandings about genes at this time, and this produces confusion in clients who approach practitioners of natural medicine. Acting safely and ethically on all levels is crucial for the health of the client.

Allopathic medicine is concerned with the modality of medical genetics. This is the diagnosis and management of hereditary disorders and the use of gene testing to identify and treat some of the symptoms. The overwhelming theme is that these conditions are life-long and therefore not curable. Natural medicine in contrast concerns itself more with nutrigenomics. This is the knowledge of how nutrition and lifestyle affect genetic expression and how this can be manipulated to effect positive changes to quality of life.

Genetic testing companies are evolving daily and there are now hundreds to choose from. The respective companies provide the majority of nutrigenomic training, encouraging bias towards SNP treating. The practitioner needs to be discerning in the use of appropriate testing/companies.

The book provides an overview of the functions of each pathway, the individual SNP functions and their inhibitors and inducers, although there are a small number of SNPs where the lack of evidence precludes the provision of such. Discussion of a complex case will follow at the end of each section. Cases always make the learning journey more realistic by providing real-life experiences and this is the main theme of the book. This is not the only way to approach a nutrigenomics case, but it does demonstrate safe practice. It also alerts the practitioner to areas that could become unsafe with unskilled recommendations. A general knowledge of the specific nutrient content of foods is assumed, as this information is widely available. For basic sound knowledge and a good starting point, *Dirty Genes* (Lynch 2018) helps the individual to initiate the identification and removal of environmental pollutants that Lynch terms soak and scrub.

A very timely paper (Collins *et al.* 2018) looking at current nutrigenomic training practice has clearly identified the variation in training and the associated bias. Collins *et al.* state that those seeking training should scrutinize the training provider for cost, duration, mode of training delivery, content and affiliations to testing companies.

The practitioner is advised to read this book in full to gain a complete picture before embarking on the use of individual sections of the book for specific clients. For example, when supporting methylation, addressing the folate and methionine pathways first may be fine for a very small minority, but those who are sick need the satellite pathways addressing first to avoid adverse events.

References

Collins J, Adamski MM, Twohig C, Murgia C (2018) Opportunities for training for nutritional professionals in nutritional genomics: What is out there? *Nutrition and Dietetics 75*, 2, 206–218. doi:10.1111/1747-0080.12398

Lynch B (2018) *Dirty Genes: A Breakthrough Programme to Treat the Root Cause of Illness and Optimize Your Health.* New York, NY: HarperCollins.

1
Background to Nutrigenomics Testing

We have Gregor Mendel to thank for our interest in genomics. He was a 19th-century Austrian monk who derived the laws of inheritance while he was conducting hybridization experiments on garden peas in the backyard of his church. Between 1856 and 1863, he cultivated and tested some 5000 pea plants. From these experiments he deduced two generalizations, which became known as Mendel's principles of heredity, or Mendelian inheritance. His ideas were published in 1866 but largely went unrecognized until 1900, long after his death. While Mendel's research was related to plants, the basic principles of heredity also apply to people and animals as the mechanisms of heredity are essentially the same for all complex life forms.

Mendel's laws of heredity

- Each physical characteristic corresponds to a single gene.
- Genes are paired. Human cells carry two copies of each chromosome and therefore two versions of each gene. We call these alleles.
- Only one gene of a pair is passed down to the next generation by each parent.

- It is equally probable that either gene will be inherited by the offspring.
- Some characteristics are dominant while others are recessive. Dominant alleles show their effects when only one allele is expressing, also known as heterozygous presentation. Recessive alleles only show their effects if both alleles are expressing.

Some milestones in history

1952: Rosalind Franklin used X-ray diffraction to produce the first images of deoxyribonucleic acid (DNA).

1951–1953: James D. Watson and Francis Crick published the first scientific paper on the double-helix structure of DNA.

1961: Marshall Nirenberg cracked the genetic code.

1986: The first identification of a mitochondrial DNA in human disease.

1990: The BRCA1 gene was discovered.

2003: The Human Genome Project announced that their completed sequence covered 99% of the genome. Forty thousand genes are known to exist; however, the function of less than half of these is known.

2005: The first genome-wide association study (GWAS) was conducted on 96 patients with age-related macular degeneration and 50 healthy controls.

2006: 23andMe was launched in California. This was owned and managed by Anne Wojcicki, wife of Google entrepreneur Sergey Brin. 23andMe is probably the best-known genetic testing company because they were able to market their product to the consumer. In 2014, 23andMe launched in the UK via online services and 600 Superdrug stores. Since 2014, they have really opened up the market for genetic profiling and as a result the service is open to anyone who is interested and at a reasonable rate. This offers a real opportunity for integrative practitioners.

Benefits of nutrigenomic testing

DTC-GT has grown exponentially in the last ten years with a corresponding increase in clinical use, especially within the integrative medicine field. A number of reasons emerge for us here. From the perspective of a client, the information gained can create a greater insight into health concerns. It can foster and deepen the concept and overall understanding of biochemical individuality. The focus can be more on health promotion rather than disease prevention. It can have a profound and empowering effect for clients. Motivation and compliance can be so much better (Tutty *et al.* 2021). After several years of regulatory challenges, the Food and Drug Administration (FDA) has recently approved direct-to-consumer marketing for ten diseases that have clear genetic risk factors (Apathy *et al.* 2018). These are not in the list of single nucleotide polymorphisms being discussed.

A number of client types are highly motivated by the thought of nutrigenomic testing because they have what they would perceive to be bad genes or a family history of chronic disease such as diabetes, heart disease, colon or other cancers, osteoporosis, dementia or cerebrovascular accidents. Some clients have a long history of ill health themselves and do not seem to improve, or they hit a plateau where they really need to personalize their health programme further. In recent times, clients who are already health-conscious such as competing athletes have become advocates of the process.

For the practitioner, the benefits are huge, too. Nutrigenomics with functional testing can inform a personalized programme. It can help to identify a client's hidden challenges while offering an opportunity for client education and empowerment. It can provide the framework for identifying potentially useful functional tests. Nutrigenomics has been at the forefront of complementary and alternative medicine (CAM) therapies for a number of years, but it was limited in scope and expensive. The availability of direct-to-consumer testing has reduced the cost, increased public demand and dictated that practitioners need to become literate in the basic concepts of nutrigenomics (Su 2013). The purpose of this book is to help the practitioner to practise safely and ethically within the field of nutrigenomics.

Public perception of nutrigenomics testing

There may be a few client concerns that we should consider. The biggest issue people face is a worry that their data will be shared. However, security or personal data has to follow GDPR guidelines, meaning all testing laboratories have to follow strict procedures to protect anonymity. Samples submitted to the laboratories are mostly labelled and registered against a barcode system rather than a name. Other concerns include that in the future there may be ramifications when applying for health insurance.

There may be a number of criticisms associated with DTC-GT, not restricted to the clinical utility of such tests. Studies have identified disparities in consumer ability to interpret these tests accurately (Caulfield & McGuire 2012; Leighton *et al.* 2012), in addition to racial disparities and social factors that could influence the understanding of genetic risk factors and also intensify inequities in testing, counselling and treatment (Smith *et al.* 2016). Inequities in genetic research may also include low minority representation and lack of awareness of testing and clinical utility in minority groups. Some older studies have identified ethnic, racial and educational disparities in awareness of genetic testing, particularly for cancer screening (Pagán *et al.* 2009; Wideroff *et al.* 2003). The Health Information National Trends Survey (HINTS) in the USA (Apathy *et al.* 2018) stated that awareness of genetic testing was at 30.6% in 2007, peaked at 48.9% in 2012 and declined to 36.5% in 2013 and 38.4% in 2014. In most years, awareness was dependent on income, education, healthcare insurance status and the presence of a regular healthcare provider. Rates of awareness for ethnic groups varied only in years 2011 and 2014. There were higher rates of awareness in pre-diagnosis cancer groups in 2011 only. Internet users were 2.6% more likely to be aware of DTC-GT, while graduates were around twice as likely. The highest awareness in demographic subgroups was 51% and this was found within the £57,500/$75,000 and above income bracket. These findings imply that there is still a great deal of education to provide in clinical practice.

Possibilities of collaborative or transdisciplinary working

Nazare *et al.* (2009) are clear in their premise that joint research in food and health provides a multitude of benefits. Nutritionists are now able to work in a transdisciplinary way using molecular and cellular biology and physiology. It is expected that they will begin to work with geneticists, molecular biologists and bioinformaticians using tools such as genomics, metabolomics and proteomics. Strategies are being developed to take us from gene expression to dietary recommendations. This is a major leap in personalized medicine although more large-scale studies are needed for validation of the benefits.

The Department of Health Genomics England is also proudly embracing the advent of genetics into medical care as part of the patient pathways approach, with Professor Sue Hill leading this project. A lot of the focus is on attaining a more personalized approach to cancer treatments through genetics (Hill 2018). However, there are also plans to offer genetic testing to every child born; this is currently being trialled at Liverpool Women's NHS Foundation Trust. Here, every new mother is offered a full genetic profile test at baby's fifth-day heel test. It is not compulsory at the moment, so uptake will no doubt depend very much on the appropriate education of prospective parents. It is highly recommended by the delivery and postnatal teams. While the NHS has been undertaking genetic testing since the 1960s for single-gene disorders, this is very new territory. The focus of these projects is still to identify the possibility of future potential illness. Integrated healthcare and applied nutrition (ICAN) practitioners are at the forefront of this knowledge, supporting the biochemistry or underlying cause of potential illness, so this is cutting-edge right now.

Clarification of basic terminology

Genomics is the attempt to look at the totality of all our genes as a dynamic system, interacting with and influencing our biochemical pathways and physiology.

Nutrigenomics is the effect of nutritional intervention on these pathways.

Epigenetics is the study of heritable changes in gene expression without a change in DNA sequence.

Some commonly used terms include:

DNA

We have two types of DNA, nuclear and mitochondrial. Both are stored within the cells and consist of sugars, phosphates and bases (nucleotides) arranged in a double-helix structure. Segments of DNA in chromosomes correspond to specific genes. Functions of DNA include management of gene expression via cell growth, cell differentiation, cell replication and cell death.

Chromosome

Thread-like gene-carrying bodies in the nucleus of the cell made mainly of DNA and protein. Each chromosome contains genes in a linear order. Chromosomes are visible only under magnification at certain stages of cell division.

Gene

A sequence of nucleotides that codes for cells to make protein and associated control sequences. Genes are actually a subset of a cell's DNA. However, while all genes are made from DNA, our entire DNA is not comprised of genes. In fact, less than 2% of a person's DNA represents active genes. The rest of the DNA appears to be involved in mediating how the genes are expressed.

Genotype or genome

This is the complete set of genetic material a person has. It is made up of many alleles. An allele is one of a pair of genes that form on a particular chromosome at a particular location. They control particular characteristics such as hair or eye colour. Human blood type is also determined by alleles inherited from each parent.

Phenotype

The result of the interactions between genes and environmental factors. This is the detectable expression of a genotype and is determined by the alleles. The presence of an allele does not mean that the trait will be expressed in the individual. This is why we need functional testing alongside genetic sequencing.[1]

Histones

With almost six feet of DNA in each cell, the challenge is to prevent it sticking out beyond. Histones are alkaline or basic pH proteins found in the nucleus of eukaryotic cells. Histones shorten these six-feet strands of DNA to about 0.09mm by wrapping up the DNA around itself into structural units called nucleosomes. Histones also play a role in gene regulation.

Bases

These are amino acids arranged in pairs, attached by hydrogen bonds. The bases are adenine (A), thymine (T), guanine (G) and cytosine (C). Adenine and thymine are connected by two hydrogen bonds, while cytosine and guanine are connected by three hydrogen bonds.

Adenine and guanine are purine bases with two carbon rings; cytosine and thymine are pyrimidine bases with only a single carbon ring. The structure of the two groups differs in that the purine bases are made up of two rings of atoms, while pyrimidine bases are made up of only one ring. The rings contain nitrogen and carbon bases, making them nitrogenous bases. Purine bases will only bond with pyrimidine bases. Thymine is an interesting base as this is replaced with uracil in ribonucleic acid (RNA) and is the only base found exclusively in DNA. Cytosine can be easily modified into other bases to carry epigenetic information. Guanosine triphosphate (GTP) acts as an energy source for cellular roles including protein synthesis and gluconeogenesis, which makes sugar out of protein.

---

1   Definitions taken from Simpkins & Williams 1989.

Single nucleotide polymorphism (SNP)

Changes in DNA allow for natural selection, with certain inherited variations in our genes allowing adaptability to a changing environment. Mother nature needs to encourage as much variety as possible in order to ensure survival of the species. Mutations occur in nature to make this possible. However, when the environment changes too rapidly, we may not have enough adaptability. Maybe this is in part why we have so many individuals suffering with chronic disease in today's world. A mutation is an inherited alteration or change in the genetic material, which clinically could be harmful to the individual. This can arise spontaneously through errors or it can be the result of exposure to mutagenic agents. It would be more likely recognized if the effects were detrimental. One or more base pairs can change and these can be major deletions, insertions or genetic rearrangements that can affect one or several genes at one time. Single nucleotide polymorphisms (SNPs) are the most common, occurring in about 1:1000 bases. Most SNPs considered in the realm of nutrigenomics will be prevalent in 20, 30 or 50% of the population.

There are also copy number variations when some DNA simply repeats itself – for example, AAGAAGAAGAAG. The number of repeats can vary considerably. This can be assessed via chromosome micro array. Segments of chromosomes are lost or gained as part of evolution and occur at conception. Most are harmless. However, where a large chunk of genetic material is lost, this can be more detrimental than if genetic material is gained. Determining the prospective harmfulness of the change depends on the size, importance of the gene and whether the gene was inherited. Large important genes and those that are inherited are said to be more problematic. Disease associated mutations can be due to the alteration of functional proteins (Kékesi *et al.* 2012; Schaefer *et al.* 2012) or non-functional missing proteins (Hanson *et al.* 2009). Differences in the copy number of a gene can decrease the level of activity of that gene.

Deficiencies and exaggerations of specific enzyme activity are linked to the expression of polymorphisms. These may be:

- absence of expression
- partial expression
- overexpression.

Alleles

Two alleles or alternative forms of a gene (SNP), one from each parental chromosome, usually determine each characteristic. If a person has a homozygous presentation, depending on the genetic company used to determine this, it can be presented in one of three ways: +/+ or vt/vt (homozygous), +/ or vt/wt (heterozygous) and –/– or wt/wt (wild type). Generally, in the UK we see the +/+ presentation on testing reports. Individuals can be homozygous for some genes and heterozygous or wild type for others. There can also be a null presentation or a deletion; GSTM1 and GSTT1 are familiar genes that fall into this category Pinheiro *et al.* (2013) found a correlation between null presentations of these two genes and type 2 or non-insulin dependent diabetes mellitus (NIDDM). In their cohort of 120 NIDDM and 147 healthy individuals, they found GSTT1 null phenotype increased the risk of NIDDM 3.5-fold with higher levels of triglycerides and very low-density lipoproteins (VLDL), while GSTM1 null was associated with higher levels of fasting glucose and HBA1c.

> **KEY POINT**
> Every significant SNP exists because, at some point in human evolution, it provided advantages for survival by enabling those with the polymorphism to adapt better to specific environmental challenges.

How to read a genetic interpretive report

Using a SNP example which most practitioners are familiar, this is how the practitioner or client is likely to view the single nucleotide polymorphism in a report.

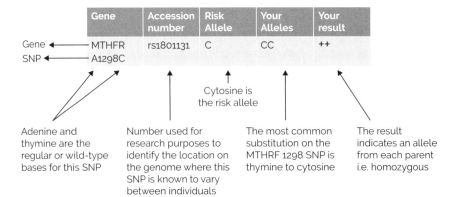

Figure 1.1 Reading a report

NB: A combination of the gene name with the position of the SNP with either the nucleotide base or the amino acids variants is generally used. Accession numbers are extremely useful to check against research articles for accuracy in interpretation of risk, efficacy of therapy, etc. However, not all earlier studies mention the accession number, so specificity may be compromised. It may be necessary to consult a number of studies to ascertain this, so that practitioners can be certain that their recommendations are valid.

For SNPs to be a useful clinical tool, they need to be modifiable via reasonable clinical intervention. We need to be able to modify their expression using clinical tools such as nutrition, lifestyle, food supplements and/or medication.

High or low penetrance

The penetrance of a gene describes the frequency in which the characteristic it controls is seen in people who carry the gene. If every person who carries the gene develops the associated disease, this is complete or 100% penetrance. In high penetrance, the trait of the allele is almost always expressed. In low penetrance, it is difficult to distinguish the effects of genetics from environmental factors. Single-gene disorders are those in which a mutation in a single gene can cause an inherited disease according to Mendel's laws. Such examples include Tay–Sachs disease, cystic fibrosis, xeroderma pigmentosa, Fragile X syndrome, sickle cell anaemia or Huntington's disease. These are beyond the remit of

(CAM) therapies. However, CAM practitioners are absolutely the best placed to support individuals with multi-factorial diseases such as arthritis that can be modified by nutrition and lifestyle change. Multiple SNPs have been identified in many of these conditions. Nutrigenomic testing alongside functional testing can be invaluable in identifying root causes and also in designing a much more personalized approach to wellness.

Available testing and interpretation

When considering genetic testing for your client or yourself, there are some considerations you need to be mindful of when recommending. We do need to be aware that the raw data from some DTC-GT companies requires interpretation via additional application software. There are a number of these interpretation applications on the market, all with their own unique perspective, some offering nutritional supplement advice for each SNP screened. This information can be very confusing and misleading, especially if a number of SNPs have been identified, as a possible intervention for one SNP may be detrimental for another SNP in the same pathway. This concept of using a supportive nutrient where a given SNP is reported is known as SNP treating, and this practice can be detrimental to clients. For example, giving a client methylfolate to support an MTHFR SNP if they are slow dopamine metabolizers can induce panic or even psychosis. This will be discussed in more detail in the 'Neurotransmitter' section in Chapter 5.

Any genetic tests should always be combined with a full in-depth clinical history and functional testing. This has never been more important, as Moscarello *et al.* (2018) report concerns regarding cases where patients had used DTC-GT. Patients had then associated individual genes with perceived conditions such as Ehler Danlos syndrome, idiopathic recurrent myocarditis and arrhythmogenic right ventricular cardiomyopathy. As a result patients appear to be deluging their healthcare provider with questions and demands to address the genetic predisposition. This is demonstrating patient confusion and anxiety, which is then becoming a burden to the healthcare system. Health professionals are concerned that false positives and non-genetics provider misunder-standing are leading to misleading interpretation and possible misman-agement. However, the study clearly points out that the SNPs identified in the study cases did not correspond to clinical history.

Another confusion arises from lack of regulation of DTC-GT, and this is that the different testing companies identify their own range of SNPs with their own accession codes or reference SNP cluster identifi-cation code (rsid). This means they may be measuring the same gene(s) at different points, so the effects of expression may be inconsistent with the evidence base. This becomes evident if the consumer analyzes their raw data via a number of the interpretation application software sites. The companies are rather vague about how they agree on the particular SNPs they are using; however, they do all have a scientific research team, and the decision to include a SNP appears to be based on the identification of three good genome-wide association studies (GWAS) (Uffelmann *et al.* 2021). It is early days in the nutrigenomic milieu, so some form of standardization needs to occur (Webster 2010; Ortiz *et al.* 2009). It is necessary for practitioners to regularly consult with the evidence base to ensure they are working in a consistent manner with SNPs and rsids.

There are also a number of key companies who provide their own genetic test and interpretation without the need for interpretation though an application. Many of these tests offer a very narrow range of SNPs. This can mean more tests are required to build a holistic picture in those who are sick, and this, of course, greatly increases the cost to the consumer or client. Unfortunately for practitioners, these companies are experts at marketing, so they can cajole both practitioners and the general public into very expensive testing that may not be appropriate for the client. Practitioners need to be discerning with their homework, research the companies and decide on the test based on the health of the client and the test that offers the broadest range of SNPs with the best evidence base. The evidence is changing almost daily, so the practitioner needs to be abreast of current trends. Practitioners can keep abreast of current trends by following reputable professional bodies such as the Nutrition Society, the British Association for Nutrition and Lifestyle Medicine (BANT) and the National Center for Biotechnological Information (NCBI).

Further considerations and possible limitations

For those who prefer to have their data analyzed ready for use, there are a number of companies who provide this service. The practitioner is advised to research fully before committing. While they all provide interpretation, it is not always possible to cross-reference the SNPs they measure. The practitioner needs to know the rsid for any SNPs they are considering and to be able to cross-reference with the evidence base.

There are limitations also to genetic testing itself that cannot be ignored. These tests cannot tell you if the client is sick, for example. To use genetic testing results without functional testing and full history would be unethical and deemed as SNP treating. Genetic testing cannot identify functional imbalances or diagnose disease. For optimal effectiveness and measurable outcomes, genetic testing must be combined with a functional assessment even when used for primary prevention. One of the most useful tests to combine with genetics is a urinary organic acids test. The choice of testing company would be dependent on the presentation of the case as they each have strengths within their individual organic acid profiles. It is not the intention of this book to discuss functional test interpretation as this will be undertaken in another book in the series; however, practitioners will be alerted to relevant markers on appropriate tests where they support determining genetic expression. Practitioners are advised strongly to undertake some form of nutrigenomics training within an integrative framework before using nutrigenomic tests.

Sample collection

Methods to obtain DNA samples range from saliva to buccal swabs to serum. For the most part, saliva and buccal swabs are the most common form of testing. For those who cannot produce enough saliva, this can be a challenge, and for those with mental health conditions such as anxiety or psychosis; bloodletting may also be problematic. Buccal (from the inside of the cheek) swabs appear to be gaining popularity in the UK. Hu *et al.* (2012) studied the types of sampling in relation to the quality of DNA extracted. They found that saliva was more likely to be infected with bacteria from the teeth and this could limit the number of markers seen on analysis. They presented a threshold of 31.3% of amplifiable DNA in saliva, which would produce a call rate of at least 96%. The call rate is the proportion of study subjects where the SNP data is not missing.

Arbitrio *et al.* (2016) compared saliva to blood sampling using the Drug Metabolism Enzyme and Transporters (DMET™) platform. This is a system of DNA sequencing used to assess pharmacogenomic drug metabolism to support precision medicine or patient-tailored therapies such as appropriate chemotherapy approaches. The authors concluded that blood sampling was best when using genomics to decide drug intervention. However, it may not affect the DTC-GT services at practitioner and client level.

References

Apathy NC, Menser T, Keeran LM *et al.* (2018) Trends and gaps in awareness of direct-to-consumer genetic tests from 2007 to 2014. *American Journal of Preventive Medicine 54*, 6, 806–813. doi:10.1016/j.amepre.2018.02.013

Arbitrio M, Martino MTD, Scionti F *et al.* (2016) DMET™ (Drug Metabolism Enzymes and Transporters): A pharmacogenomic platform for precision medicine. *Oncotarget 7*, 33, 54028–54050. doi:10.18632/oncotarget.9927

Caulfield T, McGuire AL (2012) Direct-to-consumer genetic testing: perceptions, problems, and policy responses. *Annual Review of Medicine 63*, 23–33. doi:10.1146/annurev-med-062110-123753

Hanson AD, Pribat A, Waller JC *et al.* (2009) 'Unknown' proteins and 'orphan' enzymes: The missing half of the engineering parts list – and how to find it. *The Biochemical Journal 425*, 1, 1–11. doi:10.1042/BJ20091328

Hill S (2018) The genomic revolution: Its future. Blog post, 23 March. NHS England. www.england.nhs.uk/blog/genomic-revolution

Hu Y, Ehli EA, Nelson K *et al.* (2012) Genotyping performance between saliva and blood-derived genomic DNAs on the DMET array: A comparison. *PLOS ONE 7*, 3, e33968. doi:10.1371/journal.pone.0033968

Kékesi KA, Juhász G, Simor A *et al.* (2012) Altered functional protein networks in the prefrontal cortex and amygdala of victims of suicide. *PLOS ONE 7*, 12, e50532. doi:10.1371/journal.pone.0050532

Leighton JW, Valverde K, Bernhardt BA (2012) The general public's understanding and perception of direct-to-consumer genetic test results. *Public Health Genomics 15*, 1, 11–21.

Moscarello T, Murray B, Reuter C *et al.* (2018) Direct-to-consumer raw genetic data and third-party interpretation services: More burden than bargain? *Genetics in Medicine 21*, 539–541. www.nature.com/articles/s41436-018-0097-2

Nazare J, Disse E, Vidal H *et al.* (2009) Link between food and health: From gene expression to nutritional recommendations. *Food Quality and Preference 20*, 8, 537–538. doi:10.1016/j.foodqual.2009.03.003

Ortiz AP, López M, Flores LT *et al.* (2011) Awareness of direct-to-consumer genetic tests and use of genetic tests among Puerto Rican adults, 2009. *Preventing Chronic Disease 8*, 5, A110.

Pagán JA, Su D, Li L *et al.* (2009) Racial and ethnic disparities in awareness of genetic testing for cancer risk. *American Journal of Preventive Medicine 37*, 6, 524–530.

Pinheiro DS, Rocha Filho CR, Mundim CA *et al.* (2013) Evaluation of glutathione S-transferase *GSTM1* and *GSTT1* deletion polymorphisms on type-2 diabetes mellitus risk. *PLOS ONE 8*, 10, e76262. doi:10.1371/journal.pone.0076262

Schaefer C, Bromberg Y, Achten D *et al.* (2012) Disease-related mutations predicted to impact protein function. *BMC Genomics 13*, Suppl. 4, S11. doi:10.1186/1471-2164-13-S4-S11

Simpkins J, Williams JI (1989) *Advanced Biology*. London: Collins Educational.

Smith CE, Fullerton SMK, Dookeran A *et al.* (2016) Using genetic technologies to reduce, rather than widen, health disparities. *Health Affairs 35*, 8, 1367–1373.

Su P (2013) Direct-to-consumer genetic testing: A comprehensive view. *The Yale Journal of Biology and Medicine 86*, 3, 359–365.

Tutty E, Hickerton C, Terrill B *et al.* (2021) The expectations and realities of nutrigenomic testing in australia: A qualitative study. *Health Expect 24*, 2, 670–686. doi: 10.1111/hex.13216

Uffelmann E, Huang QQ, Munung NS *et al.* (2021) Genome-wide association studies. *Nat Rev Methods Primers 1*, 59. doi:10.1038/s43586-021-00056-9

Webster PC (2010) Regulation of genetic tests unnecessary, government says. *CMAJ : Canadian Medical Association Journal 182*, 16, 1715–1716. doi:10.1503/cmaj.109-3686

Wideroff L, Vadaparampil ST, Breen N *et al.* (2003) Awareness of genetic testing for increased cancer risk in the year 2000 National Health Interview Survey. *Community Genetics 6*, 3, 147–156.

2
Why Has Ella's Case Been Chosen?

Ella is a complex case, used to demonstrate how a case might be approached in the different sections of the nutrigenomic profiles. Ella was chosen because she has polymorphisms in all methylation pathways, so her case is able to demonstrate how practitioners can work in those areas. In the biopterin cycle, there is a key learning about dopamine trapping that could not be demonstrated using this case, so a separate mini case has been provided, printed *in italics* for clarity. It needs to be pointed out that this is one way a case can be approached, but practitioners will need to be discerning when the analysis of the immediate and ongoing needs of the client differ from this profile.

Ella's case also required the integration of nutrigenomics with another complimentary medicine modality, that of network care. It therefore demonstrates multidisciplinary working where necessary. Numerous practitioners had seen Ella over the years. She gained benefit from some, but overall her belief was that she couldn't be helped. It was therefore important to take a much wider approach, which for some practitioners may be too esoteric. The wider approach was taken from the works of Dr Dietrich Klinghardt (the 5 levels of healing) and Dr Donald Epstein (elements of reorganizational healing). These models are discussed in Chapter 8 so they do not detract from the main theme. Practitioners who would enjoy a new frame of reference are invited to read this chapter.

Ella's timeline and case brief

Ella is 50 years old and has come to see her practitioner with a variety of health issues as can be seen on her timeline. She is a very shy and sensitive person who has struggled with most aspects of life to date. She is very successful in her own right, but despite her success she never feels good enough. No matter if she had 1000 messages in support, she would focus on the one negative comment. As a child, Ella was always told she was 'too sensitive' or that she must improve her behaviour or performance. She has carried this framework into her adult life.

Family history: Many first- and second-degree relatives had cancers (breast, colon, lung), dementia, multiple sclerosis, Hashimoto's thyroiditis, atopy (asthma, hay fever, eczema) and anxiety.

Birth history: Ella was the first child; her mother was 19 at the time. She was a natural conception and born at 43 weeks' gestation. Her mother was involved in a road traffic accident (RTA) – a tram hit her while cycling, when Ella was around seven months in utero. After a long and protracted labour, she was delivered by emergency Caesarean section. Both were in need of postpartum care, so were separated. Her mother was found to have pelvic dysplasia afterwards, possibly as a result of the RTA. Ella was bottle-fed, as this was fashionable at the time.

Age 3 months: Ella contracted amoebic dysentery lasting four weeks. It was assumed that her father had contracted this in Malaya where he had been stationed in the armed forces. The amoeba was passed from husband to wife who was subsequently identified by medics as a carrier.

Age 3: Having been a late walker at the age of 16 months, complained of aches and pains in joints and muscles.

Age 5: Commenced school where she was noted to be a highly sensitive child.

Age 6: Ella's first brother was born. Shortly after his birth Ella was diagnosed with psoriatic arthritis. Ella was prescribed non-steroidal anti-inflammatory drugs (NSAIDs), coal tar baths daily, followed by ultraviolet light therapy and dithranol in Lassar's paste to lesions. When not attending hospital for these treatments, she would be treated with various maintenance topical treatments between the ages of 6 and 26 years. These included dithranol in Lassar's paste, coal tar creams, various emollients. Also steroids both plain and combined with vitamin D that were alternated according to skin condition, (Dovobet and Dovonex) and Dermovate, one of the strongest topical steroids. The Dermovate seemed to be the best solution for Ella and she used this for eight years continuously during her teens and early 20s.

Age 9: Birth of second brother. Mother drinking heavily.

Age 12: Death of grandmother followed by grandfather 13 months later. This had a huge impact on Ella's skin and mental health. It is worth noting that up until the age of 13 years Ella's family lived in a very old, rented cottage with an outside toilet and no central heating. This was next door to an ice-cream factory, on land that was previously a lake.

Age 14: Ella commenced menses. Her cycles were irregular with dysmenorrhoea and menorrhagia. She was prescribed a number of different forms of the contraceptive pill to alleviate her symptoms but these caused depression, headaches, severe fatigue and weight gain. She persisted because she did have resolution of her menstrual issues. Also severe hay fever and other seasonal allergies began surfacing at this time.

Age 16: Seriously underachieving at school. Ella suffered with depression and anxiety and was hospitalized for severe psoriasis and psoriatic arthritis at this time. The psoriatic arthritis resolved a year later but the psoriasis continued. Following hospitalization, Ella suffered constantly with vaginitis, severe vaginal discharge and thrush. This was ongoing until her late 20s.

Age 17: Ran away from home and lived with boyfriend's family.

Age 18: Entered a career in the caring professions.

Age 25: Diagnosed with fibrocystic breast disease.

Age 28: Ella married. She was seen by her GP with amenorrhoea of ten months' duration due to long-term contraceptive use. Seasonal allergies seemed to improve on discontinuation of the pill. Light sensitivity seemed to have been an issue since the age of 14 years.

Ella associated this with her seasonal allergies and it remained an ongoing problem. She also had a rebound flare of her psoriasis due to sudden discontinuation of topical steroids prior to attempting to conceive. This was managed with dietary changes such as reducing sugar, starchy carbohydrates and stimulants, and the use of topical emollients. Also stress-reduction techniques.

Age 29: Late miscarriage at 20 weeks. Foetus was malformed and estimated to be around 14 weeks' gestation in size and development. Dilation and curettage procedure was immediately performed to cleanse the womb to help future conception and any subsequent pregnancy.

Age 30: Birth of Ella's first child. Pregnancy was difficult; Ella was plagued with extreme fatigue, iron deficiency anaemia, nausea, heartburn and reflux. This child was later diagnosed with high-functioning autism. Ella suffered a post-partum haemorrhage after delivery. This required two separate surgical interventions on consecutive days and she had 7 units of blood transfused. Following the birth recovery, Ella's health improved markedly.

Age 32: Birth of second child. This pregnancy was uneventful; in fact, Ella glowed, was in the best of health throughout, continuing to work in her clinical research role 30 hours weekly until 38 weeks' gestation. Spontaneous labour at 40 weeks produced a healthy second child in three hours, with no medicinal intervention.

Age 35–45: Immense stress due to eldest child's additional educational and health needs, running a home and career.

Age 42: HPA axis dysfunction (low salivary cortisol on all four markers), borderline low T4 and T3 with normal TSH, no ABO antibodies. It is important to note that the term adrenal fatigue is no longer considered very helpful, although at the time it was very prominent as a possible cause for fatigue-related conditions.

Adrenal fatigue is defined as a low salivary cortisol state as a result of lifestyle choices. However, the symptoms of adrenal fatigue such as brain fog, low energy, depression, salt and sweet cravings could also be a symptom of other conditions. A systematic review of 58 studies (Cadegiani & Kater 2016) concluded that adrenal fatigue is not a medical condition. The more updated term is hypothalamus pituitary adrenal (HPA) axis dysfunction. This is because the adrenal glands form part of the HPA axis, which is stimulated by and governs the stress response (Dunlavey 2018).

Age 45: Diagnosed with coeliac disease. Started working with naturopathic doctors. Placed on a gluten-free diet.

Age 46: Diagnosed with myalgic encephalitis (ME)/chronic fatigue, due to mould intolerance. The NHS team diagnosed the ME. The mould was assessed on organic acids, followed by urine mycotoxins testing and clinical presentation of becoming sick very soon after mould exposure on three separate occasions. Mould had also been found in a stool sample, tested by NHS gastroenterologists. The mould intolerance was determined to be a major factor underlying her ME by her naturopathic doctor at the time.

Age 47: Mould and mycotoxin exposure leading to pneumonia. Ella was bedbound for eight weeks and given intravenous phospholipid exchange therapy (described in Chapter 3) with phenylbutyrate. This began to turn Ella's health around, but cost prohibited continuation of this approach.

PRACTITIONER NOTES

Sodium phenylbutyrate is a pro-drug generally used as an ammonia scavenger for individuals with urea cycle disorders. It is metabolized in the body to phenylacetate. This combines with glutamine, becoming phenylacetlyglutamine, which is rapidly excreted via the kidneys. Metabolism through the urea cycle is unnecessary. As it is metabolized, it scavenges ammonia. It is available in granules and intravenous form on the NHS. However, a worldwide team of doctors, under the guidance of Dr Patricia Kane, use phenylbutyrate as a component of phospholipid exchange therapy. This will be discussed in Chapter 3.

Age 50: Symptoms at first presentation included the feeling of walking in treacle, severe brain fatigue requiring 3–4 power naps daily, brain 'shutting down' mid-sentence. Ella had overall low mood with underlying anxiety/frustration. She suffered serious reactions to high-histamine/mould products such as tomatoes, cheese and cinnamon; according to Ella, the tomato and cheese were life-long issues.

Ella tested strongly positive for urinary kryptopyrroluria (KPU) also called haemopyrrollactamuria (HPU). Please note these terms are interchangeable with the term pyrroluria but they are measuring slightly different markers. There is no current consensus as to which marker is the ideal.

Kryptopyrroluria is not a recognized diagnosis in the UK. In the 1950s, all psychiatric patients were screened for KPU, but due to advances in allopathic treatments, possibly the variance in testing and difficulties in prevention of degradation of KPU in the urine sample (pyrroles are sensitive to heat, light and oxygen), it has become unfavourable as a consideration. Pfeiffer (1975) found that 30% of patients with a diagnosis of schizophrenia were suffering from KPU and that supporting these patients brought forth a vast improvement, often very quickly. KPU is the mauve factor that builds up in urine as a result of stress. It attracts aldehydes such as B6, and as zinc is a cofactor for B6, this is lost in urine too, along with manganese. Some sources also suggest the loss of biotin and chromium. Ongoing B6 and zinc deficiency or KPU manifests in a triad of impairments in neurotransmitters, hormones and gut function, with the potential addition of heavy-metal toxicity. It was always believed that KPU was transmitted genetically mainly via the female bloodline, but more recently it has been observed clinically manifesting post-trauma. Practitioners are also identifying it more post-COVID-19.

Without B6, haem cannot be formed so any enzyme that requires haem will be compromised. This includes all the CYP450 enzymes. This means the whole of detoxification and methylation is affected. Haemoglobin cannot be made either, so oxygen cannot be carried around the body effectively. B6 and zinc are required as enzyme support throughout the methylation system, as will be demonstrated. To this end, Dr Klinghardt would advocate supporting KPU before addressing methylation pathways. Klinghardt has been a huge proponent for evaluation of KPU and addressing PKU and its impact on sulphation prior to addressing other methylation pathways.

Current medical diagnoses

- Myalgic encephalitis/chronic fatigue.
- Psoriasis.
- Psoriatic arthritis, controlled with diet and lifestyle (see below).
- Perimenopausal.
- Coeliac disease.

Awaiting further gastroenterology assessment for a diagnosis of gastroparesis. Symptoms include gastro-oesophageal reflux, heaviness after eating, chronic abdominal pain, high bloating, early satiety, weight loss and significant loss of energy after eating.

Current medications

None. Ella had excessive side effects to all medications such as NSAIDs, contraceptives and antidepressants, so she preferred not to take them.

She had undertaken many rounds of topical treatments for her psoriasis including coal tar, dithranol in Lassar's paste, vitamin D analogues and many high-strength topical steroids long-term. Ella discontinued these, believing the steroids to be contributing to her fatigue. Following a period of rebound exacerbation, she was at this point experiencing some degree of calming with natural topical creams as emollients and dietary restriction.

Current supplementation

A previous therapist had recommended:

- betaine hydrochloride 700mg x 3 per meal and 1 with snacks to support protein digestion (Guilliams & Drake 2020)
- beetroot complex with taurine x 2 per meal to support bile flow (Spiridonov 2012; Yamanaka *et al.* 1986)
- sodium and potassium bicarbonate x 2 daily to support bowel pH for maximum digestive enzyme function and microbiome diversity (Jakab *et al.* 2012)
- coenzyme Q10 300mg daily to support mitochondrial energy (Neergheen *et al.* 2017)
- multi-strain probiotic 5 billion x 3 daily to balance microbiome and aid bowel detoxification (Shimizu 2012).

Current diet

- Organic; gluten-, casein-, soy- and nightshade-free, low histamine.
- Restricted to five foods resulting from self-diagnosed intolerances – white rice, frozen fish, carrots, kale, frozen peas.

NB: Fish is a high-histamine food; however, when frozen at source, it often hasn't had the degradation time to build up the histamine, so some can tolerate it.

The main aim of the first appointment with Ella was to establish which genes were expressing, how her pathways might be compromised and in which order to address the metabolic pathways to give Ella maximum benefit to reduce her levels of anxiety. It was established that Ella had undertaken many programmes of microbiome rebalancing and gut restoration with a number of practitioners, interspersed with her own efforts, but her health continued to decline. This was her reason for wanting to consult purely on a nutrigenomic basis. Ella's genes and gene expression are discussed at the end of each designated pathway section. There was a serious clinical concern with regard to her extremely limited diet and major digestive symptoms of stomach pains and cramps, slow gastric emptying, sleepy after meals, stomach upsets when taking antimicrobials, undigested food in stools even when taking betaine and digestive enzymes, nausea when eating fats, and pain between the shoulder blades. Ella also had an extremely restricted diet/fear of food, so it was imperative to relieve her anxiety in order to increase her food choices.

It was therefore decided to refer Ella for Network Spinal Analysis to see if this could help her anxiety and her gut motility. Network Spinal Analysis is a specialized form of gentle chiropractic care that works to 'free' the spine to enable its natural somatic wave, which in turn allows the body to come back into parasympathetic dominance for healing to occur. It is based around the work of Dr Donald Epstein called reorganizational healing. For practitioners who would like to learn more, Epstein's model has been discussed in detail in Chapter 8.

Ella's health plan: KPU

Ella was not keen to introduce new foods at this stage and a trusting relationship needed establishing, so the decision was made to continue her current supplement regime with the addition of one supplement to replace the loss of nutrients resulting from the KPU, and also to begin to support the transsulphuration pathway (see Chapter 5) with the use of Epsom salts baths and molybdenum. The rationale for this is that all channels of elimination will need to be open before commencement of a programme that potentially detoxifies the liver and cell membranes enzymatically. In the interim period, Epsom salts, once dissolved in water, provide magnesium and sulphate ions. The body naturally makes sulphate during methylation but this seems impaired in some (Hartzell & Seneff 2012). Epsom salts encourage detoxification by drawing out impurities from the layers of the skin via reverse osmosis (Rudolph 1917). Gröber et al. (2017) also reviewed a number of articles claiming that transdermal delivery of magnesium via Epsom salts baths raises blood levels of magnesium, which is crucial for the production of adenosine triphosphate (ATP). As a result, the approach has been used in allopathic medicine for many years as pain relief. The autism community has also used this approach for many years with excellent results, providing much anecdotal evidence. Allopathic medicine has also used it orally as a bitter salt designed to 'purge' and humans do have a bitter receptor called TAS2R7 for the purpose of detection of bitter salts (Behrens *et al.* 2019).

Supplements

- Betaine hydrochloride 700mgs x 3 per meal a 1 with snacks to support protein digestion (Guilliams & Drake 2020).
- Beetroot complex with taurine x 2 per meal acting as a chola-gogue to support bile flow (Spiridonov 2012; Yamanaka *et al.* 1986).
- Sodium and potassium bicarbonate x 2 daily to support bowel pH for maximum digestive enzyme function (Jakab *et al.* 2012).
- Coenzyme Q10 300mgs daily to support mitochondrial energy (Neergheen *et al.* 2017).
- Multi-strain probiotic 5 billion x 3 daily to balance microbiome and aid bowel detoxification (Shimizu 2012).

At this point a combination supplement containing B6, zinc, manganese, biotin, calcium, molybdenum, boron, magnesium (to address KPU) was slowly added to Ella's programme (Forsgren & Klinghardt 2017).

We will revisit Ella's case at the end of each section.

References

Behrens M, Redel U, Blank K *et al.* (2019) The human bitter taste receptor TAS2R7 facilitates the detection of bitter salts. *Biochemical and Biophysical Research Communications 512*, 4, 877–881. doi:10.1016/j. bbrc.2019.03.139

Cadegiani FA, Kater CE (2016) Adrenal fatigue does not exist: A systematic review. *BMC Endocrine Disorders 16*, 1, 48. doi:10.1186/ s12902-016-0128-4

Dunlavey CJ (2018) Introduction to the hypothalamic-pituitary-adrenal axis: Healthy and dysregulated stress responses, developmental stress and neurodegeneration. *Journal of Undergraduate Neuroscience Education 16*, 2, R59–R60.

Forsgren S, Klinghardt D (2017) Kryptopyrroluria (aka hemopyrrollactamuria): A major piece of the puzzle in overcoming chronic Lyme disease. *Townsend Letter*, July 2017. www.townsendletter.com/July2017/ krypto0717.html

Gröber U, Werner T, Vormann J *et al.* (2017) Myth or reality – transdermal magnesium? *Nutrients 9*, 8, 813. doi:10.3390/nu9080813

Guilliams TG, Drake LE (2020) Meal-time supplementation with betaine HCl for functional hypochlorhydria: What is the evidence? *Integrative Medicine (Encinitas) 19*, 1, 32–36.

Hartzell S, Seneff S (2012) Impaired sulfate metabolism and epigenetics: Is there a link in autism? *Entropy 14*, 10, 1953–1977. doi:10.3390/e14101953

Jakab RL, Collaco AM & Ameen NA (2012) Cell-specific effects of luminal acid, bicarbonate, cAMP, and carbachol on transporter trafficking in the intestine. *American Journal of Physiology. Gastrointestinal and Liver Physiology 303*, 8, G937–G950. doi:10.1152/ajpgi.00452.2011

Neergheen V, Chalasani A, Wainwright L *et al.* (2017) Coenzyme Q10 in the treatment of mitochondrial disease. *Journal of Inborn Errors of Metabolism and Screening 5*, 1–8. doi:10.1177/2326409817707771

Pfeiffer CC (1975) *Mental and Elemental Nutrients: A Physician's Guide to Nutrition and Health Care.* New Haven, CT: Keats Publishing.

Rudolf RD (1917) The use of Epsom salts, historically considered. *Canadian Medical Association Journal 7*, 12, 1069–1071.

Shimizu M. (2012) Modulation of intestinal functions by dietary substances: An effective approach to health promotion. *Journal of Traditional and Complementary Medicine 2*, 2, 81–83. doi:10.1016/ s2225-4110(16)30080-3

Spiridonov NA (2012) Mechanisms of action of herbal cholagogues. *Medicinal and Aromatic Plants 1*, 5. doi:10.4172/2167-0412.1000107

Yamanaka Y, Tsuji K, Ichikawa T (1986) Stimulation of chenodeoxycholic acid excretion in hypercholesterolemic mice by dietary taurine. *Journal of Nutrition Science and Vitaminology (Tokyo) 32*, 3, 287–296. doi:10.3177/jnsv.32.287

3
Assimilation

As we are integrating nutrigenomics into an integrative framework, it would be prudent to commence our journey with assimilation. Assimilation is the process of digestion and absorption of food and nutrients by the body. Some of the SNPs associated closely with assimilation include FUT2, BCMO1, TCN1 and 2, ATG16L1, IRGM, HLA, HLA-DQ2, HLA-DQ8, PEMT and DAO. Some SNPs will resurface at other relevant points but they will be discussed in full at the most appropriate point.

Fucosyltransferase: FUT1, 2 and 3

The FUT2 gene (the most common) encodes (provides instructions for making) the enzyme galactoside 2-L-fucosyltransferase. This protein is found in the stack of the Golgi apparatus, an organelle where proteins made in the cell are glycosylated and folded. This is a very interesting enzyme, found in the gastrointestinal tract and the lungs. It helps to create part of the H antigen, which is the precursor of the ABO antigens. Blood-type antigens are secreted into all organs with a mucous lining, so this would include the gastrointestinal tract, reproductive, respiratory and urinary systems. FUT2 therefore controls the amount of these secretions from secretor glands (Saboor *et al.* 2014).

The H antigen is a short sequence of sugars or oligosaccharides found on many body cells. It attaches to the cell membrane of red blood cells and is also found in in plasma and in the body's secretions. The H antigen must be made before the body can make the A and B antibodies (the two dominant antibodies of the ABO blood group). When the A or B antigen is produced H activity ceases in the chain. This reciprocal relationship determines the amount of H, A or B on the cell.

H ANTIGEN CLARIFICATION

H is produced by the combination of fucose sugar residue and a pre-existing oligosaccharide. In very rare cases, a person can have a deletion or a double homozygous expression of the genes for both H and ABO; this is known as the Bombay phenotype. These individuals tend to be of Asian origin and, as a result, cannot be given blood from any other type except another Bombay phenotype. This is due to a deletion or double homozygous expression of both H genes also known as FUT1 (Khan 2019). Lack or deletion of these two genes means individuals have a very strong anti-H, anti-A and anti-B antigen, and this renders the incompatibility. This is therefore different to the FUT secretor/non-secretor status that will be discussed in relation to assimilation.

FUT2 typically results in the Lewis antigen Lea– Leb+ (secretor) status. Mourant (1946) first described the Lewisa (Lea) antigen and Andresen (1948) described the Lewisb (Leb). Red blood cells lacking in these Lea and Leb antigens will take them up from the surrounding plasma. Equally, red cells expressing either Lea or Leb will give these up to plasma where they are lacking. Lewis antigens are located on type 1 glycosphingolipids that are absorbed on to the red cells from plasma. They are not therefore intrinsic to red cells and therefore not, strictly speaking, a red cell blood group (Saboor *et al.* 2014).

    When we discuss secretor/non-secretor status in nutrigenomics, secretors are those with no mutation or wild card –/– presentation. D'Adamo and Whitney (2002), supported by Azad *et al.* (2018) sees heterozygous presentation +/– as a partial secretor and homozygous presentation +/+ as a non-secretor.

So what does secretor status mean? The original evidence was born out of Peter D'Adamo's research, in particular his book *Live Right for Your Type.* There are a number of interesting alleles of FUT2 but originally D'Adamo focused on secretor/non-secretor status or Lewis antigen presentation. FUT2 wild type (–/–) (G) are said to be secretors while non-secretors or Lewis antigen positive have AA or homozygous presentation (+/+) alleles at rs601338 and the more recent rs200157007-TT (Mottram *et al.* 2017).

Many health issues have been linked to non-secretor status (Le^a+ Le^b–) such as dysbiosis, intestinal hyperpermeability and susceptibility to inflammatory bowel disease (Wacklin *et al.* 2014). This may in fact be due to altered mucin structure that subsequently affects microbial adhesion. These individuals lack diversity, richness and abundance of microbiota, especially the *Bifidobacteria* strains. Sometimes an over-abundance of other strains such as *Clostridia sphenoides* may be seen. This has been associated with IBS (Wacklin *et al.* 2011). They may also be susceptible to rotavirus, *Campylobacter jeuni* (Wu *et al.* 2017) and *Helicobacter pylori* (Koda *et al.* 2001).

However, resistance to norovirus infection in non-secretors has also been identified. A double Lewis phenotype (Le^a+ Le^b+) due to expression of FUT3 genes is very rarely seen in Western populations but a little more common in Asian communities (Corvelo *et al.* 2013). Some conditions also appear to create a change in the Lewis blood group. Generally speaking, around 20% of Caucasians are said to be non-secretors (Saboor *et al.* 2014). The advantage of being a secretor may be the propensity towards a more stable and diverse microbiome as secretors have a steady supply of blood-type antigens in the mucus to allow for protection against pathogens and lectins from the environment. This is due to the constant food supply for the commensal bacteria within the gut.

The activity of alkaline phosphatase within the serum and the intestines has been strongly correlated with secretor status; non-secretors (FUT2 +/+) have the highest levels of alkaline phosphatase irrespective of their ABO blood group. Secretor status is completely independent of ABO status, so one can be a type-O secretor or non-secretor. The H antigen attached to the ABO (ABO-H) can therefore be used as a marker for secretor status. However, since the availability of genetic testing, the presentation of FUT2 –/– (wild type) has been accepted as evidence of secretor status. The FUT2 secretor status can be tested as a stand-alone test from www.4yourtype.com.

Table 3.1: Secretor/non-secretor

Body system	Secretors	Non-secretors
Circulation		Factor VIII and vWF (especially group O)
	Slow clotting times	Shorter bleeding times
		Platelet aggregation
		Type As at risk for atheroma and cardiovascular disease
Digestive system		Periodontitis
	Dental cavities (group A)	Dental cavities
		Digestive symptoms
		H. pylori, duodenal and gastric ulcers.
		Coeliac disease
		Crohn's disease
		Clostridium difficile, Salmonella
Respiratory system	Protection to environmental insults	Asthma in coal miners
	Some protection from cigarette smoking	Risk of snoring
	Risk of chronic obstructive pulmonary disease	

Immune	Levels of IgG and IgA antibodies	Risk of autoimmune conditions
		Risk of recurrent urinary tract infections
		Risk of persistent Candida, fails to prevent attachment (type 0)
Hormonal		Risk of diabetes (especially adult-onset type 2)
		Risk of heart complications from diabetes (men)
Alcohol		Risk of alcoholism
		Alcohol exerts a negative effect on lung function and a risk of heart disease

vWF = von Willeband factor antigen.

Source: D'Adamo & Kelly 2001

Non-secretors have been shown to be far more susceptible to many forms of autoimmune disease such as Crohn's disease and non-coeliac gluten sensitivity (Forni *et al.* 2014; Nylund *et al.* 2016). They also have less resistance to low-grade infections such as yeast overgrowth or streptococcal infections (Azad *et al.* 2018), *H. pylori* (Moran 2008) and necrotizing enterocolitis (NEC) in preterm infants with severe outcomes (Morrow *et al.* 2011). In the Morrow study of 410 infants, there were 26 deaths, 30 cases of NEC and 96 cases of sepsis in preterm infants of 32 weeks' gestation and below. Low secretor phenotype was associated with (P <.05) NEC and (P =.05) with gram-negative sepsis.

Blood type O none-secretors are often the victim of bacterial over-growth of the stomach, leading to serious conditions such as Barrett's oesophagus and chronic upper stomach and oesophageal inflammation (Thompson 2011). This appears to be due in part to the inability to secrete ABO antibodies but also poor production of bifidobacteria in the large intestine (Wacklin *et al.* 2011). This, of course, has widespread ramifications, so in addition to the conditions already discussed, this could manifest as infections or inflammation of any system covered by a mucous membrane – that is, lungs, gastrointestinal tract, reproductive system and/or urinary system. It could lead to low B12 status, more commonly related to the rs602662 allele (Tanwar *et al.* 2013; Surendran *et al.* 2018), which, of course, has ramifications for methylation status (Zinck *et al.* 2015), when accompanied by other SNPs, as will be seen later.

Homozygous FUT2 +/+ has also been associated with the lack of development of bifidobacteria in breast-fed infants. Lewis *et al.* (2015) found that infants fed by non-secretor mothers were delayed in establishing bifidobacteria-laden microbiota. They postulate that the delay may be due to the infant having difficulty in acquiring a species of bifidobacteria able to consume the specific milk oligosaccharides delivered in the breast milk. This has led to some interesting research on the beneficial properties of human milk oligosaccharides (HMOs), the first prebiotic for infants (Seppo *et al.* 2017). In a review of the likely forward trend of HMOs, Ray *et al.* (2019) discuss types of HMOs, factors determining variation, the role as a prebiotic, antimicrobial properties, immune impact and growth and survival. The authors conclude that while HMOs present the next frontier in neonatal nutrition where breast feeding is not possible, clinical data should justify the species, quantity and time period required for supplementation. Cabrera-Rubio *et al.* (2019) discuss the differences in HMOs in breast milk determined by secretor status. *Lactobacillus* spp., *Streptococcus* spp., *Enterococcus* spp. and *Bifidobacteria* spp. were lower in non-secretors. This is, however, only a pilot study as this is emerging research.

HMOs are unconjugated complex carbohydrates found in breast milk but completely absent in formula milk. HMOs are said to reach the colon where they act as a prebiotic, balancing the early microbiome (Jantscher-Krenn & Bode 2012). They are thought to protect humans against NIDDM (Xiao *et al.* 2018) due to beneficial effects within the microbiota, such as the generation of short-chain fatty acids (SCFAs) and their action on T cells. Currently there are long-term studies being performed on the general population.

Possible interventions based on FUT2 genetic expression
Nutrient cofactors to support FUT2 enzyme activity
Including probiotics, specifically bifidobacteria (Giampaoli *et al.* 2020), prebiotics, oligoribonucleotides (short fragments of RNA that may be used to alter the function of RNAs or DNAs to which they hybridize (cross-breed)) (Aldi *et al.* 2015).

Helpful inducers of FUT2 enzyme activity
Polyphenols (Kohlmeier *et al.* 2018). Non-secretor dietary modifications (Giampaoli *et al.* 2020).

Unhelpful inhibitors that reduce FUT2 enzyme activity
Ethanol (Bell *et al.* 2009).

Drug interactions/substrates (can exacerbate expression of the gene or be responsible for switching the gene on)
Antibiotics, steroids and NSAIDs are known to have a negative impact on intestinal epithelial barrier function (Chelakkot *et al.* 2018). Although there is no evidence to suggest they exacerbate FUT2 expression, it would seem prudent to consider them in the overall case presentation.

PRACTITIONER NOTES

In this instance, the FUT2 +/+ and +/– has been widely associated as determining non-secretor status with a reduction in microbiome diversity, specifically bifidobacteria (Wacklin *et al.* 2011). However, in order to practise safely, it is recommended that practitioners use functional stool testing and a thorough history to determine the need for intervention.

Human leukocyte antigen: HLA-B27, HLA-DQ2 and HLA-DQ8

These genes encode for a protein that plays a crucial role within the immune system. Human leukocyte antigen (HLA) complexes play a critical role in helping the immune system to distinguish between friend or foe, or indeed distinguish between the body's own proteins and those from foreign viruses and bacteria. There are many HLA genes with differing risk factors. The focus in this section is simply on those associated with the case presented. The HLA-DQ2 gene is part of the major histocompatibility complex (MHC) class II and this gene provides instructions for making proteins on the cell surface. These proteins then attach to peptides outside the cell. MHC class II proteins present these peptides to the immune system and, if seen as foreign, this triggers an immune response to attack the pathogen. HLA-DQ2 and HLA-DQ8 are most often known for their contribution to the development of coeliac disease. However, they do have associations with other conditions. A transcription factor is a protein that regulates gene expression by turning the gene on or off so that the gene is expressed at the correct time, in the correct cell and in the correct way. This occurs due to the transcription factor controlling the rate of transcription from DNA to messenger RNA when it binds to a specific gene sequence. Transcription factors regulate cell growth, division and death throughout the human lifespan. HLA-DQ2 and HLA-DQ8 are also part of the same complex although research has been more focused on HLA-DQ2. Polymorphisms in the HLA genes have been associated with various diseases. Cozzolino *et al.* (2018) found a higher incidence of HLA-DQ2 and HLA-DQ8 SNPs in mothers of full-term stillborn infants and suboptimal foetal growth. Cutaneous lupus erythematous (CLE), particularly at loci rs2187668, rs9267531, rs4410767 and rs3094084 (Kunz *et al.* 2015), may infer an autoimmune propensity. Some studies found a major role for HLA-DQB1 and HLA-DRB1 in type 1 diabetes (Raha *et al.* 2013), while Kiani *et al.* (2015) found HLA-DQA1 genes were accompanied by nine other SNPs in their type 1 diabetes study, implying that HLA should not be taken as a propensity towards type 1 diabetes unless all other associated genes are expressing. Bastos *et al.* (2017) found HLA-DQA2 to be more associated with coeliac disease while HLA-DQ8 was more akin to those with type 1 diabetes. For integrative practitioners, there is also the possibility of non-coeliac gluten sensitivity (NCGS) (Czaja-Bulsa 2015). HLA-B27 has so far not been identified in the UK-based genetic profiles but can be measured on a simple venous blood test. Expression of this gene is associated with autoimmune conditions such as psoriatic arthritis.

Possible interventions based on HLA genetic expression
Nutrient cofactors to support HLA enzyme activity
Human milk oligosaccharides (Castanys-Muñoz *et al.* 2016; Xiao *et al.* 2019).

Helpful inducers that increase HLA enzyme activity
Unknown.

Unhelpful inhibitors that reduce HLA enzyme activity
Gluten. Clients therefore need to avoid all forms of gluten (wheat, rye, barley, oats and their derivatives).

Drug interactions/substrates (can exacerbate expression of the gene or be responsible for switching the gene on)
Lapatinib (biological therapy – tyrosine kinase inhibitor used as a targeted treatment for HER2-related breast cancers).

Possible functional testing to determine expression of HLA genes

- Functional immunology and autoimmunity testing.
- Intestinal hyperpermeability.
- Stool testing for microbial diversity and specific microbial populations such as the aforementioned *Bifidobacteria* spp., *Streptococcus* spp., *Lactobacillus* spp. and *Enterococcus* spp. which may impact on immune function, in particular autoimmunity (Ahmad *et al.* 2006; Choo 2007) and under-nutrition (Iqbal *et al.* 2019).

Possible approaches

- Gluten-free diet.
- Supporting functional aspects of digestion using digestive algorithm, comprising full tracking of gastrointestinal symptoms associated with possible low stomach acid, low digestive enzymes and poor bile flow (Downing & Pemberton 2014, p.120).
- Human identical milk oligosaccharides (HIMO) (Coulet *et al.* 2014; Garrido *et al.* 2016) as they become available.

Histamine

Histamine is produced by basophils and mast cells. All other body cells secrete histamine following synthesis but do not store it intracellularly according to Barcik *et al.* (2017). Prior to secretion, histamine can be metabolized via methylation by histamine-N-methyltransferase (HNMT) to N-methylhistamine, or by DAO to imidazole acetic acid, inactivating the histamine, thereby preventing cell danger response (Naviaux 2019, 2014). DAO is responsible for neutralizing extracellular histamine while HNMT metabolizes intracellular histamine from within the cytosol (Klocker *et al.* 2005).

Histamine has a number of roles within the body. It is an excitatory neurotransmitter, helping us to pay attention. It stimulates gastric acid, improving digestion and bowel movement. Histamine is also responsible for the delivery of blood and nutrients to the tissues and creates permeability in the capillaries to allow more white cells and proteins to engage with pathogens as part of immune defence. When someone with a high level of histamine scratches themselves, the resulting huge red wheel on the skin is due to the release of histamine. This reaction is also responsible for hives, itching, stuffy nose and general inflammation associated with allergies and propensity to allergic-like symptoms. Histamine needs to be balanced: too much increases the incidence of intolerance, where there can be too much or a turbulent blood flow, too much attention and no ability to switch off, vasodilation and increased gut permeability, or even miscarriage.

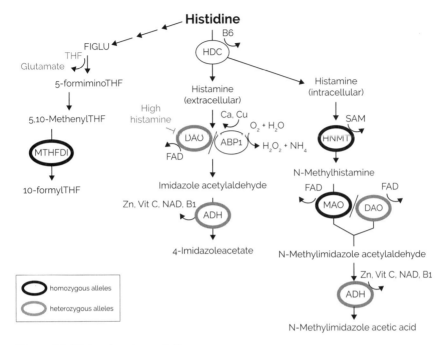

Figure 3.1: Histamine degradation
Key: HDC = histamine decarboxylase, HNMT = histamine N-methyltransferase, MAO = monoamineoxidase inhibitor B, ADH = alcohol dehydrogenase, DAO = diamineoxidase, ABP1 = actin binding protein 1, NH4 =ammonium, Cu = copper, Ca = calcium, H_2O_2 = hydrogen peroxide, Zn = zinc, NAD = nicotinamide adenine dinucleotide, FAD = flavin adenine dinucleotide, SAM = S-adenosylmethionine, CoA = coenzyme A.

There are a number of symptoms associated with histamine:

- headaches and migraines
- difficulty falling asleep, easy arousal, very light sleeping
- hypertension
- vertigo/dizziness
- arrhythmia/tachycardia
- difficulty regulating body temperature
- hives
- fatigue
- anxiety
- nausea and vomiting
- abdominal cramps

- flushing
- nasal congestion, sneezing, difficulty breathing
- abnormal menstrual cycle including lengthy or shorter cycles with dysmenorrhea or menorrhagia
- tissue swelling
- history of need for antihistamines
- history of hay fever, asthma, atopy.

Causes of high histamine and also mast cell activation may include allergies (IgE reactions), bacterial overgrowth of the gut, intestinal hyperpermeability or DAO deficiency.

Some foods are very high histamine liberators too, such as tomato, pickled or canned foods, smoked foods, ferments and shellfish, some nuts and chocolate. There are a number of available food lists, and individuals do tend to react to different ones, which can confuse.

Foods that are high in histamine

- Fermented dairy products such as aged cheese, kefir and yogurt. Sour cream and buttermilk.
- Fermented vegetables such as sauerkraut, kimchi and pickles, soy products.
- Kombucha.
- Cured meats such as sausages, salami and fermented ham.
- Alcoholic beverages.
- Fermented grains such as sourdough bread.
- Tomato.
- Aubergine.
- Spinach.
- Fish, including salted or canned such as sardines and tuna.
- Vinegar.
- Ketchup.

Foods that promote histamine
Pineapple, banana, citrus fruit, strawberries, papaya, nuts, spices, legumes, cocoa, seafood, egg white and food additives. NB: While this

list provides the most common foods, reactions will vary according to individual biochemistry and exposure to other factors such as mould.

Histamine relevant polymorphisms

Diamine oxidase: DAO

The diamine oxidase (DAO) gene, also known as AOC1, encodes for a paroxysmal enzyme D-amino acid oxidase, which oxidizes creating ammonia and hydrogen peroxide. In the gut, it breaks down histamine although the exact mechanism is still eluding scientists. The enzyme used flavin adenine dinucleotide (FAD) as its side group. Because histamine release is body-wide, we do need to consider other SNPs in the pathway. DAO is not presented in the latest version of some DTC-GT, so you may need to check this independently with a functional diagnostic lab. DAO also appears to be responsible for the breakdown of glycoxylate, metabolized in the TCA cycle from isocitrate lyase and from pathogenic yeast in the gut. Low levels of DAO can therefore predispose to higher levels of oxalates. Practitioners should therefore be mindful of recommending high doses of glycine when clients present with expressing DAO SNPs as glycine is converted to serine in the glycoxylate pathway.

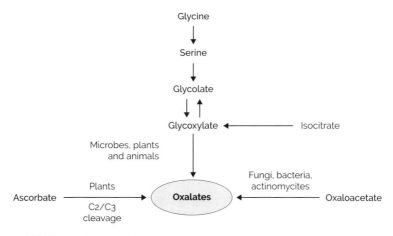

Figure 3.2 Glycoxylate pathway
Reproduced from Chakraborty et al. 2013 by permission of the American Society of Plant Biologists

> ## PRACTITIONER NOTES
>
> Histamine intolerance is very tricky to isolate as it can be confused with mast cell activation disorder (MCAD) and biotoxin illness such as mould. If the client is TH2 dominant, there is also a higher likelihood of them being affected by histamine.

Dysbiosis is a major determinant of histamine intolerance and mast cell activation (Lu & Huang 2017). However, natural lactobacillus residents such as *Lactobacillus reuteri* are also histamine liberators (Greifova *et al.* 2018). Other gut microbes such as *Bifidobacterium longum* and *Bifidobacterium infantis* demonstrate antihistamine effects (Dev *et al.* 2008). Certain strains of probiotic bacteria are known to reduce histamine in the gut; although there is no comprehensive definitive list currently, these are discussed below.

Testing for histamine intolerance can be extremely precarious due to the incredible homeostatic mechanism, so it is of the utmost importance to attain a full and thorough clinical history. Histamine rises acutely and falls again around an hour after the event. This means ideally testing for serum histamine needs to be undertaken as soon as possible after the reaction. To distinguish between histamine and mast cell activation, consider serum tryptase testing. Tryptase is an enzyme released from mast cells, along with histamine, as part of the normal immune response. Levels of tryptase rise within 15 minutes when mast cells are activated, peaking at 1–2 hours and returning to normal several hours after the allergic reaction. Levels would be significantly and persistently elevated in mastocytosis. Those with a positive rheumatoid factor may also have raised tryptase. As with serum histamine testing, a sample taken at the wrong time can result in normal findings even though the individual has many symptoms.

1 and 3-methylhistidine (MHis) on the organic acids profile could be useful as an overall guide as this rises in response to muscle breakdown. It can also be raised from soy ingestion or a heavy intake of meat-based dietary protein, neither of which was relevant to Ella. Muscle breakdown is a characteristic symptom of high histamine/mast cell activation

disorder (Afrin *et al.* 2017). I see this marker raised in many individuals with histamine issues. MHis is derived from the hydrolysis of anserine from meat, specifically poultry. Since it is not metabolized by human tissue, most of it is excreted in urine. Histidine is also methylated to form histamine. In addition, histidine is also broken down to histamine by bacteria of the Enterobacteriaceae group (*Klebsiella, E. coli, Proteus* and *Salmonella*). While MHis can determine a carnivore from a vegetarian, it may also indirectly lead the practitioner to explore histamine further.

Possible interventions based on DAO genetic expression
Nutrient cofactors to support DAO enzyme activity
(and therefore histamine breakdown)
Gelatin, riboflavin (D'Adamo 2014), copper, calcium, water, oxygen (Lynch 2018), iron, cobalamin, vitamin C (Cohen 2015), magnesium (Nishio *et al.* 1987).

Helpful inducers that increase DAO enzyme activity
Hydrogen peroxide from mitochondrial respiration especially in the gut, lungs and thyroid; and ammonia from the oxidation of DAO and gut microbiome (Liu *et al.* 2018; Lynch 2018).

Unhelpful inhibitors that reduce DAO enzyme activity
Glycine, estradiol (D'Adamo 2014), amiloride (Lynch 2018).

Drug interactions/substrates (can reduce expression
of the gene or be responsible for switching the gene
off) preventing the breakdown of histamine
Diuretics, hormone replacement therapies (HRT), monoamine oxidase inhibitors (MAOIs), antiepileptic drugs (AEDs), statins and ibuprofen (Cohen 2015).

Practical advice

- Check ammonia levels that may be produced in the gut, not being converted to urea or resulting from high protein intake. This may be an indication of liver or kidney disease. High levels of ammonia are toxic to the brain and may cause brain damage, coma or even death.

- Find the root cause of the high histamine such as low stomach acid, gut dysbiosis, intestinal hyperpermeability, allergies. Initiate strategies to reduce ammonia if raised. Recall that an expressing DAO SNP creates ammonia when oxidized.
- Butyrate (Canani *et al.* 2011) can reduce ammonia produced in the gut.
- Protein may need to be restricted, especially animal protein (Griffin & Bradshaw 2019).
- Branched-chain amino acids to help mediate the transport of histidine through the blood brain barrier (Dam *et al.* 2011).
- Carnitine may possibly help but this is a very small study (Nojiri *et al.* 2018).
- Check drug interactions and refer for GP review as necessary.
- Support gut function as indicated by stool testing.

Possible approaches for histamine issues

- Find the root cause for raised histamine.
- Advise low-histamine diet temporarily until root cause has been addressed.
- Encouraging an anti-inflammatory diet aids the client towards tolerance of some histamine-promoting foods.
- Encourage an array of good-quality proteins (Wollin *et al.* 2017) as proteins have been shown to increase DAO activity, omitting fish initially then assessing for tolerance later according to case. Some can tolerate frozen fish as histamine rises as a result of amine degradation. Some can tolerate oily fish as a result of high levels of omega 3 providing anti-inflammatory effects.
- Advise good levels of oily fish (Wollin *et al.* 2017) to moderate inflammation after the initial removal.
- Increase intake of omega 9 oils (Wollin *et al.* 2017) as omega 9 from olive oil has been shown to increase DAO levels by as much as 500%. Above all, ensure the balance of raw omega 6 to 3 (linoleic: alpha linolenic) is balanced in a 4:1 ratio to support cell

membranes. This will be discussed in more detail in 'Cell membrane integrity' in Chapter 5.

- Reduce or eliminate alcohol intake (Manzotti *et al.* 2016) as alcohol blocks DAO, and also ALDH enzymes are required to be effective in order to metabolize alcohol to support functioning of the DAO enzyme and to break down the alcohol already in the body as a result of possible yeast overgrowth.

Advise antihistamine probiotics:

- *Lactobacillus rhamnosus* GG especially for stabilizing mast cells (Forsythe *et al.* 2012; Wang *et al.* 2012; Oksaharju *et al.* 2011).
- *Lactobacillus plantarum* (Capozzi *et al.* 2012) helps break down several biogenic amines including tyramine and histamine.
- *Lactobacillus reuteri* whilst increasing histamine also suppresses tumor necrosis factor in a unique way (Thomas *et al.* 2012; Indrio *et al.* 2011).
- *Bifidobacterium infantis* by suppression of H1 receptors and the expression of histidine decarboxylase (Dev *et al.* 2008).
- *Bifidobacterium longum* (Takeda *et al.* 2009) and BB536 (Roselli *et al.* 2009) helps histamine degradation and supports genes/enzymes that hold the gastrointestinal tight junctions together, thereby reducing the incidence of aberrant histamine release.
- *Lactobacillus casei* Shirota (Barrett *et al.* 2008).
- *Eschericia coli* Nissle 1917 (Henker *et al.* 2008).
- VSL#3 (Toh *et al.* 2012).

DAO support:

- Consider other genes that may be involved, such as MTHFR, MAOB, HNMT, PEMT, ALDH2 and ALDH3A2 (Lynch 2018), MAOB, HDC, HRH, ALDH7 (Kucher & Cherevko 2018). As the evidence base expands, there may be others.
- Consider the age and status of the client as DOA expression varies during the monthly cycle – being higher during the luteal phase, low during the follicular phase and high during pregnancy.

High oestrogen can be consistent with high histamine and DAO enzyme impairment. Oestrogen up-regulates mast cells while down-regulating DAO activity. However, the placenta makes a huge amount of DAO during pregnancy. This is why we may see less allergic-type reactions during pregnancy (Maintz *et al.* 2008).

- Consider mopping up the histamine in the early days with binders such as clinoptilolite (MANC®) (Kraljević Pavelić *et al.* 2018).
- Consider a DAO supplement (Manzotti *et al.* 2016) such as Histamine Block, GI Hist or nanomulsified Hista-Aid. These are generally derived from porcine kidney (Maintz & Novak 2007). Purchase from a reputable source as there are many substandard products claiming to be DAO on the market.
- Be aware of nutrient deficiencies such as B6, zinc or copper as these support DAO.
- A vicious cycle may be evident if DAO deficiency produces a lot of symptoms that can inhibit HNMT activity (Ahrens *et al.* 2002).
- DAO blocking medications (Lynch 2017, 2018; Cohen 2015):
  - anti-inflammatory/antipyretic drugs (aspirin, ibuprofen, paracetamol, codeine)
  - antidepressants (duloxetine, venlafaxine, fluoxetine, sertraline)
  - immune modulators (adalimumab, etanercept hydroxychloroquine)
  - antiarrhythmic (propranolol, metaprolol, diltiazem hydrochloride, amlodipine)
  - antihistamines (fexofenadine, cetirizine, diphenhydramine)
  - histamine H2 blockers (cimetidine, famotidine, ranitidine)
  - antiseizure medications (sodium valproate, carbamazepine, lamotrigine, levitiracetam, oxcarbazepine, ethosuximide, topiramate)
  - statins (atorvastatin, fluvastatin, pravastatin, rosuvastatin, simvastatin).

Histidine decarboxylase (HDC)

Histidine decarboxylase encodes for the enzyme decarboxylase. This is the rate-limiting enzyme that converts L-histidine to histamine in mast cells, using pyridoxal-5-phosphate as a cofactor. A number of natural products have been reviewed for their potential to inhibit this gene or to stabilize mast cells, preventing excessive release of histamine (see below). When a polymorphism occurs here and is expressing, it can have a deregulating effect on consistent levels of histamine.

Studies have identified the rs17740607 and rs2073440 alleles in relation to excessive histamine release and chronic heart failure (CHF) from up-regulation of the HDC enzyme. In contrast, He *et al.* (2015) found numerous associations with rs1740607 and a protective mechanism in CHF, implying down-regulation of this allele and a reduction in histamine. However, histamine is needed for the brain to focus and to stay awake, so the H1 to H4 receptors in the hypothalamus also assist with regulation. Too little histamine has been investigated in relation to narcolepsy (Scammell & Mochizuki 2009) but was found to be inconclusive as high levels of histamine were also evident in narcolepsy. The authors purported the reason to be the short half-life of histamine, which is between five and 30 minutes. Karagiannidis *et al.* (2013) found overexpression of the two alleles rs854150 and rs1894236 in a large-scale study of 520 nuclear families from seven European populations, with Tourette syndrome. This work supported a strong hypothesis for histamine-induced Tourette syndrome.

Possible interventions based on HDC genetic expression
Nutrient cofactors to support HDC enzyme activity
Pyridoxine (Lynch 2018).

Inducers that may increase HDC enzyme activity (helpful or unhelpful according to enzyme expression)
Catecholamines, hormones made by the adrenal glands such as dopamine, noradrenaline and adrenaline that can also serve as neurotransmitters; benzene (found in crude oil and used to make plastics, resins, rubber and other synthetic materials); inflammation; lipopolysaccharides; bacteria; histamine-containing foods – putrescine, spermine, spermidine (polyamines from putrefying meat) (Lynch 2018).

Inhibitors that may reduce HDC enzyme activity or stabilize mast cells (helpful or unhelpful according to enzyme expression)
Vitamin C, providing oxalates are not high (Padayatty & Levine 2016); *Bifidobacterium longum* and *B. infantis* (Dev *et al.* 2008); pancreatic enzymes (Maintz & Novak 2007); luteolin (Theoharides 2009); epigallo-catechin gallate (Du *et al.* 2012) and rutin (Ganeshpurkar & Saluja (2017).

Drug interactions/substrates that can reduce or prevent enzyme activity associated with the gene:
B6 inhibitors such as the contraceptive pill, fexofenadine (Zhao *et al.* 2009), diphenhydramine.

Practical advice

- Where this gene is expressing, it is advisable to check for mould in the history.
- Advise how to remove all environmental exposure to plastics where possible.
- Ensure good levels of B6 and HPA axis support if further testing supports this.
- Be aware that B6 supports the production of DAO enzyme but also increases HDC, so testing for the need for B6 and introducing slowly is advisable.
- Support digestive health and methylation as appropriate.

Histamine N-methyltransferase (HNMT)

HNMT encodes for the histamine N-methyltransferase enzyme and is also used as a neurotransmitter in the brain. The enzyme regulates histamine by breaking it down on an intracellular level. It tends to be down-regulated when the SNP is expressing, meaning histamine is not being broken down. Chronic histamine intolerance is said to be as a result of HNMT enzyme deficiency rather than DAO deficiency (Yoshi-kawa *et al.* 2019). The highest levels are found in the bronchi, trachea, liver and kidneys. Having a high concentration in the liver, HNMT degrades histamine that has been generated during normal bodily functions, especially within mast cells. Histamine in the bronchial epithelium is also degraded by HNMT (Yamauchi *et al.* 1994). Ingestion of high-histamine foods may trigger bronchoconstriction and asthma attacks. HNMT is the only pathway known to terminate the neurotransmission actions of histamine in the central nervous systems of humans. It does so by transferring a methyl group from S-adenosyl-L-methionine to histamine (N-methylation). The methyl group donor for HNMT is SAMe, which is not available as a supplement in the UK but is available elsewhere and is made in the methylation cycle. Optimizing methylation can therefore be hugely beneficial for incidence of histamine intolerance. This will be discussed further in the methylation section.

Possible interventions and considerations based on HNMT gene expression
Cofactors to support HNMT enzyme activity
S-adenosylmethionine (Lynch 2018), a methyl donor produced in the methionine cycle.

Helpful inducers that increase HNMT enzyme activity
Folinic acid, magnesium, pantothenic acid, thiamine, pyridoxine, turmeric (D'Adamo 2014).

Unhelpful inhibitors that reduce HNMT enzyme activity
Nicotine, caffeine (Lynch 2018).

Drug interactions/substrates (can exacerbate expression of the gene or be responsible for switching the gene on)
Diphenhydramine hydrochloride (antihistamine), amodiaquine (antimalarial), metoprine (HMT inhibitor).

Practical advice

- Reduce caffeine intake and advise cessation of smoking.
- Check for drug interactions and refer to GP for review if needed.
- Support gut health and methylation as needed.

Monoamine oxidase B (MAOB)

MAOB encodes for the enzyme monoamine oxidase in the outer mitochondrial membrane. The MAOB enzyme degrades the amines in the dopamine pathway, noradrenaline, adrenaline and dopamine. MAOB is more abundant in serotonergic and histaminergic neurones, tends to be over-expressed (+/+ or +/−) and its activity is significantly increased in the brain as a result of ageing (Shih *et al.* 2011), meaning neurotransmitters are broken down more quickly. This gene/enzyme has a twin, MAOA, which we will meet in the 'Neurotransmitter' section in Chapter 5. Higher levels of MAOB have been linked with Alzheimer's and Parkinson's disease due to the elevation of reactive oxygen species produced by elevated MAOB, in turn creating cellular damage (Nagatsu & Sawada 2006). As MOAB levels increase with age, this may suggest a role for its involvement in late diagnosis of neurological disease and cognitive decline (Kumar & Andersen 2004).

The nutrient cofactor for MAOB is flavin adenine dinucleotide (FAD), one of the enzyme-activated forms of riboflavin. FAD is also very important in many areas of the methylation cycle, especially in the recycling of glutathione and in folate conversion. FAD is also required for the conversion of retinol to retinoic acid in the skin, which enhances skin cell proliferation, although the mechanism is unclear (Hirano & Namihira 2017). It is therefore used in many anti-ageing creams (Kong *et al.* 2016). One of the key symptoms of riboflavin deficiency is light sensitivity, so it might be advisable to explore this when taking a case history. Low levels of riboflavin are often seen on organic acid profiles.

Possible interventions based on MAOB genetic expression

Nutrient cofactors to support MAOB enzyme activity
Riboflavin (FAD), progesterone (D'Adamo 2014).

Unhelpful inducers that increase the activity of the MAOB enzyme
Curcumin, oestrogen (D'Adamo 2014).

Helpful inhibitors that reduce MAOB enzyme activity
MAO inhibitor medications such as rasagiline, selegiline and safinamide (used to treat Parkinson's disease). Hypericum (St John's Wort) (Herraiz & Guillén 2018).

Drug interactions/substrates (can exacerbate expression of the gene or be responsible for switching the gene on)
HRT, oral contraceptives, methotrexate, potassium-sparing diuretics (amiloride, triamterene, eplerenone, spironolactone; tricyclics (amitriptyline, clomipramine, imipramine, lofepramide and nortriptyline). Tricyclic antidepressants are no longer being prescribed as a first-line treatment for depression but they can be used for nerve pain (Cohen 2015).

Practical advice
This gene tends to be over-expressed, resulting in higher levels of oxidative stress, so please check for factors that may induce expression such as excessive oestrogen, reducing extraneous sources of oestrogen such as plastics and healthcare products.

Balance blood glucose levels to help balance oestrogen. The rise in oestrogen during the first phase of the menstrual cycle increases sensitivity to insulin. Following ovulation in the luteal phase, rising levels of progesterone increase insulin resistance. During the final week of the menstrual cycle, progesterone levels drop, leaving oestrogen unopposed. Where there is insulin resistance, a susceptible person may be predisposed to the symptoms of premenstrual syndrome and carcinogenesis (Suba 2012).

Check for drug interactions and refer to GP for medication review as necessary.

Support the gene with nutrient cofactors as needed.

Transcobalamin TCN1 and 2

TCN1 encodes a member of the vitamin B12-binding protein family. Also known as R binders, these may be expressed in various body secretions and tissues. The protein is a major constituent of secondary granules in neutrophils. Of the two vitamin B12-binding proteins, TCN1 rs526934 appears to be the one most researched. TCN2 rs9606756 and rs1801198 are also prevalent and have been associated with decreased levels of B12 and frailty. Due to the fact that TCN1 transports B12 into cells from the bloodstream, there is a suggestion from Amy Yasko (2014) that lithium orotate as a low-dose mineral supplement would be advantageous when urinary methylmalonic acid (MMA) and/or homocysteine is high (Marshall 2015). Lithium appears to play an important role of activating MTR and MTRR, which is a critical juncture in driving the production of methyl groups. It is also important for transporting B12 into the cells. The mechanism of action of lithium is still under investigation. However, Guzman (2019) suggests neuroprotective and neurotransmission modulation.

Be aware of clients who are on long-term proton pump inhibitors (PPIs) or those with positive antibodies to intrinsic factor, as these may contribute to poor B12 absorption in the small intestine (Matteini *et al.* 2010). The book *Could It Be B12?* by Pacholok and Stuart (2011) purports that a deficiency of B12 can lead to body-wide effects including serious neurological damage but appears to be markedly under-diagnosed which may be due to the use of serum B12 as a marker for B12 deficiency. Holotranscobalamin (HoloTC) (Nexo & Hoffmann-Lücke 2011) or MMA (Hannibal *et al.* 2016) appear to be more sensitive markers.

Possible interventions based on TCN genetic expression
Nutrient cofactors to support TCN enzyme activity
Cobalamin.

Helpful inducers that increase TCN enzyme activity
Unknown.

Unhelpful inhibitors that reduce TCN enzyme
activity of B12 assimilation
A lack of intrinsic factor.

Drug interactions/substrates (can exacerbate expression of the gene or be responsible for switching the gene off)
Proton pump inhibitors, antacids.

Practical advice

Recommend GP testing for B12 levels. Standard serum B12 levels are not representative of active B12. However, it is important that the GP is made aware if B12 deficiency is suspected or proton pump inhibitors are suspected of reducing B12 uptake.

Supplement B12 if levels of active B12 are supportive or consider lithium orotate (the mineral not the medication) if serum levels are high and active levels are low (Menegas *et al.* 2020; Schrauzer *et al.* 1992).

Phosphatidylethanolamine methyltransferase (PEMT)

PEMT encodes the enzyme that converts phosphatidylethanolamine (PE) to phosphatidylcholine (PC) by methylation in the liver. Where there is limited folate metabolism (due to MTHFR, MTHFD1 expression), methyl trapping (due to TCN, FOLR1, MAOA expression) or increased requirement for homocysteine recycling (due to MTR, MTRR, BHMT-08, BHMT-02 expression), there will be propensity towards poor conversion of PE to PC, and therefore a need to consume more preformed PC. Reduced function of this gene (+/+ or +/−) can increase the risk of alcohol toxicity from toxic aldehydes and ammonia produced in the gut. PC is a major constituent of cell membranes, found in the outer surface of the cell. It plays a role in cell signalling and in the activation of other enzymes.

PEMT is another of those interesting and important genes. Practitioners speak passionately about intestinal permeability or leaky gut and leaky blood–brain barriers, but they don't often discuss leaky cell membranes. If a leaky gut/leaky blood–brain barrier is evident, then appreciation for the wider picture is necessary. It is very important that our cell membranes are intact and fully working, so they need adequate PC to produce the phospholipid bilayer. Practitioners can try to repair the gut barrier or blood–brain barrier, but if the cell is poorly functioning, then overall healing may be limited. We will discuss this more in the methylation section where it rightfully belongs. Low PC has also been recognized as a potential issue in inflammatory conditions such as chronic active ulcerative colitis (Stremmel *et al.* 2005), especially at the distal colon (Karner *et al.* 2014) as PC is an essential component of the mucosal barrier. Karner *et al.* studied 156 patients from 24 ambulatory referral centres in Lithuania, Germany and Romania. Their double-blind placebo-controlled superiority study identified significant improvement in patients who were treated with LT-02, a newly designed modified-release PC. These were patients who previously failed mesalazine treatment. PC is also influential in bile formation and bile flow (Boyer 2013). Poor bile flow has been linked to many disorders of the digestive tract and poor detoxification (Chai *et al.* 2015).

Possible interventions based on PEMT genetic expression
Nutrient cofactors to support PEMT enzyme activity
Folate, S-adenosylmethionine (Lynch 2018).

Helpful inducers that increase PEMT enzyme activity
Choline, oestrogen, cortisol (Lynch 2018).

Unhelpful inhibitors that reduce PEMT enzyme activity
(and therefore reduce production of PC)
Disrupted methylation (especially around the methyltransferase area of the methionine cycle), expressing MHHFD1 and/or MTHFR polymorphism (Lynch 2018).

Drug interactions/substrates (can exacerbate expression of the gene or be responsible for switching the gene on)
Tamoxifen (Lynch 2017).

Practical advice
If this gene is expressing, there will be a requirement for PC to be given as an oral supplement. PC liquid may be more suitable for those with upper gastrointestinal symptoms and capsules for those with symptoms lower down in the bowel. PC is a major component of the bowel mucosa

and has been evaluated for treatment of ulcerative colitis (Karner *et al.* 2014) where mesalazine refractory conditions have occurred.

Please also see the intravenous version of PC (PLX therapy), later in this chapter, used by doctors when cell membranes are compromised in a serious way or the client has incurred substantial toxic exposure. However, also note that the PC used intravenously only contains PC, whereas the oral PC liquid and capsules should contain the full spectrum of phospholipids. These are PC, phosphatidylinositol (PI), phosphatidylethanolamine (PE), phosphatidylserine (PS) and phosphatidylamine (PA).

All phospholipids have specific functions and specific target organs in the body. PE has been identified as protective of degeneration dopaminergic neurones in Parkinson's disease (Patel & Witt 2017; Wang *et al.* 2014). PI is crucial for lung health where a surfactant (a lipoprotein complex) is a crucial requirement for gas exchange (Agudelo *et al.* 2020). PS is known to support the production of myelin sheath and healthy nerve cell membranes (Glade & Smith 2015). PC has numerous health benefits including cognition (Whiley *et al.* 2014), gallbladder support (Kasbo *et al.* 2003), liver and intestinal barrier function (Chen *et al.* 2019) and for the formation and replenishment of the gut mucosal layer (Korytowski *et al.* 2017).

Betacarotene monooxygenase 1 (BCMO1)

The BCMO1 (sometimes known as BCO1) gene instructs the betacarotene monooxygenase 1 enzyme to convert betacarotene to vitamin A. The retinol form of vitamin A is fat-soluble and very important for cell differentiation, mucosal tolerance, embryonic development, skin, vision and cell differentiation, among other roles. Those who carry an expressing T allele at rs12934922 or rs7501331 have a BCMO1 enzyme that is about 60% less active than those who carry the A and C alleles at the same positions. As retinol is fat-soluble, absorption is very much dependent on good bile flow. Optimizing bile flow is crucial when digestion is compromised and BCMO1 and PEMT are expressing.

Possible interventions based on BCMO1 genetic expression
Nutrient cofactors to support enzyme activity of BCMO1
Hesperidin (Poulaert *et al.* 2014).

Helpful inducers that increase BCMO1 enzyme activity
Betacarotene, lutein and/or zeaxanthin.

Unhelpful inhibitors that reduce BCMO1 enzyme activity
Trichostatin A (histone deactylase inhibitor), bisphenol-A, tretinoin (topical vitamin A derivative), testosterone.

Practical advice

- Check for extraneous source of gene inhibitors such as bisphenol-A in plastics, topical vitamin A use and testosterone medication.
- Support gene activity with hesperidin, lutein or zeaxanthin.
- If necessary test and advise on vitamin A supplementation. Oil-based forms are said to be less toxic and better assimilated (Myhre *et al.* 2003).

Alcohol dehydrogenase ADH

ADH encodes for the enzyme alcohol dehydrogenase. ADH was first isolated from *Saccharomyces cerevisiae* in 1937 (Negelein & Wulff 1937). The ADH1B, sometimes seen as ALDH1, gene shows two variants of SNPs, which can either lead to a raised level of histidine or arginine. With the histidine version, the ADH enzyme is a much more efficient catalyzer of the conversion of ethanol into acetaldehyde which may confer a predisposition to the effects of alcohol damage to tissues such as intestinal hyperpermeability, dysglycaemia, memory impairment and sleepiness, also alcohol-related cancers (NIAAA 2007). Conversion of acetaldehyde to acetic acid is the last stage of alcohol breakdown via ALDH2. Those with the histidine variant alleles rs1229984 AG and rs1229984 AA are sensitive to alcohol, thereby conferring less susceptibility to alcoholism (Bierut *et al.* 2012). This gene is of special interest when dealing with a client with long-term fungal/yeast overgrowth as yeast overgrowth is known to increase levels of acetaldehyde (Marttila *et al.* 2013). Those with the arginine variant may convert arginine to nitric oxide much more quickly than usual. Nitric oxide (NO) is extremely beneficial in the correct amounts as it confers protection against heart disease, hypertension and inflammation, especially within the gastrointestinal tract. NO is therefore well known to increase blood flow so is often taken as a supplement to improve sports performance. However, too much arginine or NO can result in worsening of herpes flares, increased risk of death following myocardial infraction (heart attack) and hypotension. It appears to be very unusual to see high levels of NO unless supplementing (Bescós *et al.* 2012).

Possible interventions based on ADH genetic expression
Nutrient cofactors to support ADH enzyme activity
Haem.

Helpful inducers that increase ADH enzyme activity
Ethanol (D'Adamo 2014), zinc, vitamin C, NAD, thiamine (Lynch 2018).

Unhelpful inhibitors that reduce ADH enzyme activity
Selenium, estradiol (D'Adamo 2014).

Practical advice

- Eliminate or at least reduce alcohol intake.
- Support overall digestive health to reduce levels of acetaldehyde created by pathogens.
- Consider nutrient cofactors to support enzyme activity after testing for appropriate requirements.

ELLA'S MYCOTOXIN PROFILE

Recall that Ella had a recent history of mould-induced pneumonia. It was also evident on Ella's organic acid results that mould may still be preventing her health improvement. Levels of furan-2,5-dicarboxylic and furancarbonylglycene were both high, which are associated with *Aspergillus* overgrowth. Some experts report that mycotoxins can prevent the breakdown of histamine by blocking the action of enzymes such as HNMT. The evidence is not supportive of this idea at this point in time. However, it is well known that mycotoxins can stimulate mast cell activation (Kritas *et al.* 2018) so the net result may be comparative. It is not known why the mast cells are not switching off, but given all the toxins in today's environment from processed food, chemicals, heavy metals, infections, fragrances, etc., it isn't a surprise. Ella's urine mycotoxin profile, as discussed below, highlighted moderate levels of ochratoxin A, sterigmatocystin and verrucarin.

Ochratoxin A (OTA) is nephrotoxic, immunotoxic and carcinogenic, so it was important to pay attention to this. This toxin can significantly reduce dopamine levels in the brain, thereby contributing to the development of neurodegenerative disease such as Alzheimer's and Parkinson's. Ella was struggling with her brain function. She was requiring as many as four power naps of 20–30 minutes daily to allow her to function throughout the day. This was thought to be due to low levels of dopamine, creating narcolepsy (Burgess *et al.* 2010) that was confirmed on neurotransmitter testing. She also reported that she would be holding a conversation with a colleague and suddenly would lose the entire thread of the conversation, which would come to a complete halt mid-sentence. For a high achiever, this was immensely stressful, causing Ella health anxiety around possible diagnosis of Alzheimer's disease or dementia. Ella required a lot of psychological support at this time.

Exposure can be from contaminated foods such as grapes, cereals, dairy, spices, wine, dried vine fruit and coffee. It can also be from water-damaged buildings. Ella was a regular spice user but had no known intake of the other foods. Her exposure was undoubtedly from repeated exposure in water-damaged buildings as determined in Ella's timeline and case brief (see Chapter 2).

Sterigmatocystin (STC)
Closely related to aflotoxins, STC is produced from several species of mould such as *Aspergillus*, *Penicillium* and *Bipolaris*. It has been found in

the dust from damp carpets and is also a known contaminant of many foods such as grains, corn, bread, cheese, spices, coffee beans, soybeans, pistachio nuts and animal feed.

Raised levels of STC are well known to excessively increase levels of oxidative stress, causing a depletion of glutathione and other antioxidants, especially in the liver (Fountain *et al.* 2016)

Verrucarin A

Verrucarin A is a macrocytic trichothecene mycotoxin produced from specific species of moulds, namely *Stachybotrys*, *Fusarium* and *Myrothecium*. It is most often the result of water-damaged buildings, although occasionally can be found in contaminated grain. This mycotoxin produces reactive oxygen species in excessive amounts that then disrupt mitochondrial function. It causes damage to human cells by inhibiting protein and DNA synthesis (Bin-Umer *et al.* 2011).

Intranasal and transdermal glutathione may be helpful when combined with bile acid sequestrants to bind the GI toxins, making them unavailable for reabsorption. Sequestrants are best considered for food-related exposure, with bentonite clay (Nones *et al.* 2016), modified citrus pectin (Zheng *et al.* 2008), activated charcoal (Tack *et al.* 2011), chlorophyll (Simonich *et al.* 2007) and/or cholestyramine being the optimal choices for verrucarin A exposure. Humic and fulvic acid appear also to bind up glyphosate (Gildea *et al.* 2017). Most of the evidence originates from animal husbandry, with little pertaining to direct application in human trials. Ahlberg *et al.* (2019) compared the use of lactic acid-producing bacteria (LAB) to natural sequestrants in their animal study on food safety aspects of aflotoxin binding. They found binders to be preferable to LAB. It might be logical to assume that binding up toxins in the GI tract might also bind up valuable minerals. However, studies have shown this to be a mistaken belief (Chu *et al.* 2013; Katsoulos *et al.* 2009).

It is important to stress the need to assess and initiate mould renovation where necessary. In Ella's case, her primary exposures were believed to be external to her home. However, specialist environmental assessment identified water damage Ella was previously unaware of. A shower she had newly fitted when she moved into her current home five years previously had a continual leak that had run between the stud partition walls, completely destroying the base support. Two walls and the floor had to be taken out and replaced. Ella also used a propolis diffuser (Temiz *et al.* 2013; Matny 2015).

ELLA'S HISTAMINE SNPS AND POSSIBLE MOULD IMPACT

Ella's CYP SNPs included DAO, HNMT, MAO, MTHFD1 and ADH. These would likely express in the presence of mycotoxin exposure but in addition Ella's mould exposure had triggered mast cell cytokine immune response (Kritas *et al.* 2018). It was therefore important at this point to also consider Ella's histamine pathway SNPs.

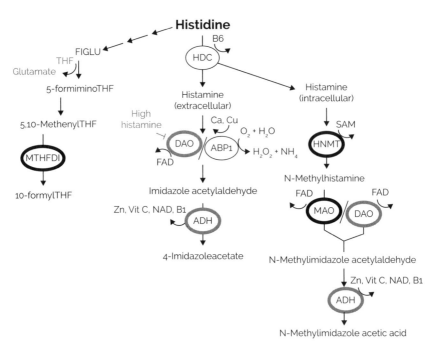

Figure 3.3 Ella's histamine SNPs
Key: MTHFD1, HNMT and MAOB are all homozygous +/+ presentation (black outline); DAO and ADH are both heterozygous +/– presentation (grey outline).

A standard blood tryptase result returned a borderline result for Ella. Raised tryptase is a measure of mast cell degranulation as a result of anaphylaxis. Being a larger protein than histamine, tryptase has a much longer serum half-life. It would therefore be difficult to ascertain a positive result unless three samples were taken in the immediate time period of the exposure, four hours after the exposure and 24 hours after exposure according to NICE clinical guidelines 183 (2014). However, Ella's history and her histamine pathway SNPs allowed us to assume at least a mould allergy or intolerance as evidence is mounting that mould exposure predisposes to mast cell activation as a result of its impact on certain SNPs. The most important SNPs are DAO, HNMT, MAOB and ADH (Conti *et al.* 2018; Kritas *et al.* 2018; Ratnaseelan *et al.* 2018).

In Ella's case, support was aimed at removing the source of exposure and repairing cell membranes. The exposure was found to be from repeated short-term exposures, exacerbated by a hidden long-term shower leak in her home. Remediation of the water damage was necessary in addition to supporting detoxification of the OTA.

ELLA'S HEALTH PLAN: HISTAMINE

Ella remained very restricted in her food intake although she was ready to try introducing simple foods that would support her digestion. She was responding well to the network spinal analysis (NSA) and the KPU support (see 'Ella's health plan: KPU' in Chapter 2) in that her anxiety was reducing but not maintaining between sessions. She was mindful of being constantly 'triggered' into anxiety without knowing why, so other tools were suggested such as Sensate and HeartMath (see Appendix). She was keen to have a face-to-face HeartMath session so this was provided. She then took this tool to help her in the NSA sessions. The KPU supplement was also being increased slowly.

Steps were taken to remove all xenoestrogens such as plastics, bisphenol-A, cling film and pesticides (Fernandez & Russo 2010). Also, synthetic personal care products and toiletries were exchanged for natural solutions. A plan for mould renovation at Ella's home was also commenced.

It was recommended to increase fibre intake with the use of soluble fibres such as linseed, chickpeas and lentils. Fibre is known to reduce absorption or oestrogens by their action on the microbiome while simultaneously increasing excretion from the gastrointestinal tract (Harnden & Blackwell 2016). These were introduced very slowly and all pre-soaked before cooking to reduce the amount of phytates, so that absorption of nutrients could be optimized. This approach was also to prevent further absorption of oestrogenic chemicals into the bloodstream and promote excretion via the bile and stool (Flower *et al.* 2014). A small amount of fermented soy products was also trialled and rejected as this caused pruritus and bowel inflammation, seen as raised calprotectin (Bjarnason 2017). Asafoetida was added to the cooking fluid for the pulses to help reduce incidence of flatulence (Mahendra & Bisht 2012). Peppermint, ginger (Haniadka *et al.* 2013), cumin and fennel (Rahmy *et al.* 2019) were also recommended for their ability to support digestion.

Glucosinolates precursors were provided in the form of cruciferous vegetables such as broccoli, Brussels sprouts, cabbage and cauliflower. These caused excessive bloating, suggesting possible SIBO or trans-sulphuration difficulties. Epsom salts baths and molybdenum (see Chapter 5) allowed a gradual introduction of cruciferous vegetables. Ella was also advised to take regular small portions of broccoli sprouts as an added bonus (Upadhyaya *et al.* 2018). She managed a small amount of these, preferring them to the other cruciferous suggestions.

It would have been necessary also to remove all extrinsic sugars and stimulants and to ensure a good balance of proteins, complex carbohydrates and essential fats to balance blood glucose levels in order to help regulate oestrogen further. However, Ella was so restricted and afraid of food that the balance was already being achieved. Ella was peri-menopausal at this time.

Gentle rebounding on a trampet ensuring feet remained in contact with the trampet was recommended. Ella agreed this would be manageable at 5–10 minutes three times weekly. When it wasn't manageable, Ella would undertake simple feet flexing and extending exercises and ankle rotations. This would support lymph drainage (Cogoli 1991) and help reduce some of her stress response due to endorphin release (Daneshvar *et al.* 2019).

On receipt of the mycotoxin profile result and discontinuation of intravenous phospholipid exchange therapy, it was decided to maintain levels of phosphatidylcholine via the oral route. Essential fatty acids were also delivered via an activated nut- and seed-based smoothie with the addition of specific essential fatty acids and the PC. The ratio of fatty acids was in accordance with Ella's red blood cell fatty acid profile. The particular test used was one that highlighted specific deficiencies and excesses of a range of omega 3, 6 and 9 fatty acids. It also gave indications of how to rebalance these by either burning off (transfats, very long-chain fats and medium-chain), building (all essential fatty acids plus non-essentials that are defined as low) or balancing (all eicosanoids and their precursors). Practitioner and patient receive a report consistent with their role, which is then personalized by the practitioner.

Removal of the mycotoxin load was initiated with a combination of indole-3-carbinol (I3c) (Ishibashi *et al.* 2012), methylation support and a combination of clinoptilolite (Zeolite) (Kraljević Pavelić *et al.* 2018) and activated charcoal binders/sequestrants. As I3c is a NRF2 up-regulator (Saw *et al.* 2011), this had an immediate positive effect on Ella's energy levels, possibly due to its impact on the glutathione system (Harvey *et al.* 2009). I3c may also be used in this manner to assist bile movement (Ishibashi *et al.* 2012). As such, it was necessary to strictly time the ingestion of I3c and sequestrants so that the sequestrants could mop up the toxic bile as the I3c stimulated it. Sequestrants need to be taken half an hour before the I3c and food eaten 15 minutes after the I3c. This was quite a time-focused approach that required a lot of support during the eight-week period.

Ella's supplement programme included the following for 8 weeks

- Betaine HCL + pepsin 700mgs caps x 3 per meal to assist protein digestion (Guilliams & Drake 2020).
- Digestive enzymes x 1 per meal (Ianiro *et al.* 2016).
- KPU complex.
- Bifidobacteria x 2 daily (antihistamine and microbiome rebalancing).

- *Lactobacillus plantarum, L. rhamnosus, L. salivaricus* x 1 daily (anti-histamine and microbiome rebalancing).
- Clinoptilolite (MANC®) to bind mycotoxins (Kraljević Pavelić *et al.* 2018).
- Liposomal glutathione to support NRF2, ROS (Guilford & Hope 2014) as NRF2 is inhibited by OTA (Kaczmarek *et al.* 2019).
- I3C for eight weeks followed by broccoli seed extract taken as a powder in water to support NRF2 cellular protection and micro-biome diversity (Kaczmarek *et al.* 2019; Dinkova-Kostova *et al.* 2017).
- It was also noted that a small dose of extra riboflavin was very helpful in reducing some of Ella's anxiety.

Riboflavin is a precursor to the riboflavin adenine dinucleotide and flavin mononucleotide, and these two enzymes are crucial for many enzymes within the methylation system. As can be seen from her SNPs, FAD is useful to support DAO and MAO, which are highly linked to anxiety. However, it also supports the conversion of oxidized glutathione to its reduced version. High amounts of oxidized glutathione can also be responsible for anxiety (Steenkamp *et al.* 2017). Ella's need for riboflavin was high on her organic acids test.

PRACTITIONER NOTES

Other possible therapeutic agents could include:

- Cholestyramine (bile acid sequestrants), charcoal, clay, chlorella (broad-spectrum toxin binders) (Hope 2013), phenylalanine which prevents OTA absorption from food and stimulates chol-ecystokinin feedback loop (Hira *et al.* 2008) which may support excretion of toxins from gallbladder and liver.
- Antioxidants: vitamins A, E, C, N-acetyl-cysteine (Guilford & Hope 2014), rosmarinic acid (Moghtader *et al.* 2011).
- Binders: bentonite or zeolite have been shown to reduce absorption of OTA (Gulfam *et al.* 2018; Var *et al.* 2008).

> – Some studies have also shown OTA in sweat, which supports the use of saunas to increase secretion of OTA (Hope and Hope 2012).

Lymphatic congestion

Following successful removal of the mycotoxins, as confirmed by a follow-up urine mycotoxin profile, Ella was struggling with very heavy legs. She reported that she felt as if she was walking in treacle. This symptom was one that directed the consultation findings towards the possibility of stagnant lymph. Given Ella's earlier long-term relationship with yeast and mould, it would make sense that many of the gut toxins may now be in her general lymph system. It was felt important to cleanse this system to prevent more recurrences of microbial overgrowth and to support Ella's brain health, as will be discussed in the 'Neurotransmitter' section in Chapter 5. There is good evidence to support lymphatic cleansing in neurological disease (Sun *et al.* 2018), and although Ella does not appear to fall into the category of neurological disease, there were clear indications of brain fog and brain exhaustion.

Other signs of lymphatic congestion might include:

- dry skin
- cold extremities
- fluid retention
- bloating
- itchy skin
- feeling tired
- rings become tight on fingers
- early-morning stiffness and/or soreness.

Underlying causes of lymphatic congestion include:

- stress
- digestive imbalances – the quality of the villi is important for assimilation, detoxification, lymph detoxification and immunity (Douillard 2017, pp.133–152)

- iodine deficiency – iodine supports lymph at the cellular level (Fields 2014).

The work of Dr John Douillard was the consulted influence behind this stage of Ella's journey. The rationale for consulting Dr Douillard was to gain an understanding of the use of kitchari as a healing food for Ella. Kitchari is a hulled mung bean and white basmati rice recipe often fed to those with poor constitution as a revival food or to reset digestion. It is also used to wean babies. It was important to supply Ella with more nutrient diversity, in an easy-to-digest formula, while not negatively affecting her gut with high-histamine foods such as bone broth and ferments, all of which caused Ella symptoms of intestinal inflammation. Kitchari is noted to have been used in Indian and Ayurveda medicine since around 1500 BC and is regarded as a most cherished food. The yellow split pea is often mistaken for the split mung bean, but the mung bean is roughly half the size of the split pea. It is important to make this distinction.

Hulled mung beans, according to Ganesan and Xu (2018), are said to contain an array of nutritional benefits including antioxidant, antimicrobial and antidiabetic, antihypertensive, anti-inflammatory and lipid metabolism alongside antitumour effects. They contain high quantities of manganese, magnesium, folate, copper, potassium, zinc and various B vitamins. These are all important nutrients for the SNPs Ella presents in this section. White rice would be contraindicated in a Western approach due to its possible impact on blood glucose. The health benefits of ingesting brown rice in preference to white are clear in the evidence. However, brown rice is also well known for its high content of phytates, which can, of course, reduce absorption of nutrients in the gut and also reduce enzyme activity for protein digestion (Perera *et al.* 2018). Brown rice also contains lectins, which may be responsible for some allergic reactions (Salazar *et al.* 2013) as they are glycoproteins and as such they bind up glucosamine. The amount of rice in the dish is minimal and can be omitted or replaced with vegetables (see recipe below).

Kitchari can be cooked on top of the stove within an hour, or slow-cooked with warming spices to improve digestion in Ayurvedic medicine. Some doctors would advocate pressure-cooking to completely remove lectins (Gundry 2019). However, although long-term evidence exists for the negative impact of lectins on autoimmunity and inflammation (Kumar *et al.* 2012), no evidence exists currently that supports a particular cooking method for their removal. Soaking, cooking and fermenting, to name a few methods, may reduce the amount of lectins. Hulled mung beans (moong dahl) contain very little lectin prior to cooking.

This dish provides a nutrient-dense food with high soluble fibre that encourages improved gut motility, rebalances microbiome and encourages detoxification and excretion of toxins from gut-associated lymphoid tissue (GALT) and the gallbladder using a process called lipophilic-mediated detoxification (Herron & Fagan 2002). When combined with a good early-morning supply of ghee to pull the toxins out of GALT, this method is said to be very effective clinically (Douillard 2017, pp.133–152). However, there are no studies to my knowledge that have supported this in Western practice. There are contradicting published works on the risk–benefit ratio with regard to lipid metabolism and cardiovascular risk with ghee intake. However, Sharma *et al.* (2010) identified significant improvements in subjects with psoriasis due to the ability of ghee to lower secretion of leukotrienes, prostaglandin and thromboxane, as these are arachidonic acid metabolites. Based on these studies and Ella's fatty acid result determining a need for saturated fats, organic goats ghee was introduced very slowly and tolerated well.

Health benefits of spices contained in kitchari

- Ginger: antioxidant, anti-inflammatory, anti-nausea, anticancer, antiplatelet, antidiabetic (Bode & Dong 2011).
- Turmeric: antioxidant, anti-inflammatory, decreases inflammatory cytokines and vascular endothelial growth factor. Can be supportive in arthritic conditions, metabolic syndrome, anxiety and hyperlipidaemia (Hewlings & Kalman 2017).
- Coriander: improvement of ileum microflora (Hosseinzadeh *et al.* 2014), antimicrobial, antioxidant, antidiabetic, anxiolytic, antidepressant, antiseizure, antimutagenic, antihypertensive, anti-inflammatory, neuroprotective and diuretic (Sahib *et al.* 2013).

- Cumin: antioxidant, antidiabetic, antihypertensive, neuroprotective, antimicrobial, antiviral, antiparasitic, antifungal, anticancer, increased sperm motility, anti-toxicological properties (Yimer *et al.* 2019).
- Mustard seeds: antimicrobial, antioxidant (Rahman *et al.* 2018).
- Asafoetida: relaxant, neuroprotective, digestive enzyme, memory enhancer, antioxidant, antispasmodic, hypotensive, hepatoprotective, anticancer, antitoxicity, antiobesity, anthelmintic (Amalraj & Gopi 2016).
- Fennel: health benefits have been seen in menopausal women (Saghafi *et al.* 2017). It has been used to improve visual acuity, stomach pains, vomiting, nausea, chronic fever, internal obstructions, urinary tract disorders, chronic diarrhoea, catarrh, cataracts, infantile colic and as an emmenagogue to stimulate menstrual flow (Mahboubi 2019).
- Fenugreek: antioxidant, glucose- and cholesterol-lowering, fever, vomiting, poor appetite, antifungal, antibacterial (Nagulapalli *et al.* 2017).

KITCHARI RECIPE (ADAPTED FROM DOUILLARD 2017)
Ingredients

1 cup split yellow mung dahl
¼ to ½ cup white basmati rice
8 cups water (or home-made sodium-free vegetable broth)
1 tsp fresh ginger, finely grated
½ tsp turmeric powder or 1 tsp fresh turmeric, finely grated
½ tsp coriander powder or 1 tsp seeds
½ tsp cumin powder or 1 tsp seeds
½ tsp mustard seeds
1 pinch hing (asafoetida)
½ tsp Himalayan salt
1 small handful fresh coriander

Directions

Rinse mung dahl and rice together a few times until water runs clean.

Toast the spices (optional) for 2–5 minutes to enhance the flavour.

In a large saucepan, combine the rice, beans, water and spices.

Cover and bring to the boil, reduce heat and simmer for 30–45 minutes, until the rice and dahl are very soft. This needs to look like a soup.

Garnish with salt and fresh coriander.

Ella was more than happy to cook one pot of food daily and eat kitchari for every meal, including early-morning ghee for two weeks. Interestingly, it was more difficult to get Ella to reintroduce foods after the two weeks as she was just beginning to reap the benefits. The addition of more vegetables and low-sugar fruit allowed her increased variety within the kitchari recipe. Ella found the kitchari to be very supportive for her digestion and she continued to carry it in a flask for lunchtime most days after the initial two weeks, as an ongoing part of her programme.

The addition of lymph-supporting herbs such as ginger and manjistha powder, sold as a dried bitter herbal food product (*Rubia cordifolia Linn*), in the form of daily teas was also helpful (Rabb 2018). Lifestyle adaptations included rebounding for ten minutes daily and deep breathing techniques in the form of HeartMath techniques as already taught. The addition of a few sessions of lymphatic drainage also helped (Yuan *et al.* 2015).

Lifestyle interventions

Ella was consistent with rebounding and was able to increase slowly to ten minutes three times weekly.

Ella joined a walking group in her local area. The group was mostly retired individuals who preferred to amble rather than compete, so this ensured she had contact with her community and received the health benefits of being in nature without getting exhausted (Seymour 2016).

Further HeartMath techniques were taught to Ella, specifically the quick coherence technique and heart lock-in. These were taught to improve heart rate variability (HRV) as a marker for resilience (Hartmann *et al.* 2019). Ella was encouraged to measure her own HRV regularly. Once she mastered the techniques, it would be easy for her to incorporate them into her activities of daily living.

NSA chiropractic care was continued. Ella found this particularly helpful, reporting less congestion in her solar plexus area and a slight increase in gastric emptying (less fullness after meals). She also reported her anxiety levels diminishing, although this wasn't being sustained between appointments at this time.

Autophagy genes related to Crohn's disease and inflammatory bowel disorder

ATG1 16l 1, GTpaseM (IRGM), NOD2

These genes will be discussed collectively because they are all immune-related, forming a cluster of genes that have been found to be clinically relevant in conditions such as Crohn's disease. Autophagy-related 16L1 and IRGM are two of the genes that are supportive for the immune system, very much dependent on good levels of macrophages. Autophagy is the natural process of building and repair of the body cells. Autophagy can destroy bacteria and viruses after an infection and also mop up damaged proteins and organelles that create ageing; in effect, these genes increase autophagy so they are anti-ageing genes. However, when the gene is expressing, this benefit is lost. They were discovered initially in the 1960s, but Yoshinori Ohsumi was awarded the Nobel Prize in 2016 for his work in identifying the mechanisms behind autophagy. An improved understanding of Parkinson's disease and dementia has occurred as a result. In 2007, Hampe *et al.* found in their genome-wide association study (GWAS) a disease association between ATG1 16L1 (rs2241880) and NOD2, also known as CARD15 genes in Crohn's disease, which has been replicated many times (Büning *et al.* 2007).

According to Cadwell *et al.* (2010), IRGM expression and a viral infection could predispose to Crohn's disease. The Cadwell study compared mice with ATG16L1 and either an activated or a non-activated form of murine norovirus. Paneth cell abnormalities such as aberrant granule size and distribution were seen in the activated viral group, thereby producing a significantly altered intestinal injury response. The inactivated virus did not produce these abnormalities. IRGM has been extensively studied in relation to viral load such as HIV, measles, mumps and hepatitis C (Grégoire *et al.* 2011), so it would be prudent to bring the two aspects together now. Intermittent or short-term fasting is said to enhance autophagy (Mehrdad *et al.* 2010).

Tests to consider that would ascertain gene expression

- Comprehensive stool testing.
- DNA-based stool testing.
- SigA.
- Organic acids – relevant markers include yeast, bacteria, clostridia and oxalates.
- B12 and folate, homocysteine or methylation test options (see the methylation section in Chapter 5), because high homocysteine impairs autophagy (Tripathi *et al.* 2016).

Possible approaches to digestive wellness

- The 5R (see box below) approach according to presenting signs, symptoms and functional test results.
- Fermented foods such as kefir, kombucha, kimchi, beet kvass, sauerkraut (not with high histamine).
- High histamine: *Bifidobacteria* (Schink *et al.* 2018), *Lactobacillus plantarum* (Kung *et al.* 2017), *L. rhamnosus* (Oksaharju *et al.* 2011) and *L. salivaricus* (Wang *et al.* 2015), *Saccharomyces boulardii* (Moré & Vandenplas 2018).
- Human milk oligosaccharides (HMO) encourage *Bifidobacteria* acting as a prebiotic (Castanys-Muñoz *et al.* 2016).
- It is important not to forget lifestyle and stress as stress inhibits digestion.

THE 5R APPROACH TO DIGESTIVE HEALTH

Remove

Any digestive irritants such as poorly tolerated foods, over-the-counter medications and supplements, stress, infections (bacterial, viral, yeast, parasitic).

Replace

Betaine HCL, bile salts, digestive enzymes, bicarbonate of soda, bitter foods to stimulate digestion and/or nutrients to address imbalances.

Repopulate

Prebiotic and probiotic foods such as onions, garlic, leeks, apples and bananas. Fermented foods such as yogurt, sauerkraut, kombucha and kimchi.

Repair

Anti-inflammatory foods and foods containing vitamins A, C, D and E and zinc. Foods rich in amino acids such as bone broth. Supplements such as L-glutamine, collagen, aloe vera, slippery elm and/or marshmallow root.

Rebalance

Stress management, sleep hygiene, exercise, engaging in activities that make one happy, improving relationships.

ELLA'S CASE: ASSIMILATION

As indicated, Ella had long-term issues with dysbiosis, testing positive for many pathogens at different points in time. She was infected with *Klebsiella pneumoniae*, *Pseudomonas*, *Candida albicans* and *C. parapsilosis*, mould and *Blastocystis homini* at this time. The *Candida* species proved difficult to eradicate and she struggled with detoxification of the metabolites when initiating an Institute for Functional Medicine–designed 4R (IFM 2010) approach with herbal antimicrobials. General liver support was only partially helpful, so cycling between antimicrobials and gut healing was enabling some progress; however, this was slow.

Ella's genetic profile showed the following gut related polymorphisms:

Table 3.2: Ella's digestive SNPs and functional markers

SNPs	Issue	Expression	Support
FUT2 +/+	Non-secretor	Dysbiosis (Stool testing, organic acids) Lewis +ve	Bifidobacteria, Lactobaccillus plantarum, L. rhamnosus, L. salivaricus, Saccharomyces boulardii
BCMO1 +/–	Less able to convert betacarotene to vitamin A	Malabsorption (organic acids) serum fat-soluble vitamins	May require fat-soluble vitamin A Dose according to testing Therapeutic range 4000iu females, 5000iu males[1]
PEMT +/+	Poor conversion PE to PC Cell membranes, liver, etc.	PE and PC (organic acids)	Phosphatidylcholine (Vance 2014)
DOA +/+	Poor breakdown of histamine in the gut	Clinical history, plasma DAO levels	Porcine kidney-based DAO support, clinoptilolite (MANC®), low-histamine diet initially
HNMT +/+	Could be less able to break down histamine intracellularly	History	Improve methylation later for SAMe PC to stabilize cell membranes

cont.

---

1   Vitamin A dosing is age dependent (Mann & Truswell 2007) with therapeutic dosage set at 4000–5000iu for adults (IFM 2005). Practitioners should be aware of potential toxicity (Olson *et al.* 2019).

SNPs	Issue	Expression	Support
MAOB +/+	Slow MAO = food cravings, breaks down serotonin too quickly	5-HIAA (organic acids)	Riboflavin-5-phosphate
PON1 +/+	Less able to break down glyphosate	Assume	Organic food

Ella's organic acid results

Ella had moderate levels of bacteria (DHPPA, 3-HPA, hippuric acid), yeast (arabinose, 5-HIAA, citramalic acid) and mould (furan 2,5-dicarboxylic) with high malabsorption markers (PAA).

It is evident that Ella has some expression on her FUT2, which would have slowed down her ability to detoxify within the gut. She needed an organic diet due to her poor ability to detoxify glyphosate and she also needed to exchange her general probiotics for bifidobacteria initially with the later addition of *Lactobacillus plantarum*, *salivaricus* and *rhamnosus*, as these are notably antihistamine (Toh *et al.* 2012). There wasn't a marker on her organic acid test for glyphosate, though measures of glyphosate on DNA can be identified as DNA adducts in some specialist laboratory tests. Also, there is now a urine glyphosate test available that can be added to the OAT profile. Ella had not seriously considered her mould intolerance prior to the pneumonia. At the time of the pneumonia insult, she was working in a mouldy environment and had suffered two previous mould exposures in previous years. She recognized the characteristic dry, unproductive cough of mould exposure but wasn't too worried. However, in addition to this, she inadvertently ate food containing high-fructose corn syrup, which set off an allergic reaction requiring hospital admission. She became worse when given antibiotics for the pneumonia. From her own research on specific social media forums, she knew to find a doctor with experience of intravenous phospholipid exchange therapy in order to stabilize her cell membranes and that was her turning point to improved health.

PHOSPHOLIPID EXCHANGE (PLX) THERAPY

Related to expression of the PEMT gene and to expression of genes within the methionine cycle, especially methyltransferase genes.

PLX is outside the remit of nutrition therapists. However, it can be a very useful therapy in severe cases of toxicity, chronic unremitting disease and neurological impairment. The therapy is in line with Naviaux's (2014, 2019) theory of cell danger response. It is said to detoxify and restabilize the cell membrane (see section 'Cell membrane integrity' in Chapter 5). Drs Ed and Patricia Kane have largely undertaken the research behind this therapy at the Neurolipid Research Foundation. The therapy includes intravenous (IV) delivery of PC alongside B12, folinic acid and phenylbutyrate and/or other nutrients specific to the individual. The IV therapies are delivered alongside a neurolipid keto diet plan known as the PK protocol. Lipids are delivered in a power drink according to the individual's fatty acid analysis from Kennedy Krieger laboratories in the USA. The diet plan is produced from a basic blood chemistry report called BBB1 arranged through a functional blood-testing laboratory and analyzed by Body Bio. Dr Patricia Kane has a team of doctors worldwide who provide the complete service; three of these doctors are resident in London, UK.

Exposure to mould can down-regulate expression of DAO and HNMT as the toxins reduce enzyme function, thereby preventing the breakdown of histamine (Yoshikawa *et al.* 2019). High-fructose corn syrup is one of the highest histamine and mould combinations, so given her previous exposures this was too great for her body. HNMT is expressed body-wide but the heaviest expression is within the brain, lungs and bronchial epithelium – hence histamine being related to asthma. Yoshikawa *et al.* (2019) also speculate that future development of HNMT inhibitors could prove useful in controlling certain types of brain dysfunction such as Parkinson's and attention deficit hyperactivity disorder (ADHD). Ella's mother and sister were atopic with asthma and chronic obstructive airway disease (COPD). The excessive histamine and mast cell activation from the combined insult was too great for Ella and her body hurtled into a cell danger response (Naviaux 2014, 2019). As her 1-methylhistidine was over 3000, this was accepted alongside her history as a histamine marker; histamine and intestinal hyperpermeability are co-dependent (Potts *et al.* 2016). With this in mind and in order to ensure some healing of cell membranes and gut, it was decided to use clinoptilolite binders to help bind up both the mould (Prasai *et al.* 2017) and the histamine in the gut. Clinoptilolite is a microporous alumino-silicate mineral. This reduced Ella's inflammation quite markedly and allowed a slightly wider variety of foods into her regime. There is a general apprehension towards the use of binders in that they are believed to also bind up valuable minerals. However, Prasai *et al.* (2017) found quite the opposite. Ella's experience was that her night-time cramps, restless legs and early-morning anxiety diminished within a few days, suggesting more availability of magnesium and electrolytes, so this was pleasing. In addition to binding up the toxins, Ella's functional digestion was assessed according to Downing and Pemberton's algorithm (Downing & Pemberton 2014, p.120). Ella's digestion was not strong enough to cope with a paleo or more ketogenic approach alongside the PLX therapy, so the nutritional approach used was focused on 80% plant diet ensuring good levels of protein, as this was more likely to provide Ella with microbial diversity according to Toribio-Mateus (2018). Ella was encouraged to take liquid PC and balanced oil with a 4:1 ratio of omega 6 to 3 together during the IV PLX stage.

Ella was already being supported with betaine hydrochloride, digestive enzymes and bile support (beetroot and taurine). Her general probiotic was exchanged for specific histamine-reducing probiotics (*Bifidobacteria*, *Lactobacillus plantarum*, *L. rhamnosus* and *L. salivaricus*). Antimicrobials were not considered at this time as Ella had reacted badly to those previously due to poor detoxification. This will be discussed further in Chapter 4.

Supplements

- Betaine hydrochloride 700mgs x 3 per meal and 1 with snacks to support protein assimilation (Guilliams & Drake 2020).

- Beetroot complex with taurine x 2 per meal to support bile flow (Ash 2008).
- Sodium and potassium bicarbonate x 2 daily between meals, to support small bowel pH and enzyme activity (this also lifted her energy after lunch) (Jakab *et al.* 2012).
- KPU combination product continued.
- Coenzyme Q10 300mgs daily for mitochondrial energy and anti-oxidant (Quinzii & Hirano 2010; Sinatra *et al.* 2003).
- *Lactobacillus plantarum* (Arasu *et al.* 2016), *L. rhamnosus* (Segers & Lebeer 2014) and *L. salivaricus* (Neville & O'Toole 2010), *Bifidobac-terium* (O'Callaghan and Van Sinderen 2016) and *Saccharomyces boulardii* (Kelesidis & Pothoulakis 2012) in a combined product x 1–2 daily as tolerated. These were all chosen for their antihista-mine effects.
- A porcine kidney combination was added to support DAO enzyme activity while rebalancing gut microbiome (Kettner *et al.* 2020).
- PC liquid 5ml daily to repair and protect cell membranes from histamine cell danger response (Hagemann *et al.* 2019).

Lifestyle interventions

Time out in nature was recommended for 20 minutes three times weekly. Ella chose to sit in her garden barefoot with a book and no electronic gadgets or to take a walk in the local woodland (Marselle *et al.* 2019).

Very gentle exercise in the form of Dru yoga and/or gentle Pilates was recommended to help Ella generate oxygen circulating to help her become more alert and lift her moods (Yeh *et al.* 2017). Ella also continued her gentle rebounding for 30 minutes three times weekly (Bhattacharya *et al.* 1980). She sometimes combined this with being outside to gain double the benefit.

Ella continued with her twice-weekly entrainments with the NSA chiropractor. She was noticing that her anxiety levels were reducing significantly and this was maintaining for about 2–3 days. Her spine felt more flexible, allowing her to undertake Dru yoga and she reported feel-ing more open internally around her solar plexus (stomach, duodenum, gallbladder and pancreas area. Ella was also becoming very aware of some of the emotions or situations and/or phrases that would trigger her anxiety, so she was dealing with those through the NSA and its sister therapy, Somato Respiratory Integration techniques taught within the NSA.

References

Agudelo CW, Samaha G, Garcia-Arcos I (2020) Alveolar lipids in pulmonary disease. A review. *Lipids in Health and Disease 19*, 1, 122. doi:10.1186/s12944-020-01278-8

Afrin LB, Self S, Menk J *et al.* (2017) Characterization of mast cell activation syndrome. *The American Journal of the Medical Sciences 353*, 3, 207–215. doi:10.1016/j.amjms.2016.12.013

Ahlberg S, Randolph D, Okoth S *et al.* (2019) Aflatoxin binders in foods for human consumption: Can this be promoted safely and ethically? *Toxins 11*, 7, 410. doi:10.3390/toxins11070410

Ahmad T, Marshall SE, Jewell D (2006) Genetics of inflammatory bowel disease: The role of the HLA complex. *World Journal of Gastroenterology 12*, 23, 3628–3635. doi:10.3748/wjg.v12.i23.3628

Ahrens F, Gabel G, Garz B *et al.* (2002) Release and permeation of histamine are affected by diamine oxidase in the pig large intestine. *Inflammation Research 51*, S83–S84.

Aldi S, Capone A, Giovampaola CD *et al.* (2015) Identification of a novel, alpha2-fucosylation-dependent uptake system in highly proliferative cells. *Tissue and Cell 47*, 1, 33–38. doi:10.1016/j.tice.2014.10.007

Amalraj A, Gopi S (2016) Biological activities and medicinal properties of Asafoetida: A review. *Journal of Traditional and Complementary Medicine 7*, 3, 347–359. doi:10.1016/j.jtcme.2016.11.004

Andresen PH (1948) The blood group system L: A new blood group L2. A case of epistasy within the blood groups. *Acta Pathologica et Microbiologica Scandinavica 25*, 728–731.

Arasu MV, Al-Dhabi NA, Ilavenil S *et al.* (2016) *In vitro* importance of probiotic *Lactobacillus plantarum* related to medical field. *Saudi Journal of Biological Sciences 23*, 1 (Supplement), S6–S10. doi:10.1016/j.sjbs.2015.09.022

Ash M (2008) Bile acid functional tests and protocols. www.clinicaleducation.org/wp-content/uploads/BileAcidTestsAndProtocols.pdf.

Azad MB, Wade KH, Timpson NJ (2018) *FUT2* secretor genotype and susceptibility to infections and chronic conditions in the ALSPAC cohort [version 2; peer review: 2 approved]. *Wellcome Open Research 3*, 65. doi:10.12688/wellcomeopenres.14636.2

Barcik W, Wawrzyniak M, Akdis CA, O'Mahony L (2017) Immune regulation by histamine and histamine-secreting bacteria. *Current Opinion in Immunology 48*, 108–113. doi:10.1016/j.coi.2017.08.011

Barrett JS *et al.* (2008) Probiotic effects on intestinal fermentation patterns in patients with irritable bowel syndrome. *World Journal of Gastroenterology 14*, 5020–5024.

Bastos MD, Kowalski TW, Puñales M *et al.* (2017) Search for DQ2.5 and DQ8 alleles using a lower cost technique in patients with type 1 diabetes and celiac disease in a population of southern Brazil. *Archives of Endocrinology and Metabolism 61*, 6, 550–555. doi:10.1590/2359-3997000000282.

Bell RL, Kimpel MW, McClintick JN *et al.* (2009) Gene expression changes in the nucleus accumbens of alcohol-preferring rats following chronic ethanol consumption. *Pharmacology Biochemistry and Behavior 94*, 1, 131–147. doi:10.1016/j.pbb.2009.07.019

Bescós R, Sureda A, Tur JA *et al.* (2012) The effect of nitric-oxide-related supplements on human performance. *Sports Medicine 42*, 99–117. doi:10.2165/11596860-000000000-00000

Bhattacharya A, McCutcheon EP, Shvartz E *et al.* (1980) Body acceleration distribution and O2 uptake in humans during running and jumping. *Journal of Applied Physiology: Respiratory, Environmental and Exercise Physiology 49*, 5, 881–887. doi:10.1152/jappl.1980.49.5.881

Bierut LJ, Goate AM, Breslau N *et al.* (2012) ADH1B is associated with alcohol dependence and alcohol consumption in populations of European and African ancestry. *Molecular Psychiatry 17*, 4, 445–450. doi:10.1038/mp.2011.124

Bin-Umer MA, McLaughlin JE, Basu D *et al.* (2011) Trichothecene mycotoxins inhibit mitochondrial translation – implication for the mechanism of toxicity. *Toxins 3*, 12, 1484-1501.

Bjarnason I (2017) The use of fecal calprotectin in inflammatory bowel disease. *Gastroenterology and Hepatology 13*, 1, 53–56.

Bode AM, Dong Z (2011) The Amazing and Mighty Ginger. In: IFF Benzie, S Wachtel-Galor (eds) *Herbal Medicine: Biomolecular and Clinical Aspects*, 2nd edn. Boca Raton, FL: CRC Press. www.ncbi.nlm.nih.gov/books/NBK92775

Boyer JL (2013) Bile formation and secretion. *Comprehensive Physiology 3*, 3, 1035–1078. doi:10.1002/cphy.c120027

Büning C, Durmus T, Molnar T *et al.* (2007) A study in three European IBD cohorts confirms that the *ATG16L1* c.898A > G (p.Thr300Ala) variant is a susceptibility factor for Crohn's disease. *Journal of Crohn's and Colitis 1*, 2, 70–76. doi:10.1016/j.crohns.2007.08.001

Burgess CR, Tse G, Gillis L *et al.* (2010) Dopaminergic regulation of sleep and cataplexy in a murine model of narcolepsy. *Sleep 33*, 10, 1295–1304. doi:10.1093/sleep/33.10.1295

Cabrera-Rubio R, Kunz C, Rudloff S *et al.* (2019) Association of maternal secretor status and human milk oligosaccharides with milk microbiota: An observational pilot study. *Journal of Pediatric Gastroenterology and Nutrition 68*, 2, 256–263. doi:10.1097/MPG.0000000000002216

Cadwell K, Patel KK, Maloney NS *et al.* (2010) Virus-plus-susceptibility gene interaction determines Crohn's disease gene Atg16L1 phenotypes in intestine. *Cell 141*, 7, 1135–1145. doi:10.1016/j.cell.2010.05.009

Canani RB, Costanzo MD, Leone L *et al.* (2011) Potential beneficial effects of butyrate in intestinal and extraintestinal diseases. *World Journal of Gastroenterology 17*, 12, 1519–1528. doi:10.3748/wjg.v17.i12.1519

Capozzi V, Russo P, Ladero V *et al.* (2012) Biogenic amines degradation by Lactobacillus plantarum: Toward a potential application in wine. *Frontiers in Microbiology*. doi:10.3389/fmicb.2012.00122

Castanys-Muñoz E, Martin MJ, Vazquez E (2016) Building a beneficial microbiome from birth. *Advances in Nutrition 7*, 2, 323–330. doi:10.3945/an.115.010694

Chai J, Feng X, Zhang L *et al.* (2015) Hepatic expression of detoxification enzymes is decreased in human obstructive cholestasis due to gallstone biliary obstruction. *PLOS ONE 10*, 3, e0120055. doi:10.1371/journal.pone.0120055

Chakraborty N, Ghosh R, Ghosh S *et al.* (2013) Reduction of oxalate levels in tomato fruit and consequent metabolic remodeling following overexpression of a fungal oxalate decarboxylase. *Plant Physiology 162*, 1, 364–378. doi:10.1104/pp.112.209197

Chelakkot C, Ghim J, Ryu SH (2018) Mechanisms regulating intestinal barrier integrity and its pathological implications. *Experimental and Molecular Medicine 50*, 8, 1–9. doi:10.1038/s12276-018-0126-x

Chen M, Huang H, Zhou P *et al.* (2019) Oral phosphatidylcholine improves intestinal barrier function in drug-induced liver injury in rats. *Gastroenterology Research and Practice*, 8723460. doi:10.1155/2019/8723460

Choo SY (2007) The HLA system: Genetics, immunology, clinical testing, and clinical implications. *Yonsei Medical Journal 48*, 1, 11–23. doi:10.3349/ymj.2007.48.1.11

Chu GM, Kim JH, Kim HY *et al.* (2013) Effects of bamboo charcoal on the growth performance, blood characteristics and noxious gas emission in fattening pigs. *Journal of Applied Animal Research 41*, 1, 48–55. doi:10.1080/09712119.2012.738219

Cogoli A (1991) Changes observed in lymphocyte behavior during gravitational unloading. *ASGSB Bulletin 4*, 2, 107–115.

Cohen S (2015) Medication-induced SNPs. Available from: https://shop.suzycohen.com/products/medication-induced-snps-video

Conti P, Tettamanti L, Mastrangelo F *et al.* (2018) Impact of fungi on immune responses. *Clinical Therapeutics 40*, 6, 885–888. doi:10.1016/j.clinthera.2018.04.010

Corvelo TC de O *et al.* (2013) The Lewis histo-blood group system: molecular analysis of the 59T>G, 508G>A, and 1067T>A polymorphisms in an Amazonian population. *PLOS One 8*, 7, e69908. doi:10.1371/journal.pone.0069908

Coulet M, Phothirath P, Allais L *et al.* (2014) Pre-clinical safety evaluation of the synthetic human milk, nature-identical, oligosaccharide 2'-O-Fucosyllactose (2'FL). *Regulatory Toxicology and Pharmacology 68*, 1, 59–69. doi:10.1016/j.yrtph.2013.11.005

Cozzolino M, Serena C, Calabró AS *et al.* (2018) Human leukocyte antigen DQ2/DQ8 positivity in women with history of stillbirth. *American Journal of Reproductive Immunology 80*, 5, e13038. doi:10.1111/aji.13038

Czaja-Bulsa G (2015) Non coeliac gluten sensitivity: A new disease with gluten intolerance. *Clinical Nutrition 34*, 2, 189–194. doi:10.1016/j.clnu.2014.08.012

D'Adamo P (2014) Opus23 practitioner only database. www.datapunk.net/opus23/dashboard.pl

D'Adamo PJ, Kelly GS (2001) Metabolic and immunologic consequences of ABH secretor and Lewis subtype status. *Alternative Medicine Review 6*, 4, 390–405.

D'Adamo PJ, Whitney C (2002) *Live Right for Your Type*. Penguin Books.

Dam G, Keiding S, Munk OL *et al.* (2011) Branched-chain amino acids increase arterial blood ammonia in spite of enhanced intrinsic muscle ammonia metabolism in patients with cirrhosis and healthy subjects. *American Journal of Physiology: Gastrointestinal Liver Physiology 301*, G269–G277. doi:10.1152/ajpgi.00062.2011

Daneshvar P, Ghasemi G, Zolaktaf V *et al.* (2019) Comparison of the effect of 8-week rebound therapy-based exercise program and weight-supported exercises on the range of motion, proprioception, and the quality of life in patients with Parkinson's disease. *International Journal of Preventive Medicine 10*, 1, 131. doi:10.4103/ijpvm.IJPVM_527_18

Dev S, Mizuguchi H, Das AK *et al.* (2008) Suppression of histamine signaling by probiotic Lac-B: A possible mechanism of its anti-allergic effect. *Journal of Pharmacological Sciences 107*, 159–166.

Dinkova-Kostova AT, Fahey JW, Kostov RV *et al.* (2017) KEAP1 and done? Targeting the NRF2 pathway with sulforaphane. *Trends in Food Science and Technology 69*, B, 257–269. doi:10.1016/j.tifs.2017.02.002

Douillard J (2017) *Eat Wheat: A Scientifically Proven Approach to Safely Bring Gluten and Wheat Back into Your Diet*. New York, NY: Morgan James Publishing.

Downing D, Pemberton A (2014) *The Vitamin Cure for Digestive Disease*. Laguna Beach, CA: Basic Health Publications.

Du GJ; Zhang Z, Wen XD *et al.* (2012). Epigallocatechin gallate (EGCG) is the most effective cancer chemopreventive polyphenol in green tea. *Nutrients 4*, 11, 1679–1691. doi:10.3390/nu4111679

Fernandez SV, Russo J (2010) Estrogen and xenoestrogens in breast cancer. *Toxicologic Pathology 38*, 1, 110–122. doi:10.1177/0192623309354108

Fields J (2014) Iodine deficiency. The Healing Gardens. http://thehealinggardens.org/images/PDFs/article-archives/IodineDeficiency.pdf

Flower G, Fritz H, Balneaves LG *et al.* (2014) Flax and breast cancer: A systematic review. *Integrative Cancer Therapies*, 181–192. doi:10.1177/1534735413502076

Forni D, Cleynen I, Ferrante M *et al.* (2014) ABO histo-blood group might modulate predisposition to Crohn's disease and affect disease behavior. *Journal of Crohn's and Colitis 8*, 6, 489–494. doi:10.1016/j.crohns.2013.10.014

Forsythe P, Wang B, Khambati I et al. (2012) Systemic effects of ingested *Lactobacillus rhamnosus*: Inhibition of mast cell membrane potassium (IKCa) current and degranulation. *PLOS ONE 7*, 7, e41234. doi:10.1371/journal.pone.0041234

Fountain JC, Bajaj P, Nayak SN et al. (2016) Responses of *Aspergillus flavus* to oxidative stress are related to fungal development regulator, antioxidant enzyme, and secondary metabolite biosynthetic gene expression. *Frontiers in Microbiology 7*, 2048. doi:10.3389/fmicb.2016.02048

Ganesan K, Xu B (2018) A critical review on phytochemical profile and health promoting effects of mung bean (Vigna radiata). *Food Science and Human Wellness 7*, 1, 11–33.

Ganeshpurkar A, Saluja AK (2017) The pharmacological potential of rutin. *Saudi Pharmaceutical Journal 25*, 2, 149–164. doi:10.1016/j.jsps.2016.04.025

Garrido D, Ruiz-Moyano S, Kirmiz N et al. (2016) A novel gene cluster allows preferential utilization of fucosylated milk oligosaccharides in *Bifidobacterium longum* subsp. *longum* SC596. *Scientific Reports 6*, 35045. doi:10.1038/srep35045

Giampaoli O, Conta G, Calvani R et al. (2020) Can the FUT2 *non-secretor* phenotype associated with gut microbiota increase the children susceptibility for type 1 diabetes? A mini review. *Frontiers in Nutrition 7*, 606171. doi:10.3389/fnut.2020.606171

Gildea JJ, Roberts DA, Bush Z (2017) Protective effects of lignite extract supplement on intestinal barrier function in glyphosate-mediated tight junction injury. *Journal of Clinical Nutrition and Dietetics 3*, 1. doi:10.4172/2472-1921.100035

Glade MJ, Smith K (2015) Phosphatidylserine and the human brain. *Nutrition 31*, 6, 781–786. doi:10.1016/j.nut.2014.10.014

Greifova G, Body P, Greif G et al. (2018) Human phagocytic cell response to histamine derived from potential probiotic strains of *Lactobacillus reuteri*. *Immunobiology 223*, 1, 618–626. doi:10.1016/j.imbio.2018.07.007

Grégoire IP, Richetta C, Meyniel-Shicklin L et al. (2011) IRGM is a common target of RNA viruses that subvert the autophagy network. *PLOS Pathogens*. doi:10.1371/journal.ppat.1002422

Griffin JWD, Bradshaw PC (2019) Effects of a high protein diet and liver disease in an in silico model of human ammonia metabolism. *Theoretical Biology and Medical Modelling 16*, 11. doi:10.1186/s12976-019-0109-1

Gröber U, Werner T, Vormann J et al. (2017) Myth or reality – transdermal magnesium? *Nutrients 9*, 8, 813. doi:10.3390/nu9080813

Gundry MD (2019) 5 ways to remove lectins from your favourite foods. https://gundrymd.com/remove-lectins

Guilford FT, Hope J (2014) Deficient glutathione in the pathophysiology of mycotoxin-related illness. *Toxins 6*, 2, 608–623. doi:10.3390/toxins6020608

Guilliams TG, Drake, LE (2020) Meal-time supplementation with betaine HCl for functional hypochlorhydria: What is the evidence? *Integrative Medicine 19*, 1, 32–36.

Gulfam N, Zahoor M, Khisroom M et al. (2018) In vivo detoxification of ochratoxin A by highly porous magnetic nanocomposites prepared from coconut shell. *Brazilian Journal of Poultry Science 20*, 675–698. doi:10.1590/1806-9061-2017-0702

Guzman F (2019) Lithium's mechanism of action: An illustrated review. Open access article. https://psychopharmacologyinstitute.com/publication/lithiums-mechanism-of-action-an-illustrated-review-2212

Hagemann PM, Nsiah-Dosu S, Hundt JE et al. (2019) Modulation of mast cell reactivity by lipids: The neglected side of allergic diseases. *Frontiers in Immunology 10*, 1174. www.frontiersin.org/article/10.3389/fimmu.2019.01174

Hampe J, Franke A, Rosenstiel P et al. (2007) A genome-wide association scan of nonsynonymous SNPs identifies a susceptibility variant for Crohn disease in ATG16L1. *Nature Genetics 39*, 207–211. doi:10.1038/ng1954

Haniadka R, Saldanha E, Sunita V et al. (2013) A review of the gastroprotective effects of ginger (Zingiber officinale Roscoe). *Food and Function 4*, 6, 845–855. doi:10.1039/c3fo30337c

Hannibal L, Lysne V, Bjørke-Monsen AL et al. (2016) Biomarkers and algorithms for the diagnosis of vitamin B12 deficiency. *Frontiers in Molecular Biosciences*. doi:10.3389/fmolb.2016.00027

Harnden KK, Blackwell KL (2016) Increased fiber intake decreases premenopausal breast cancer risk. *Pediatrics 137*, 3, e20154376. doi:10.1542/peds.2015-4376

Hartmann R, Schmidt FM, Sander C *et al.* (2019) Heart rate variability as indicator of clinical state in depression. *Frontiers in Psychiatry 9*, 735. doi:10.3389/fpsyt.2018.00735

Harvey CJ, Thimmulappa RK, Singh A *et al.* (2009) Nrf2-regulated glutathione recycling independent of biosynthesis is critical for cell survival during oxidative stress. *Free Radical Biology and Medicine 46*, 4, 443–453. doi:10.1016/j.freeradbiomed.2008.10.040.

He G-H, Cai W-K, Meng J-R *et al.* (2015) Relation of polymorphism of the histidine decarboxylase gene to chronic heart failure in Han Chinese. *American Journal of Cardiology 115*, 11, 1555–1562. doi:10.1016/j.amjcard.2015.02.062

Henker J *et al.* (2008) Probiotic *Escherichia coli* Nissle 1917 (EcN) for successful remission maintenance of ulcerative colitis in children and adolescents: An open-label pilot study. *Zeitschreift für Gastroenterologie 46*, 874–875. doi:10.1055/s-2008-1027463

Herraiz T, Guillén H (2018) Monoamine oxidase-A inhibition and associated antioxidant activity in plant extracts with potential antidepressant actions. *BioMed Research International 2018*, 4810394. doi:10.1155/2018/4810394

Herron RE, Fagan JB (2002) Lipophil-mediated reduction of toxicants in humans: an evaluation of an ayurvedic detoxification procedure. *Alternative Therapies in Health and Medicine 8*, 5, 40–51.

Hewlings SJ, Kalman DS (2017) Curcumin: A review of its effects on human health. *Foods 6*, 10, 92. doi:10.3390/foods6100092

Hira T, Nakajima S, Eto Y *et al.* (2008) Calcium-sensing receptor mediates phenylalanine-induced cholecystokinin secretion in enteroendocrine STC-1 cells. *FEBS Journal 275*, 18, 4620–4626. doi:10.1111/j.1742-4658.2008.06604.x

Hirano K, Namihira M (2017) FAD influx enhances neuronal differentiation of human neural stem cells by facilitating nuclear localization of LSD1. *FEBS Open Bio 7*, 12, 1932–1942. doi:10.1002/2211-5463.12331

Hope J (2013) A review of the mechanism of injury and treatment approaches for illness resulting from exposure to water-damaged buildings, mold, and mycotoxins. *The Scientific World Journal*, 767482. doi:10.1155/2013/767482

Hope JH, Hope BE (2012) A review of the diagnosis and treatment of Ochratoxin A inhalational exposure associated with human illness and kidney disease including focal segmental glomerulosclerosis. *Journal of Environmental and Public Health*, Article ID 835059. doi:10.1155/2012/835059

Hosseinzadeh H, Alaw Qotbi AA, Seidavi A *et al.* (2014) Effects of different levels of coriander (*Coriandrum sativum*) seed powder and extract on serum biochemical parameters, microbiota, and immunity in broiler chicks. *The Scientific World Journal*, 628979. doi:10.1155/2014/628979

Ianiro G, Pecere S, Giorgio V *et al.* (2016) Digestive enzyme supplementation in gastrointestinal diseases. *Current Drug Metabolism 17*, 2, 187–193. doi: 10.2174/1389 20021702160114150137

IFM (2005) *Clinical Nutrition: A Functional Approach*, 2nd edn. Washington, DC: Institute for Functional Medicine.

IFM (2010) *Clinical Nutrition: A Functional Approach*. Washington, DC: Institute for Functional Medicine.

Indrio F *et al.* (2011) Lactobacillus reuteri accelerates gastric emptying and improves regurgitation in infants. *European Journal of Clinical Investigation 41*, 4, 417–422. doi:10.1111/j.1365-2362.2010.02425.x

Iqbal NT, Syed S, Sadiq K *et al.* (2019) Study of Environmental Enteropathy and Malnutrition (SEEM) in Pakistan: Protocols for biopsy based biomarker discovery and validation. *BMC Pediatrics 19*, 247. doi:10.1186/s12887-019-1564-x

Ishibashi H, Kuwahara T, Nakayama-Imaohji H *et al.* (2012) Effects of indole-3-carbinol and phenethyl isothiocyanate on bile and pancreatic juice excretion in rats. *Journal of Medical Investigation 59*, 3–4, 246–252. doi:10.2152/jmi.59.246

Jakab RL, Collaco AM, Ameen NA (2012) Cell-specific effects of luminal acid, bicarbonate, cAMP, and carbachol on transporter trafficking in the intestine. *American Journal of Physiology: Gastrointestinal and Liver Physiology 303*, 8, G937–G950. doi:10.1152/ajpgi.00452.2011

Jantscher-Krenn E, Bode L (2012) Human milk oligosaccharides and their potential benefits for the breast-fed neonate. *Minerva Pediatrica 64*, 1, 83–99.

Kaczmarek JL, Liu X, Charron CS *et al.* (2019) Broccoli consumption affects the human gastrointestinal microbiota. *Journal of Nutritional Biochemistry 63*, 27–34. doi:10.1016/j.jnutbio.2018.09.015

Karagiannidis I, Dehning S, Sandor P *et al.* (2013) Support of the histaminergic hypothesis in Tourette syndrome: Association of the histamine decarboxylase gene in a large sample of families. *Journal of Medical Genetics 50*, 11, 760–764. doi:10.1136/jmedgenet-2013-101637

Karner M, Kocjan A, Stein J *et al.* (2014) First multicenter study of modified release phosphatidylcholine 'LT-02' in ulcerative colitis: A randomized, placebo-controlled trial in mesalazine-refractory courses. *American Journal of Gastroenterology 109*, 7, 1041–1051. doi:10.1038/ajg.2014.104

Kasbo J, Tuchweber B, Perwaiz S *et al.* (2003) Phosphatidylcholine-enriched diet prevents gallstone formation in mice susceptible to cholelithiasis. *Journal of Lipid Research 44*, 12, 2297–2303. doi:10.1194/jlr.M300180-JLR200

Katsoulos PD, Zarogiannis S, Roubies N *et al.* (2009) Effect of long-term dietary supplementation with clinoptilolite on performance and selected serum biochemical values in dairy goats. *American Journal of Veterinary Research 70*, 3, 346–352.

Kelesidis T, Pothoulakis C (2012) Efficacy and safety of the probiotic *Saccharomyces boulardii* for the prevention and therapy of gastrointestinal disorders. *Therapeutic Advances in Gastroenterology 5*, 2, 111–125. doi:10.1177/1756283X11428502

Kettner L, Seitl I, Fischer L (2020) Evaluation of porcine diamine oxidase for the conversion of histamine in food-relevant amounts. *Journal of Food Science 85*, 3, 843–852. doi:10.1111/1750-3841.15069

Khan M (2019) Bombay Blood Group – Understanding Genetics. *International Journal of Trend in Scientific Research and Development 3*, 4, 559–561. doi:10.31142/ijtsrd23861.

Kiani AK, John P, Bhatti A *et al.* (2015) Association of 32 type 1 diabetes risk loci in Pakistani patients. *Diabetes Research and Clinical Practice 108*, 1, 137–142. doi:10.1016/j.diabres.2015.01.022

Kim NH, Jeong HJ, Kim HM (2012) Theanine is a candidate amino acid for pharmacological stabilization of mast cells. *Amino Acids 42*, 5, 1609–1618. doi:10.1007/s00726-011-0847-9

Klinghardt D (2013) Dr. Dietrich Klinghardt discusses kryptopyrroluria (Pyroluria) – Lyme induced autism. YouTube. www.youtube.com/watch?v=THZhANfFnyY

Klocker J, Mätzler SA, Huetz GN *et al.* (2005) Expression of histamine degrading enzymes in porcine tissues. *Inflammation Research 54*, Suppl 1, S54–57. doi:10.1007/s00011-004-0425-7

Koda Y, Tachida H, Pang H *et al.* (2001) Contrasting patterns of polymorphisms at the ABO-Secretor gene (FUT2) and plasma α(1,3)fucosyltransferase gene (FUT6) in human populations. *Genetics 158*, 2, 747–756.

Kohlmeier M, Chirita A, Beckett E *et al.* (2018) 13th Congress of the International Society of Nutrigenetics/Nutrigenomics. *Lifestyle Genomics 11*, 169–193. doi:10.1159/000501177

Kong R, Cui Y, Fisher GJ *et al.* (2016) A comparative study of the effects of retinol and retinoic acid on histological, molecular, and clinical properties of human skin. *Journal of Cosmetic Dermatology 15*, 49–57. https://onlinelibrary.wiley.com/doi/pdf/10.1111/jocd.12193

Korytowski A, Abuillan W, Amadei F *et al.* (2017) Accumulation of phosphatidylcholine on gut mucosal surface is not dominated by electrostatic interactions. *Biochimica et Biophysica Acta 1859*, 5, 959–65.

Kraljević Pavelić S, Simović Medica J, Gumbarević D *et al.* (2018) Critical review on zeolite clinoptilolite safety and medical applications *in vivo*. *Frontiers in Pharmacology 9*, 1350. doi:10.3389/fphar.2018.01350

Kritas SK, Gallenga CE, Ovidio CD *et al.* (2018) Impact of mold on mast cell-cytokine immune response. *Journal of Biological Regulators and Homeostatic Agents 32*, 4, 763–768.

Kucher AN, Cherevko NA (2018) Genes of the histamine pathway and common diseases. *Russian Journal of Genetics 54*, 12. doi:10.1134/S1022795418010088

Kumar MJ, Andersen JK (2004) Perspectives on MAO-B in aging and neurological disease: Where do we go from here? *Molecular Neurobiology 30*, 1, 77–89.

Kumar KK, Prakash CKL, Sumanthi J *et al.* (2012) Biological role of lectins: A review. *Journal of Orofacial Sciences 4*, 1, 20–25.

Kung HF, Lee YC, Huang YL *et al.* (2017) Degradation of histamine by *Lactobacillus plantarum* isolated from miso products. *Journal of Food Protection 80*, 10, 1682–1688.

Kunz M, König IR, Schillert A *et al.* (2015) Genome-wide association study identifies new susceptibility loci for cutaneous lupus erythematosus. *Experimental Dermatology 24*, 7, 510–515. doi:10.1111/exd.12708

Lewis ZT, Totten SM, Smilowitz JT *et al.* (2015) Maternal fucosyltransferase 2 status affects the gut bifidobacterial communities of breastfed infants. *Microbiome 3*, 13. doi:10.1186/s40168-015-0071-z

Liu J, Lkhagva E, Chung HJ *et al.* (2018) The pharmabiotic approach to treat hyperammonemia. *Nutrients 10*, 2, 140. doi:10.3390%2Fnu10020140

Lu F, Huang S (2017) The roles of mast cells in parasitic protozoan infections. *Frontiers in Immunology 8*, 363. doi:10.3389/fimmu.2017.00363

Lynch B (2017) Methylation pathway planner. SHEIcon conference 2017, Seattle, USA.

Lynch B (2018) *Dirty Genes: A Breakthrough Programme to Treat the Root Cause of Illness and Optimize Your Health*. New York, NY: HarperCollins.

Mahboubi M (2019) *Foeniculum vulgare* as valuable plant in management of women's health. *Journal of Menopausal Medicine 25*, 1, 1–14. doi:10.6118/jmm.2019.25.1.1

Mahendra P, Bisht S (2012) Ferula asafoetida: Traditional uses and pharmacological activity. *Pharmacognosy Reviews 6*, 12, 141–146. doi:10.4103/0973-7847.99948

Maintz L, Novak N (2007) Histamine and histamine intolerance. *The American Journal of Clinical Nutrition 85*, 5, 1185–1196. doi:10.1093/ajcn/85.5.1185

Maintz L, Schwarzer V, Bieber T *et al.* (2008) Effects of histamine and diamine oxidase activities on pregnancy: A critical review. *Human Reproduction Update 14*, 5, 485–495. doi:10.1093/humupd/dmn014

Mann J, Truswell AS (2007) *Essentials of Human Nutrition*, 4th edn. Oxford: Oxford University Press.

Manzotti G, Breda D, Di Gioacchino M *et al.* (2016) Serum diamine oxidase activity in patients with histamine intolerance. *International Journal of Immunopathology and Pharmacology 29*, 1, 105–111. doi:10.1177/0394632015617170

Marselle MR, Warber SL, Irvine KN (2019) Growing resilience through interaction with nature: Can group walks in nature buffer the effects of stressful life events on mental health? *International Journal of Environmental Research and Public Health 16*, 6, 986. doi:10.3390/ijerph16060986

Marshall TM (2015) Lithium as a nutrient. *Journal of American Physicians and Surgeons 20*, 4, 104–109.

Marttila E, Bowyer P, Sanglard D *et al.* (2013) Fermentative 2-carbon metabolism produces carcinogenic levels of acetaldehyde in *Candida albicans*. *Molecular Oral Microbiology 28*, 4, 281–291. doi:10.1111/omi.12024

Matny O (2015) Efficacy evaluation of Iraqi propolis against gray mold of stored orange caused by *Penicillium digitatum*. *Plant Pathology Journal 14*, 3, 153–157. doi:10.3923/ppj.2015.153.157

Matteini AM, Walston JD, Bandeen-Roche K *et al.* (2010) Transcobalamin-II variants, decreased vitamin B12 availability and increased risk of frailty. *The Journal of Nutrition, Health and Aging 14*, 1, 73–77.

Mehrdad A, Kemball CC, Flynn CT *et al.* (2010) Short-term fasting induces profound neuronal autophagy. *Autophagy 6*, 6, 702–710. doi:10.4161/auto.6.6.12376

Menegas S, Dal-Pont GC, Cararo JH *et al.* (2020) Efficacy of folic acid as an adjunct to lithium therapy on manic-like behaviors, oxidative stress and inflammatory parameters in an animal model of mania. *Metabolic Brain Disease 35*, 2, 413–425. doi:10.1007/s11011-019-00503-3

Moghtader M, Salari H, Farahamand A (2011) Evaluation of the antifungal effects of rosemary oil and comparison with synthetic borneol and fungicide on the growth of *Aspergillus flavus. Journal of Ecology and the Natural Environment 3*, 6, 210–214.

Moran AP (2008) Relevance of fucosylation and Lewis antigen expression in the bacterial gastroduodenal pathogen *Helicobacter pylori. Carbohydrate Research 343*, 12, 1952–1965.

Moré MI, Vandenplas Y (2018) *Saccharomyces boulardii* CNCM I-745 improves intestinal enzyme function: A trophic effects review. *Therapeutic Advances in Gastrointestinal Endoscopy*. doi:10.1177/1179552217752679.

Morrow AL, Meinzen-Derr J, Huang P *et al.* (2011) Fucosyltransferase 2 non-secretor and low secretor status predicts severe outcomes in premature infants. *Journal of Pediatrics 158*, 5, 745–751. doi:10.1016/j.jpeds.2010.10.043

Mottram L, Wiklund G, Larson G *et al.* (2017) *FUT2* non-secretor status is associated with altered susceptibility to symptomatic enterotoxigenic *Escherichia coli* infection in Bangladeshis. *Scientific Reports 7*, 10649. doi:10.1038/s41598-017-10854-5

Mourant AE (1946) A 'new' human blood group antigen of frequent occurrence. *Nature 158*, 237–238.

Myhre AM, Carlsen MH, Bøhn SK *et al.* (2003) Water-miscible, emulsified, and solid forms of retinol supplements are more toxic than oil-based preparations. *American Journal of Clinical Nutrition 78*, 6, 1152–1159. doi:10.1093/ajcn/78.6.1152

Nagatsu T, Sawada M (2006) Molecular mechanism of the relation of monoamine oxidase B and its inhibitors to Parkinson's disease: Possible implications of glial cells. *Journal of Neural Transmission Suppl.*, 71, 53-65.

Nagulapalli Venkata KC, Swaroop A, Bagchi D *et al.* (2017) A small plant with big benefits: Fenugreek (Trigonella foenum-graecum Linn.) for disease prevention and health promotion. *Molecular Nutrition and Food Research 61*, 6. doi:10.1002/mnfr.201600950

National Institute for Health and Care Excellence (NICE) (2014) Drug allergy: Diagnosis and management. Clinical guideline (CG183). www.nice.org.uk/guidance/cg183/chapter/1-recommendations

National Institute on Alcohol and Alcoholism (2007) Alcohol Alert, Number 72. US Department of Health and Human Services. https://pubs.niaaa.nih.gov/publications/aa72/AA72.pdf

Naviaux RK (2014) Metabolic features of the cell danger response. *Mitochondrion 16*, 7–17. doi:10.1016/j.mito.2013.08.006

Naviaux RK (2019) Metabolic features and regulation of the healing cycle – a new model for chronic disease pathogenesis and treatment. *Mitochondrion 46, 278–297*. doi:10.1016/j.mito.2018.08.001

Naviaux RK (2020) Perspective: Cell danger response biology – The new science that connects environmental health with mitochondria and the rising tide of chronic illness. *Mitochondrion 51*, 40–45. doi:10.1016/j.mito.2019.12.005

Negelein E, Wulff HJ (1937) Diphosphoryridin-proteid ackohol, acetaldehyde. *Biochemische Zeitschrift 293*, 351.

Neville BA, O'Toole PW (2010) Probiotic properties of *Lactobacillus salivarius* and closely related *Lactobacillus* species. *Future Microbiology 5*, 5, 759–774. doi:10.2217/fmb.10.35

Nexo E, Hoffmann-Lücke E (2011) Holotranscobalamin, a marker of vitamin B-12 status: analytical aspects and clinical utility. *American Journal of Clinical Nutrition 94*, 1, 359S–365S. doi:10.3945/ajcn.111.013458

Nishio A, Ishiguro S, Miyao N (1987) Specific change of histamine metabolism in acute magnesium-deficient young rats. *Drug Nutr Interact 5*, 2, 89–96.

Nojiri S, Fujiwara K, Matsuura K *et al.* (2018) L-carnitine reduces ammonia levels and alleviates covert encephalopathy: A randomized trial. *Journal of Translational Science 4*. doi:10.15761/JTS.1000220

Nones J, Nones J, Poli A *et al.* (2016) Organo-philic treatments of bentonite increase the adsorption of aflatoxin B1 and protect stem cells against cellular damage. *Colloids and Surfaces B: Biointerfaces* 145, 555–561.

Nylund L, Kaukinen K, Lindfors K (2016) The microbiota as a component of the celiac disease and non-celiac gluten sensitivity. *Clinical Nutrition Experimental* 6, 17–24. doi:10.1016/j.yclnex.2016.01.002

O'Callaghan A, van Sinderen D (2016) Bifidobacteria and their role as members of the human gut microbiota. *Frontiers in Microbiology* 7, 925. doi:10.3389/fmicb.2016.00925

Oksaharju A, Kankainen M, Kekkonen RA *et al.* (2011) Probiotic *Lactobacillus rhamnosus* downregulates FCER1 and HRH4 expression in human mast cells. *World Journal of Gastroenterology* 17, 6, 750–759. doi:10.3748/wjg.v17.i6.750

Olson JM, Ameer MA, Goyal A (2019) Vitamin A toxicity. *StatPearls*. www.ncbi.nlm.nih.gov/books/NBK532916

Pacholok SM, Stuart JJ (2011) *Could It Be B12? An Epidemic of Misdiagnoses*. Fresno, CA: Quill Driver Books.

Padayatty SJ, Levine M (2016) Vitamin C: The known and the unknown and Goldilocks. *Oral Diseases* 22, 6, 463–493. doi:10.1111/odi.12446

Patel D, Witt SN (2017) Ethanolamine and phosphatidylethanolamine: Partners in health and disease. *Oxidative Medicine and Cellular Longevity* 2017, 4829180. doi:10.115

Perera I, Seneweera S, Hirotsu N. (2018) Manipulating the phytic acid content of rice grain toward improving micronutrient bioavailability. *Rice* 11, 1, 4. doi:10.1186/s12284-018-0200-y

Pfeiffer CC (1975) *Mental and Elemental Nutrients, A Physician's Guide to Nutrition and Health Care*. New Haven, CT: Keats Publishing.

Potts RA, Tiffany CM, Pakpour N *et al.* (2016) Mast cells and histamine alter intestinal permeability during malaria parasite infection. *Immunobiology* 221, 3, 468–474. doi:10.1016/j.imbio.2015.11.003

Poulaert M, Gunata Z, During A *et al.* (2014) Hesperidin increases intestinal β,β-carotene 15-15' mono-oxygenase 1 (BCMO1) activity in Mongolian gerbils (*Meriones unguiculatus*) fed with β-carotene-free diet. *Food Chemistry* 159, 477–485. doi:10.1016/j.foodchem.2014.03.018

Prasai TP, Walsh KB, Bhattarai SP *et al.* (2017) Zeolite food supplementation reduces abundance of enterobacteria. *Microbiological Research* 195, 24–30. doi:10.1016/j.micres.2016.11.006

Quinzii CM, Hirano M (2010) Coenzyme Q and mitochondrial disease. *Developmental Disabilities Research Reviews* 16, 2, 183–188. doi:10.1002/ddrr.108

Rabb UN (2018) Pharmacology of Shothahara Dravyas – a literary survey. *Journal of Ayurveda and Integrated Medical Sciences* 3, 5. doi:10.21760/jaims.v3i5.13828

Raha O, Sarkar B, Lakkakula BV *et al.* (2013) HLA class II SNP interactions and the association with type 1 diabetes mellitus in Bengali speaking patients of Eastern India. *Journal of Biomedical Science* 20, 12. doi:10.1186/1423-0127-20-12

Rahman M, Khatun A, Liu L *et al.* (2018) Brassicaceae mustards: Traditional and agronomic uses in Australia and New Zealand. *Molecules* 23, 1, 231. doi:10.3390/molecules23010231

Rahmy HAF, Bana EI, Bordent HM *et al.* (2019) Effect of caraway, fennel and Melissa addition on *in vitro* rumen fermentation and gas production. *Pakistan Journal of Biological Sciences* 22, 2, 67–72. doi:10.3923/pjbs.2019.67.72

Ratnaseelan AM, Tsilioni I, Theoharides TC (2018) Effects of mycotoxins on neuropsy-chiatric symptoms and immune processes. *Clinical Therapeutics* 40, 6, 903–917.

Ray C, Kerketta JA, Rao S *et al.* (2019) Human milk oligosaccharides: The journey ahead. *International Journal of Paediatrics* 2019, 2390240. doi:10.1155/2019/2390240

Roselli M, Finamore A, Nuccitelli S *et al.* (2009) Prevention of TNBS-induced colitis by different *Lactobacillus* and *Bifidobacterium* strains is associated with as expansion of γδT and regulatory T cells of intestinal intraepithelial lymphocytes. *Inflammatory Bowel Diseases* 15, 10, 1526–1536.

Saboor M, Ullah A, Qamar K *et al.* (2014) Frequency of ABH secretors and non secretors: A cross-sectional study in Karachi. *Pakistan Journal of Medical Sciences 30*, 1, 189–193. doi:10.12669/pjms.301.4194

Saghafi N, Ghazanfarpour M, Khadivzadeh T *et al.* (2017) The effect of *Foeniculum vulgare* (fennel) on body composition in postmenopausal women with excess weight: A double-blind randomized placebo-controlled trial. *Journal of Menopausal Medicine 23*, 3, 166–171. doi:10.6118/jmm.2017.23.3.166

Sahib NG, Anwar F, Gilani AH *et al.* (2013) Coriander (*Coriandrum sativum* L.): A potential source of high-value components for functional foods and nutraceuticals – a review. *Phytotherapy Research 27*, 10, 1439–1456. doi:10.1002/ptr.4897

Salazar F, Sewell HF, Shakib F *et al.* (2013) The role of lectins in allergic sensitization and allergic disease. *Journal of Allergy and Clinical Immunology 132*, 1, 27–36. doi:10.1016/j.jaci.2013.02.001

Saw CL, Cintron M, Wu TY *et al.* (2011) Pharmacodynamics of dietary phytochemical indoles I3C and DIM: Induction of Nrf2-mediated phase II drug metabolizing and antioxidant genes and synergism with isothiocyanates. *Biopharmaceutics and Drug Disposition 32*, 5, 289–300. doi:10.1002/bdd.759

Segers ME, Lebeer S (2014) Towards a better understanding of *Lactobacillus rhamnosus* GG – host interactions. *Microbial Cell Factories 13*, Suppl 1, S7. doi:10.1186/1475-2859-13-S1-S7

Seymour V (2016) The human–nature relationship and its impact on health: A critical review. *Frontiers in Public Health*. doi:10.3389/fpubh.2016.00260

Scammell TE, Mochizuki T (2009) Is low histamine a fundamental cause of sleepiness in narcolepsy and idiopathic hypersomnia? *Sleep 32*, 2, 133–134.

Schink M, Konturek PC, Tietz E *et al.* (2018) Microbial patterns in patients with histamine intolerance. *Journal of Physiology and Pharmacology 69*, 4. doi:10.26402/jpp.2018.4.09

Schrauzer GN, Shrestha KP, Flores-Arce MF (1992) Lithium in scalp hair of adults, students, and violent criminals. Effects of supplementation and evidence for interactions of lithium with vitamin B12 and with other trace elements. *Biological Trace Element Research 34*, 2, 161–176. doi:10.1007/BF02785244

Seppo Antti E, Autran CA, Bode L *et al.* (2017) Human milk oligosaccharides and development of cow's milk allergy in infants. *Journal of Allergy and Clinical Immunology 139*, 2, 708–711.

Sharma H, Zhang X, Dwivedi C (2010) The effect of ghee (clarified butter) on serum lipid levels and microsomal lipid peroxidation. *AYU 31*, 2, 134–140. doi:10.4103/0974-8520.72361

Shih JC. Wu JB, Chen K (2011) Transcriptional regulation and multiple functions of MAO genes. *Journal of Neural Transmission 118*, 7, 979–986. doi:10.1007/s00702-010-0562-9

Simonich MT, Egner PA, Roebuck BD *et al.* (2007) Natural chlorophyll inhibits aflatoxin B_1-induced multi-organ carcinogenesis in the rat. *Carcinogenesis 28*, 6, 1294–1302. doi:10.1093/carcin/bgm027

Sinatra DS, Sinatra ST, Heyser CJ (2003) The effects of coenzyme Q10 on locomotor and behavioral activity in young and aged C57BL/6 mice. *Biofactors 18*, 1–4, 283–287. doi:10.1002/biof.5520180232

Steenkamp LR, Hough CM, Reus VI *et al.* (2017) Severity of anxiety – but not depression – is associated with oxidative stress in major depressive disorder. *Journal of Affective Disorders 219*, 193–200.

Stremmel W, Merle U, Zahn A *et al.* (2005) Retarded release phosphatidylcholine benefits patients with chronic active ulcerative colitis. *Gut 54*, 7, 966–971. doi:10.1136/gut.2004.052316

Suba Z (2012) Interplay between insulin resistance and estrogen deficiency as co-activators in carcinogenesis. *Pathology and Oncology Research 18*, 2, 123–133. doi:10.1007/s12253-011-9466-8

Sun BL, Wang L, Yang T *et al.* (2018) Lymphatic drainage system of the brain: A novel target for intervention of neurological diseases. *Progress in Neurobiology 163–164*, 118–143. doi:10.1016/j.pneurobio.2017.08.007

Surendran S, Adaikalakoteswari A, Saravanan P et al. (2018) An update on vitamin B12-related gene polymorphisms and B12 status. *Genes and Nutrition 13*, 2. doi:10.1186/s12263-018-0591-9

Tack J, Miner P, Fischer L et al. (2011) Randomised clinical trial: The safety and efficacy of AST-120 in non-constipating irritable bowel syndrome – a double-blind, placebo-controlled study. *Alimentary Pharmacology and Therapeutics 34*. doi:10.1111/j.1365-2036.2011.04818

Takeda Y, Nakase H, Namba K et al. (2009) Upregulation of T-bet and tight junction molecules by *Bifidobactrium longum* improves colonic inflammation of ulcerative colitis. *Inflammatory Bowel Diseases 15*, 11, 1617–1618. doi:10.1002/ibd.20861

Tanwar VS, Chand MP, Kumar J et al. (2013) Common variant in FUT2 gene is associated with levels of vitamin B12 in Indian population. *Gene 515*, 1, 224–228. doi:10.1016/j.gene.2012.11.021

Temiz A, Mumcu AŞ, Tüylü AÖ et al. (2013) Antifungal activity of propolis samples collected from different geographical regions of Turkey against two food-related molds, Aspergillus versicolor and Penicillium aurantiogriseum (in English). *Gıda 38*, 3, 135–142.

Theoharides TC (2009) Luteolin as a therapeutic option for multiple sclerosis. *Journal of Neuroinflammation 6*, 29. doi:10.1186/1742-2094-6-29

Thomas CM, Hong T, van Pijkeren JP et al. (2012) Histamine derived from probiotic *Lactobacillus reuteri* suppresses TNF via modulation of PKA and ERK signalling. *PLOS ONE 7*, 2, e31951. doi:10.1371/journal.pone.0031951

Thompson R (2011) Blood group linked to risk of cancer in patients with Barrett esophagus. *Nature Reviews Gastroenterology and Hepatology 8*, 475. doi:10.1038/nrgastro.2011.129

Toh ZQ, Anzela A, Tang MLK et al. (2012) Probiotic therapy as a novel approach for allergic disease. *Frontiers in Pharmacology 3*, 171. doi:10.3389/fphar.2012.00171

Toribio-Mateus M (2018) Harnessing the power of microbiome assessment tools as part of neuroprotective nutrition and lifestyle medicine interventions. *Microorganisms 6*, 2, 35. doi:10.3390/microorganisms6020035

Tripathi M, Zhang CW, Singh BK et al. (2016) Hyperhomocysteinemia causes ER stress and impaired autophagy that is reversed by vitamin B supplementation. *Cell Death and Disease 7*, 12, e2513. doi:10.1038/cddis.2016.374

Upadhyaya P, Zarth AT, Fujioka N et al. (2018) Identification and analysis of a mercapturic acid conjugate of indole-3-methyl isothiocyanate in the urine of humans who consumed cruciferous vegetables. *Journal of Chromatography B 1072*, 341–346. doi:10.1016/j.jchromb.2017.12.001

Vance DE (2014) Phospholipid methylation in mammals: From biochemistry to physiological function. *Biochimica et Biophysica Acta 1838*, 6, 1477–1487. doi:10.1016/j.bbamem.2013.10.018

Var I, Kabak B, Erginkaya Z (2008) Reduction in ochratoxin A levels in white wine, following treatment with activated carbon and sodium bentonite. *Food Control 19*, 6, 592–598. doi:10.1016/j.foodcont.2007.06.013

Wacklin P, Mäkivuokko H, Alakulppi N et al. (2011) Secretor genotype (*FUT2 gene*) is strongly associated with the composition of *Bifidobacteria* in the human intestine. *PLOS ONE 6*, 5, e20113. doi:10.1371/journal.pone.0020113

Wacklin P, Tuimala J, Nikkilä J et al. (2014) Faecal Microbiota composition in adults is associated with the FUT2 gene determining the secretor status. *PLOS ONE 9*, 4, e94863. doi:10.1371/journal.pone.0094863

Wang Y, Liu Y, Sidhu A et al. (2012) *Lactobacillus rhamnosus* GG culture supernatant ameliorates acute alcohol-induced intestinal permeability and liver injury. *American Journal of Physiology: Gastrointestinal and Liver Physiology 303*, 1, G32–G41.

Wang S, Zhang S, Liou L-C et al. (2014) Phosphatidylethanolamine deficiency disrupts α-synuclein homeostasis in yeast and worm models of Parkinson disease. *PNAS 111*, 38, E3976–E3985. doi:10.1073/pnas.1411694111

Wang XH, Ren HY, Wang W et al. (2015) Evaluation of key factors influencing histamine formation and accumulation in fermented sausages. *Journal of Food Safety 35*, 3, 395–402.

Whiley L, Sen A, Heaton J *et al.* (2014) Evidence of altered phosphatidylcholine metabolism in Alzheimer's disease. *Neurobiology of Aging 35*, 2, 271–278. doi:10.1016/j.neurobiolaging.2013.08.001

Wollin A, Wang X, Tso P (2017) Nutrients regulate diamine oxidase release from intestinal mucosa. *The American Physiological Society 275*, 4, R969–975. doi:10.1152/ajpregu.1998.275.4.r969

Wu H, Sun L, Lin DP *et al.* (2017) Association of fucosyltransferase 2 gene polymorphisms with inflammatory bowel disease in patients from Southeast China. *Gastroenterology Research and Practice 2017*, 4148651. doi:10.1155/2017/4148651

Xiao L, Van't Land B, Engen PA *et al.* (2018) Human milk oligosaccharides protect against the development of autoimmune diabetes in NOD-mice. *Scientific Reports* 8, 1, 3829. doi:10.1038/s41598-018-22052-y

Xiao L, Van De Worp WRPH, Stassen R *et al.* (2019) Human milk oligosaccharides promote immune tolerance via direct interactions with human dendritic cells. *European Journal of Immunology 49*, 7. 1001–1014. doi:10.1002/eji.201847971

Yamauchi KI, Sekizawa K, Suzuki H *et al.* (1994) Structure and function of human histamine N-methyltransferase: critical enzyme in histamine metabolism in airway. *American Journal of Physiology 267*, 3 Pt 1, L342–349.

Yasko A (2014) *Feel Good Nutrigenomics*. TX: Neurological Research Institute.

Yeh HP, Stone JA, Churchill SM *et al.* (2017) Physical and emotional benefits of different exercise environments designed for treadmill running. *International Journal of Environmental Research and Public Health 14*, 7, 752. doi:10.3390/ijerph14070752

Yimer EM, Tuem KB, Karim A *et al.* (2019) *Nigella sativa* L. (black cumin): A promising natural remedy for wide range of illnesses. *Evidence-Based Complementary and Alternative Medicine 2019*, 1528635. doi:10.1155/2019/1528635

Yoshikawa T, Nakamura T, Yanai K (2019) Histamine N-methyltransferase in the brain. *International Journal of Molecular Sciences 20*, 3, 737. doi:10.3390/ijms20030737

Yuan SLK, Matsutani LA, Marques AP (2015) Effectiveness of different styles of massage therapy in fibromyalgia: A systematic review and meta-analysis. *Manual Therapy 20*, 2, 257–264. doi:10.1016/j.math.2014.09.003

Zhao R, Kalvass JC, Yanni SB *et al.* (2009) Fexofenadine brain exposure and the influence of blood–brain barrier P-glycoprotein after fexofenadine and terfenadine administration. *Drug Metabolism and Disposition: The Biological Fate of Chemicals 37*, 3, 529–535. doi:10.1124/dmd.107.019893

Zheng ZY, Liang L, Fan X *et al.* (2008) The role of modified citrus pectin as an effective chelator of lead in children hospitalized with toxic lead levels. *Alternative Therapies in Health and Medicine 14*, 4, 34–39.

Zinck JW, de Groh M, MacFarlane AJ (2015) Genetic modifiers of folate, vitamin B-12, and homocysteine status in a cross-sectional study of the Canadian population. *American Journal of Clinical Nutrition 101*, 6, 1295–1304. doi:10.3945/ajcn.115.107219

4

Biotransformation and Elimination Phase 1

Liver Detoxification Polymorphisms

Before methylation is discussed, it would be pertinent to set the scene with a view of the overall mechanism for liver detoxification. This chapter will look at detoxification, the genes associated and the tools that can be used to identify gene expression before addressing the underlying cause for dysfunction.

Review of detoxification basics

Liver detoxification encompasses two phases, aptly named phase 1 and phase 2. Within these two phases are a number of enzymes that create metabolic conversions throughout the detoxification system. The class of enzymes in phase 1 include those referred to as cytochrome P450 (CYP450) enzymes. These enzymes are responsible for oxidizing lipid-soluble molecules, allowing more solubility in water for excretion as each enters the liver (Guengerich 2021).

Each CYP450 enzyme performs one of the following tasks:

- oxidation reaction
- reduction reaction
- hydrolysis reaction
- hydration reaction
- de-halogenation reaction.

In some cases – for example, caffeine – the CYP enzyme has the ability to completely clear the molecule. In most cases, however, this is not so and this is where phase 2 enzymes are needed to carry out a form of neutralization followed by elimination via the bile and faeces or via the kidneys and urine. Lipid-soluble molecules that enter phase 1 include steroid hormones, xenobiotics and fatty acids. Nutrient support for phase 1 might include B vitamins, branch-chain amino acids, flavonoids, phospholipids and glutathione (Hodges & Minich 2015). These will be discussed in more detail alongside their respective genes and enzymes.

It should be noted that metabolites of phase 1 enzymes are toxic. This area between phase 1 and phase 2 therefore produces a lot of reactive oxygen species or free radicals, which, if left uncontrolled, can create a lot of oxidative stress. This can then result in damage to cells, proteins and DNA, and in fact is one of the strongest determinants of chronic disease. The term 'pathological detoxifier' has been used to identify this type of client, although this has not been evaluated. The term identifies a person who has a fast phase 1 and a compromised phase 2. Excessive formation of reactive oxygen species can promote damage to the organ – in this case the liver. If antioxidant supply is low and environmental toxin exposure is high, even relatively harmless substances can turn into carcinogenic molecules. Phase 1 oestrogen metabolites such as 4-OH-estrones are a clear example of this. These will be discussed later in the chapter.

After phase 1 activity, the reactive intermediary metabolites enter phase 2 detoxification, where conjugation occurs. Phase 2 enzymes carry out one of the following:

- a sulphation reaction
- a glucuronidation reaction
- a glutathione conjugation reaction

- an acetylation reaction
- an amino acid conjugation reaction
- a methylation reaction.

This is in order to convert an intermediary molecule into an excretory product.

An individual's unique ability to biotransform, detoxify and eliminate endogenous and exogenous toxins depends on his or her genetic variations, the DNA of the person, gut microbiome and the interaction of these with lifestyle and diet. Susceptibility to toxicity will be more or less, according to the ability of the individual to perform these interactions well. Many environmental toxins are lipophilic, thereby only dissolving in fatty or oily substances. They need to be bioactivated by phase 1, then conjugated by phase 2 to become hydrophilic. Understanding whether a SNP is up- or down-regulated and how nutrients, medications, heavy metals and other chemicals affect the speed and direction can assist the practitioner greatly in recommending specific and appropriate interventions. Pharmacogenomics is an evolving science, but most medications or substrates will up-regulate CYP enzymes unless otherwise stated here. Although the liver is the major detoxification organ, other tissues in the body also have the ability to detoxify to a degree. Some would regard cellular membrane detoxification as phase 3 (Kane 2017).

For ease and clarity, an overall discussion will precede particular key points concerning the specific CYP enzymes.

Activation of phase 1 liver detoxification occurs with inhalation, ingestion or skin absorption of many products. Some examples are listed below.

- Medications: alcohol, nicotine, phenobarbital, sulphonamides, steroids.
- Foods: broccoli, cabbage, Brussels sprouts, charcoal-broiled meats, high-protein diet, oranges and tangerines.
- Nutrients: niacin, thiamine, vitamin C.
- Herbs: caraway and dill seeds.
- Environmental toxins: exhaust fumes, carbon tetrachloride, volatile organic compounds (paints, acrylics) and dioxin pesticides.

Grapefruit contains naringenin and furanocoumarin derivatives which both reduce the activity of CYP3A4, thereby decreasing the rate of elimination of some medications. It has been found to exponentially alter the clinical activity of those medications. Eight ounces (236ml) of grapefruit juice can have a marked effect, by as much as 30% down-regulation (Lilja *et al.* 2000), holding medications in the system and increasing side effects.

Glyphosates have also been identified as CYP450 suppressors. The herbicide is used to spray genetically modified and conventional grain crops. In the UK, this had led to the research of many pesticide residues in everyday foods and the publication of the 'dirty dozen' and 'clean fifteen' foods below

Table 4.1: Dirty dozen and clean fifteen

Dirty dozen Percentage of food with multiple chemical residues	Clean fifteen Percentage of food with multiple chemical residues
Grapefruit 97%	Beetroot 0%
Oranges 96%	Sweetcorn 0%
Lemon and lime 91%	Mushrooms 0%
Strawberries 84%	Figs 0%
Pears 84%	Rhubarb 0%
Grapes 75%	Swede 0%
Cherries 72%	Turnip 0%
Peaches 72%	Onions 1%
Parsnips 69%	Avocado 2%
Asparagus 66%	Cauliflower 3%
Apples 64%	Radish 4%
Apricots 64%	Sweet potato 6%

cont.

Dirty dozen Percentage of food with multiple chemical residues	Clean fifteen Percentage of food with multiple chemical residues
	Broad beans 8%
	Leeks 8%
	Pumpkin and squash 8%

Source: Based on 2012–2017 data for multiple residues published by the Expert Committee on Pesticide Residue (Pesticide Action Network UK 2019)

Glyphosates are said to be harmless to humans but in fact they inhibit the shikimate pathway (Zabalza *et al.* 2017) that biosynthesizes the aromatic amino acids phenylalanine, tyrosine and tryptophan. Although humans do not have a shikimate pathway, their microbiome population do. Metabolism of B vitamins and amino acids is supported by the gut microbiome, so unbalancing the microbiome with glyphosates can render humans very low on these essential nutrients, which may also reduce the amount of available neurotransmitters (Aitbali *et al.* 2018). Simultaneously, this may also negatively affect sulphation, allowing pathogens to grow (Samsel & Seneff 2015).

Children with autism are known to have metabolic markers that indicate excessive glyphosate exposure; these include serum sulphate and zinc deficiency (Samsel & Seneff 2013). Two clear associations are gut dysbiosis and disrupted sulphur metabolism (Seneff *et al.* 2012). Certain microbes do actually break down glyphosate but in fact this process triggers the release of ammonia. Children with autism and the elderly with Alzheimer's disease have significantly higher levels of ammonia (Jin *et al.* 2018). Some researchers would advocate that this is the cause for the rise in autism spectrum disorders since 1978 (Samsel & Seneff 2013). Glyphosates also affect the genes and enzymes PON1, CBS, NOS3, GST and SOD in phase 2, and also inhibit many of the CYP genes in phase 1 (Abass *et al.* 2009), often by up-regulating the nuclear receptor constitutive androstane receptor (CAR), which is a major regulator of CYP enzyme activity (Abass *et al.* 2012).

Cytochrome P450 1A1 and 1A2: CYP1A1 and CYP1A2

CYP540 1A1 and 1A2 encode for their respective CYP450 enzyme of family 1 subfamily A member 1 and member 2.

This enzyme metabolizes xenobiotic, polycyclic hydrocarbons and aflotoxins. Polycyclic hydrocarbons (PAH) emissions are generated by charcoal-grilling of meat products, exhaust fumes and cigarette smoke. When these PAH toxins are metabolized by CYP1A1, they may become carcinogenic as they are processed through the aryl hydrocarbon receptor (AhR). This AhR is critical for regulating cell homeostasis (Androutsopoulos *et al.* 2009). These CYP enzymes mostly become up-regulated when expressed, meaning faster processing of these products to their more toxic metabolites. This can create increased oxidative stress if phase 2 pathways are down-regulated or slow-running. However, according to Santes-Palacios and Romo-Mancillas *et al.* (2016), this enzyme can also be down-regulated. The SNPs rs1048943, rs1799814 and rs4746903 are the most commonly researched. A CYP enzyme may not confer a deleterious situation for the individual if the nutrition and lifestyle habits of the individual are supportive. For example, someone who regularly barbecues meat and/or smokes or is exposed to xenobiotics at work may in fact covert these compounds to highly reactive carcinogenic compounds. However, if the practitioner is successful in coaching the individual to cease smoking and avoid xenobiotic exposure as much as possible, while encouraging a diet high in glucosinolates, from cruciferous vegetables, this can become a benefit.

NB: Practitioners should always consult the latest evidence base for the particular enzyme and condition of relevance. This can be found on PubMed (https://pubmed.ncbi.nlm.nih.gov), ScienceDirect (www.sciencedirect.com) or by subscribing to specific genetics-focused journals.

If CYP 1A1 is expressing due to a high caffeine intake, oestrogen metabolite levels may rise, predisposing to possible hormone-related cancers of the prostate, breast, ovaries and testicles (Wang *et al.* 2012). Although this enzyme can activate cancer-causing substances, it is usually found to be important for their detoxification (Androutsopoulos *et al.* 2009). The rs1048943 allele has been associated with lung cancer (Liu *et al.* 2016) and hepatocellular cancer (Li *et al.* 2009). Rs4646903 has been associated with DNA damage and cancer risk (Liu 2016; He *et al.* 2014; Han *et al.* 2013)

Possible interventions based on CYP1A1 genetic expression
Nutrient cofactors to support CYP1A1 enzyme activity

- Haem (Lynch 2017).
- Resveratrol (Hodges & Minich 2015).
- Astaxanthin (Ohno *et al.* 2011).
- Fish oil and garlic oil (Chen *et al.* 2003).

Unhelpful inducers that increase CYP1A1 enzyme activity
Chargrilled/burned food, xenoestrogens, cigarette smoke and moulds (Cerliani *et al.* 2016).

Helpful inhibitors that reduce CYP1A1 enzyme activity

- Sulphorophane (Yang *et al.* 2013).
- Green tea (Williams *et al.* 2000).
- Lycopene – from tomatoes, carrots and watermelon (Wang *et al.* 2010).
- Grapefruit (naringin) (Santes-Palacios & Romo-Mancillas *et al.* 2016).
- Ginger, rosemary, oregano and holy basil as garden herbs (Mohe-bati *et al.* 2012).
- Turmeric has the properties of both up- and down-regulation of this gene (Hodges & Minich 2015).

Drug interactions/substrates (can exacerbate expression of the gene or be responsible for switching the gene on)
Antipsychotics (clozapine, haloperidol, olanzapine), muscle relaxants (cyclobenzaprine), SNRIs (duloxetine), SSRIs (fluvoxamine), tricyclic antidepressants (imipramine), NSAIDs (nabumetone, naproxen) (Lynch 2017; Cohen 2015).

Practical advice

- Check rsid numbers for expected expression and ensure this corresponds with history.
- Reduce PAHs, xenoestrogens. Advise against smoking as necessary and check for possible mould exposure. Test if necessary.
- Use dietary measures from the above list of inhibitors as needed.

PRACTITIONER NOTES

Whether SNP expression occurs in CYP enzymes is dependent on the lifestyle habits of the individual – factors such as poor diet, smoking, regular consumption of charred meat or chronic exposure to xenobiotics such as pesticides and industrial chemicals. It is an advantage if the individual can avoid smoking and xenobiotics as much as possible. Consider caffeine intake, oestrogen-mimicking foods and chemicals, genetically modified foods and foods such as grains, which are sprayed with glyphosate. Consider also the good xenoestrogens such as coffee, black tea, chocolate, soy, dairy, non-organic meat and poultry, dried apricots/dates and prunes, sesame seeds, chickpeas, beans, tempeh, alfalfa sprouts, bran, phthalates and the additive 4-hexylresorcinol (used to prevent shellfish discoloration).

There are many healthy foods in this list, so the practitioner would need to be discerning about which to remove. It would not be advisable to remove all as a recommendation.

Cytochrome P450 1B1: CYP1B1

CYP540 1B1 encodes for the CYP450 enzyme of family 1 subfamily B member 1. This gene is extrahepatic, it instructs the enzyme cytochrome P450 1B1 enzyme to oxidize estrone E1 to the carcinogenic 4-hydroxyestrogen. It also converts a number of pro-carcinogens into their activated forms (e.g. polycyclic hydrocarbons). The rs1800440 allele of

CYP1B1 has been readily associated with endometrial and other oestrogen-fuelled cancers due to up-regulation of this enzyme consistent with down-regulated or slow COMT (+/+) (Reding *et al.* 2012).

Estradiol catechol oestrogens, including 2-hydroxyestradiol and 4-hydroxyestradiol, can go through reductive-oxidative cycling and produce mutagenic free radicals. CYP and peroxidase enzymes catalyze these reactions. Oestrogen semiquinones and quinones are reactive and carcinogenic intermediate metabolites of redox cycling pathways and can cause DNA damage.

CYP1B1 metabolizes tamoxifen, xenobiotics, aflotoxins and food mutagens and also polycyclic hydrocarbons. The rs10012 allele has been more associated with colorectal and prostate cancers; again, practitioners must also check COMT down-regulation (Wang *et al.* 2011). The CYP1B1 enzyme is active in many body tissues, especially those of the eye. More than 140 gene mutations have been identified to cause early-onset glaucoma, including CYP1B1 (Reis *et al.* 2016). It is also known to inactivate certain therapeutic agents such as coffee, theophylline (COPD medication), phanacetin (pain-relieving medication) and warfarin (blood thinner/vitamin K antagonist).

Table 4.2: CYP regulation

SNP and nutrient cofactors	Substrate detoxified	Likely expression	Inhibitors of gene expression	Inducers of gene expression
CYP1A1 Heame	Heterocyclic hydrocarbons (e.g. exhaust fumes, chargrilled food, cigarette smoke), hydroxylation of oestrogens and aflotoxins	Up-regulation	Antioxidants, polyphenols, phytoestrogens, cruciferous vegetables, green tea, curcumin, vitamin E, ALA, NAC, CoQ10	Chargrilled food, xenoestrogens, cigarette smoke and moulds

CYP1B1 Heame	Hydroxylation of oestrogen and testosterone	Up-regulation	Cruciferous vegetables, grapefruit juice, indol-3-carbinol, fish oils, rosemary, calcium D-glucarate (oranges, apples, grapefruit, cruciferous vegetables), NAC, cardamom	Char-grilled/burned food, xenoes-trogens, cigarette smoke

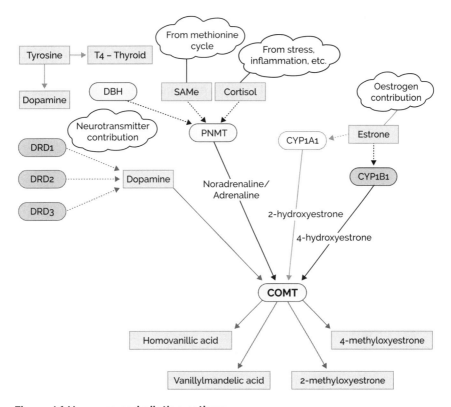

Figure 4.1 Hormone assimilation pathway
NB: Rounded labels are SNPs and rectangles are metabolic products.

Figure 4.1 demonstrates the assimilation of dopamine and oestrogen via COMT. Tyrosine is converted to L-dopa, then dopamine, which then converts to noradrenaline and adrenaline before being excreted as vanilmandelic acid. When DBH and/or COMT are down-regulated more dopamine may be excreted as homovanillic acid. Oestrone is converted to 4-hydroxyestrone by the enzyme CYB1B1, which, of course, is up-regulated when expressing. If the COMT enzyme is expressing as a slow enzyme (+/+), then dopamine, noradrenaline, adrenaline and or 4-hydroxyestrone can become trapped and therefore elevated in this pathway. This would then lead to symptoms of high levels of any or all of these metabolic products. This pathway is therefore quite important to understand when dealing with a patient who is suspected of having high levels of oestrogen and dopamine. In this scenario, psychosis is possible, if, for example, methylation is driven with high-dose folate. This has been demonstrated in the case of Edwina discussed in Chapter 5.

Possible interventions based on CYP1B1 genetic expression
Nutrient cofactors to support CYP1B1 enzyme activity
Haem.

Substrates (substances on which the CYP1B1 enzyme
acts) and inducers (regulate gene expression)
that increase activity of the enzyme

- Diesel and exhaust particles (Jacob *et al.* 2011).
- Ultraviolet light exposure (Villard *et al.* 2002).
- Biotin (Rodriguez-Melendez *et al.* 2004).
- Benzopyrene and benzofluorethine (Spink *et al.* 2008).
- Inflammatory cytokines (Šmerdová *et al.* 2014).

Inhibitors that reduce CYP1B1 enzyme activity

- Lycopene – from tomatoes, carrots and watermelon (Wang *et al.* 2010).
- Grapefruit juice (Poon *et al.* 2013).
- Quercetin (Choi *et al.* 2012). NB: Be careful with a slow COMT.
- Rosemary, ginger, holy basil, green tea, oregano (Mohebati *et al.* 2012).

PRACTITIONER NOTES

The practitioner should be concerned when evidence points clearly towards the elevation of oestrogen or intermediary oestrogen metabolites such as 2-OH-E1, 4-OH-E1, 16 alpha-OH-E1 and their ratios. For example, a high normal 16-OH-E1 with excessively high 4-OH-E1 and low 2-OH-E1 would denote a sluggish clearance. Consider the avoidance of xenoestrogens, genetically modified foods and foods exposed to glyphosate: coffee, black tea, chocolate, soy, dairy, non-organic meats and poultry, non-organic eggs, bisphenol-A, flax seed, yucca root, sports drinks or other carbonated beverages containing caffeine, dried fruits such as dates, prunes and apricots, sesame seeds, chickpeas, beans, alfalfa, tempeh, tofu and bran cereals, phthalates and 4-hexyl resorcinol – a shellfish additive to prevent discoloration (Amadasi *et al.* 2009), 4-hexyl resorcinol, which all bind oestrogen receptors. This list is not exhaustive, so please do check the evidence base if you are unsure and, of course, apply the findings of your individual case. Organic grass-fed meats, free from bovine growth hormone and antibiotics, are a must for those with over-expressed CYP1B1.

Those with over-expressed CYP1B1 and slow COMT (V158M and H62H) would appear to be more at risk for oestrogen-receptive cancers (Zhou *et al.* 2015). This is due to a particular nasty combination of fast CYP1B1 and slow COMTs; this combination, when expressing, increases the risk of 4-hydroxyestrone. However, practitioners can intervene avidly, being very careful not to drive methylation too fast until balance is achieved. Blood mean corpuscular volume is a measure of red blood cell size to indicate the possibility of macrocytic anaemia or B12 status. A high mean corpuscular volume (MCV) on standard blood work or a high methylmalonic acid might indicate that B12 is not being transported into cells to combine with methylfolate via MTHFR, MTRR and MTR (more on these later), so a small amount of lithium orotate can help (Marshall 2015). It is also important not to drive methylation with methylfolate at this point because the body may make more poorly functioning cells (Ehrlich 2019).

Methylation is the last step in a case of poor oestrogen metabolism such as this. Ensure all pathways of elimination are open first.

Cytochrome P450 2B6: CYP2B6

The CYP450 family 2 includes a number of genes such as CYP2B6, CYP2C8, CYP2C9, CYP2C19, CYP2D6 and CYP2E1. The relevant ones will be discussed in this section.

One substance metabolized by the CYP2B6 enzymes is nicotine (Chenoweth *et al.* 2016), but this is not the only substance. These enzymes catalyze many reactions involved in drug metabolism and synthesis of steroids, cholesterol and other lipids. Xenobiotics such as cyclophosphamide and ifosphomide (anticancer drugs) are also metabolized by this enzyme. There are a number of alleles for this gene including rs35303484, rs34097093, rs8192719, rs2279344, rs7260329, rs28399499, rs2279343, rs3745274, rs8192709, rs1042389 and rs36079186. These are all noted as a down-regulation or slow metabolizers of substrates. Rs3745274 is the most common and clinically useful variant. Expression here would result in vastly reduced enzyme activity (Kharasch 2017). This means drugs will stay in the system longer so we may see build-up of side effects or medication toxicity. Rs2279345 and rs2279343 are associated with higher enzyme activity and therefore a higher rate of clearance. These patients may need a higher dose of medication to achieve symptom resolution or the medication may not work (Kharasch 2017; Wang *et al.* 2011). Niu *et al.* (2011), Turpeinen *et al.* (2006) and Arellano *et al.* (2017) found many substrates associated with this enzyme, so the reader is advised to consult these works to gain a more complete list. Most allopathic medications can affect the functioning of this enzyme. However, efavirenz, a reverse transcription inhibitor used in the treatment of AIDS, can invoke central nervous system toxicity where there is gene/enzyme expression as this medication speeds up the action of CYP2B6 with successive dosing. This can lead to more serious adverse reactions over time (Röhrich *et al.* 2016).

Possible interventions based on CYP2B6 genetic expression
Nutrient cofactors to support CYP2B6 enzyme activity

- Haem (Amunugama *et al.* 2012).
- Berberine (Zhang *et al.* 2016).
- Allyl isothiocyanate; found in mustard, wasabi, radish, horse-radish (Lim *et al.* 2015).

Helpful inducers and substrates (substances on which the
CYP2B6 enzyme acts) that increase activity of the enzyme
Rifampicin, carbamazepine, phenobarbital and phenytoin (Smith 2015).
The substrates for this enzyme include artemisinin, bupropion, cyclo-phosphamide, efavirenz, ifosfamide, ketamine, meperidine, nevirapine, propofol (Indiana University School of Medicine 2018, p.450).

Unhelpful inhibitors that reduce enzyme activity
Orphenadrine (anticholinergic for Parkinson's symptoms), ticlopidine
(antiplatelet) and curcumin (Smith 2015).
 Further drug data accessed from www.drugbank.ca (Wishart *et al.*
2017; Law *et al.* 2014; Knox *et al.* 2011; Wishart *et al.* 2008; Wishart
et al. 2006).

Practical advice

- Check medications and the impact on specific alleles.
- Check environmental exposure and gut health.
- Support enzyme with foods initially.

Cytochrome P450 2C9: CYP2C9*1, *2, *3

CYP2C9 is an interesting gene. This gene encodes for its sister enzyme of
the same name; it metabolizes 15–20% of medications (Van Booven *et al.*
2010). The alleles rs1799853 and rs1057910 are down-regulations when
expressing, so this again means that if the gene is expressing, the drugs
that are assimilated by the enzyme may remain in the system too long

and the dose will need to be lowered. The rs1799853 allele down-regulates the enzyme by 50% (Van Booven *et al.* 2010). This enzyme metabolizes warfarin, angiotensin antagonists, sulphonylureas, barbiturates, potassium channel blockers and many non-steroidal anti-inflammatory agents (NSAIDs). Individuals with this genetic expression on CYP2C9*2/*3 may therefore be more prone to gastrointestinal bleeding as a result of NSAID use (Figueiras *et al.* 2016) Down-regulations in this gene can lead to many adverse drug reactions. (Rosemary *et al.* 2007). The variant has much lower frequencies in African and Asian populations compared with causations (Van Booven *et al.* 2010). The rs9332131 variant is a rare variant with a complete lack of CYP2C9 activity and has been detected in patients with adverse reactions to phenytoin (Xu *et al.* 2013).

Possible interventions and considerations based on CYP2C9 gene expression
Nutrient cofactor for CYP2C9
Haem (Daly *et al.* 2017).

Helpful inducers (activates gene expression) and substrates (substances on which the CYP2C9 enzyme acts) that increase the activity of the enzyme leading to faster drug metabolism
Medications include barbiturates (secobarbital, phenobarbital), anticonvulsants (carbamazepine), antibiotics (rifampicin); monoclonal antibodies (adalimumab, certolizumab, etanercept, golimumab and infliximab) (Smith 2015), proton pump inhibitors, antiplatelets (clopidogrel), selective serotonin reuptake inhibitors (citalopram), tricyclic antidepressants (amitriptyline, clomipramine, imipramine), muscle relaxants (carisoprodol), antimalarial (proguanil), antifungals (voriconazole), beta-blockers (labetalol) and chemotherapy drugs (cyclophosphamides). Herbal medications include St John's Wort, bisphenol-A (Xu 2017).

Unhelpful inhibitors that reduce activity of the CYP2C9 enzyme
Azole antifungals, valproic acid, apigenin, fluvoxamine, metronidazole, H1 receptor antagonists, chloramphenicol, fenofibrate, flavonols, fluvoxamine, statins and metronidazole (Lynch 2017; Cohen 2015), quercetin (Rastogi & Jana 2014), star fruit juice (Zhang *et al.* 2007).

Drug data accessed from www.drugbank.ca (Wishart *et al.* 2017, *Law et al.* 2014, Knox *et al.* 2011, *Wishart et al.* 2008, Wishart *et al.* 2006).

Practical advice
- Check alleles for potential expression and assess consistency with case history.
- Check medications and refer to GP for review of medication.
- Check iron levels and correct as necessary.
- Check nutritional intake and recommend apigenin-containing foods to rebalance expression. Examples include parsley, chamomile, artichokes, oregano, celery and vine spinach (Shankar *et al.* 2017).
- Ensure gut health is optimal.

Cytochrome P450 2C19*1, *2, *3 and *17: CYP2C19*1/2/3/17

This gene encodes the enzyme CYP2C19*1, *2 and *17 There are more than 30 variants of this gene (Arici & Özhan 2017). The CYP2C19*1 SNP produces normal enzyme activity while CYP2C19*2 produces reduced enzyme activity (rs 4244285) when expressed. The CYP2C19 17 allele rs12248560 creates an excessive up-regulation resulting in extensive metabolism of substrates (Arici & Özhan 2017). Below is an overview of the potential rate of metabolism for all expressing SNPs on this gene.

- Ultra-rapid metabolizers (*1 /*17 or *17 /*17).
- Extensive metabolizers (*1/*1).
- Intermediate metabolizers (*1 /*2, *1 /*3, or *2 /*17).
- Poor metabolizers (*2 /*2 or *2 /*3) (Yang *et al.* 2015).

Substrates metabolized by CYP19 include antidepressants, anti-epileptics (López-García *et al.* 2017), proton pump inhibitors (PPIs), antimalarials, beta-blockers, chloramphenicol, cyclophosphamide, NSAIDs, anti-retrovirals, progesterone, warfarin. As an example, a person with CYP19*17 medicated with antiplatelet medication may be at increased risk of bleeding; however, knowledge of CYP2C19 polymorphisms may offer safer medication options (Klein *et al.* 2018). PPIs are broken down too quickly, requiring higher dosages to gain effects. Poor metabolizers are prone to cardiovascular disease and an increased circulation of C-reactive protein (CRP) in women (Akasaka *et al.* 2016). Ultrafast metabolizers have an increased risk of being refractory (resistant) to PPIs (Ichikawa *et al.* 2016).

Potential interventions based on CYP2C19 genetic expression
Nutrient cofactors to support enzyme CYP2C19 function
Haem (Wei *et al.* 2008).

Inducers (activates gene expression) and substrates (substances on which the CYP2C19 enzyme acts) that increase activity of the enzyme
Antibiotics (rifampicin), antimalarial (artemisinin), anticonvulsants (carbamazepine), synthetic progestational hormones (norethisterone), corticosteroids (prednisone) and NSAIDs (aspirin).

Inhibitors that reduce CYP2C19 enzyme activity (can be helpful or unhelpful dependent on rapid or poor metabolism)
MAOA inhibitor (moclobemide), SSRI (fluvoxamine), antibiotic (chloramphenicol), anticonvulsants and PPIs (Lynch 2017; Cohen 2015), apigenin from parsley, orange, tea, camomile and onion (Wang *et al.* 2016), liquorice (*He et al.* 2015).

Drug data accessed from www.drugbank.ca (Wishart *et al.* 2017; Law *et al.* 2014; Knox *et al.* 2011; Wishart *et al.* 2008; Wishart *et al.* 2006).

Practical advice

- Check alleles for potential expression and assess consistent with case history.
- Check medications and refer to GP for review of medication.
- Check iron levels and correct if necessary.
- Check nutritional intake and recommend apigenin-containing foods to rebalance expression.
- Ensure gut health is optimal.

Cytochrome P450 2D6: CYP2D6

This gene, with its partner enzyme, is primarily expressed in the liver and in the substantia nigra portion of the central nervous system (Cheng *et al.* 2013). It is probably the most important of the pathways of phase 1 detoxification and has more than 100 alleles. It is responsible for the detoxification of xenobiotic herbicides and pesticides. It is also responsible for the metabolism of around 25% of regular medications including dextromethorphan, a key ingredient of beta-blockers, antiarrhythmic and antidepressant medications. Identification of more than 100 alleles has demonstrated a range of activity from none to ultra-rapid activity. The practitioner should therefore consult the evidence for specifics with regard to the individual case. Below is an overview of known expression of CYP2D6 SNPs.

- Normal enzyme function variants (e.g. *1 and *2).
- Reduced function variants (e.g. *9, *10, and *41).
- Non-functional variants (e.g. *3, *4, *5 and *6) (Arici *et al.* 2017; Hicks *et al.* 2013).

NB: The asterisks mean these are star-based haplotype alleles. They have been used to predict optimal dosing for 6-mercaptopurine in paediatric acute lymphoblastic leukaemia (Park *et al.* 2019).

Although CYP2D6 only accounts for 2.5% of all liver enzymes, it does assimilate 25% of medications (Reynolds *et al.* 2016). CYP2D6 metabolizes tyramine to dopamine and regenerates serotonin, and, as such, expression has been linked to disordered behaviours (Peñas-Lledó & Lierena 2014). It also inactivates neurotoxins, making it an important factor in some cases of Alzheimer's disease (Mann *et al.* 2012).

Around 75% of Europeans are said to be extensive metabolizers, less than 10% are ultrafast metabolizers, and poor and intermediate metabolizers are said to make up the other 15% of the population. A deficiency of this enzyme is inherited as an autosomal recessive trait (Bertilsson *et al.* 2002). Another term for this is a single-gene disorder, where a condition arises from the mutation of a single gene that has been passed down from both parents. Poor metabolizers are prone to being anxious and less likely to socialize (Cheng *et al.* 2013).

Homozygous (+/+) or heterozygous (+/–) allele presentation of rs1135840 in an individual would confer an up-regulation requiring non-opioids if the need for more long-term pain relief was necessary. Tramadol and morphine and its derivatives should be avoided to prevent opiate toxicity, if UGT (glucoronidation) is impaired in phase 2 (Goh *et al.* 2017). Within phase 2, opiates are conjugated to hydrophilic substances such as glycine, glucuronic acid, glutathione or sulphate.

Possible interventions based on CYP2D6 genetic expression
Nutrient cofactors to support CYP2D6 enzyme activity
Haem (Iwuoha *et al.* 2007).

Unhelpful inducers and substrates (substances on which the CYP2D6 enzyme acts) that increase activity of the enzyme
Beta-blockers, antidepressants, antipsychotics, opioid analgesics (codeine), GI serotonin receptor antagonist (ondansetron), selective oestrogen receptor modulator (tamoxifen) and others. Please consult Indiana University clinical tables for a full list and take guidance from the current evidence base (https://drug-interactions.medicine.iu.edu/MainTable.aspx).

- Curcumin (Al-Jenoobi *et al.* 2015).
- Asafoetida (Al-Jenoobi *et al.* 2014).
- Garden cress seed powder (Al-Jenoobi *et al.* 2014).

Helpful inhibitors that reduce enzyme activity
Antimalarial (chloroquine), H2 receptor antagonist (cimetidine, ranitidine), dopamine antagonist used for gastroparesis (metoclopramide), SSRIs (citalopram, paroxetine, fluoxetine, sertraline), antiarrhythmic (quinidine), synthetic opiates (methadone), stimulant drugs (cocaine) and acrylamides (from high-temperature cooking) (Lynch 2017; Cohen 2015).

Drug data accessed from www.drugbank.ca (Wishart *et al.* 2017, *Law et al.* 2014, Knox *et al.* 2011, *Wishart et al.* 2008, Wishart *et al.* 2006).

- Berberine (Kim *et al.* 2020).
- Star fruit juice (Zhang *et al.* 2007).
- Aloe vera juice (Djuv & Nilsen 2012).
- Kale (Yamasaki *et al.* 2012).
- Fennel (Langhammer & Nilsen 2014).
- Quercetin (Rastogi & Jana 2014).
- Black pepper (Livezey & Nagi 2012).
- Liquorice (He *et al.* 2015).

Practical advice

- Check medications and side effects and refer to GP for medication review if necessary.
- Check nutrient deficiencies as a result of medications.
- Advise foods for respective expression.
- Check gut health and rebalance as necessary.
- Check phase 2 liver detoxification and address imbalances.

Cytochrome P450 2E1: CYP2E1

This gene and its partner enzyme rs2070676 are located in the dopamine-containing neurons in the substantia nigra. As such, it could be important in the pathophysiology of Parkinson's disease (Shahabi *et al.* 2009), although research is still in its infancy. It has been associated with Parkinson's due to a downscaling of its mechanism of detoxifying putative neurotoxins or by increased production of reactive oxygen species, as can occur in the presence of coffee and cigarette smoke. Acrylamides, formed in the process of frying carbohydrates (crisps and chips/French fries), are absorbed readily and converted to glycidamide via epoxidation. Practitioners are advised to also check GSTM1, GSTT1, GSTP1 polymorphisms in addition. CYP2E1 overexpression has also been identified in the hippocampal region of those with drug-resistant epilepsy, suggesting sensitivity to ethanol as one possible cause (García-Suástegui *et al.* 2017).

According to Heit *et al.* (2013), CYP2E1 is involved heavily in ethanol metabolism. The central nervous system (CNS) is very sensitive to ethanol as this depresses the CNS, giving rise to behaviour changes (aggression, euphoria), poor motor control and poor memory. Alcohol dehydrogenase (ADH) and CYP2E1 are involved in the conversion of ethanol to acetaldehyde. Then acetaldehyde dehydrogenase (ALDH) converts acetaldehyde to acetate, which can then cross the blood–brain barrier to be metabolized to acetyl-CoA for the citric acid cycle. This provides safe excretion of aldehydes from the CNS.

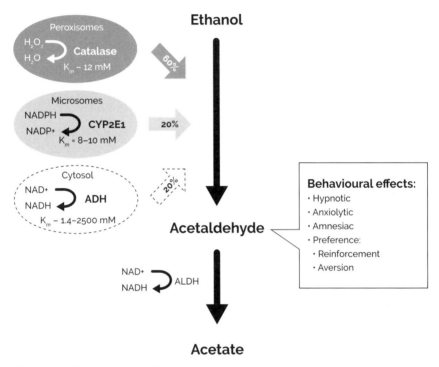

Figure 4.2: Ethanol metabolism
Source: Heit et al. (2013)

This enzyme metabolizes medications such as paracetamol, halothane and chlorzoxazone, and the xenobiotics alcohol (Heit *et al.* 2013), ketones, nitrosamines and food mutagens. It also converts ethanol to acetaldehyde, which is a known carcinogen (Cederbaum 2014; Hwang *et al.* 2012; Cederbaum 2010). Overexpression has been indicated as a factor in intestinal hyperpermeability in mice (Forsyth *et al.* 2014).

Possible interventions based on CYP2E1 genetic expression
Nutrient cofactors to support CYP2E1 enzyme activity
Haem (Cederbaum 2003).

Helpful inhibitors that reduce CYP2E1 enzyme activity
Tyrosine kinase inhibitors (midostaurin), aldehyde dehydrogenase inhibitors (antabuse/disulfiram), antibiotics (isoniazid), topical broad-spectrum antifungals (clotrimazole), synthetic cannabinoids (nabilone), platelet aggregation (ADP) inhibitor (ticlodipine), calcium channel blockers (nifedipine) and the antiepileptic (rufinamide). Acet-aldehyde is an intermediate metabolite in the metabolism of alcohol that can also be created by yeast overgrowth, alcohol, perfumes and preservatives (Lynch 2017; Cohen 2015).

- Garlic (Hodges & Minich 2015).
- Green and black tea (Yao *et al.* 2014).
- Resveratrol found in grapes, mulberries, blueberries and raspber-ries (Bedada & Neerati 2016).
- Quercetin (Surapeneni *et al.* 2014).
- Piperine found in pepper (Bedada & Boga 2017).
- Curcumin (Lee *et al.* 2013).
- Dandelion leaf (Park *et al.* 2010).

Unhelpful inducers (regulates CYP2E1 gene expression)
and substrates (substances on which the enzyme
acts) that increase activity of the enzyme
Anaesthetics, antipyretic, anti-inflammatory (paracetamol), benzene, ethanol, alcohol, nicotine, xanthine muscle relaxants (theophyl-line, chlorzoxazone), fluoroquinolone (delafloxacin), alkaloid pain relief (colchicine), glucocorticoid (dexamethasone), barbiturates (phenobarbitone).

Drug data accessed from www.drugbank.ca (Wishart *et al.* 2017, Law *et al.* 2014, Knox *et al.* 2011, Wishart *et al.* 2008, Wishart *et al.* 2006).

- Nicotine (Heit *et al.* 2013).
- Ketone bodies (Sutti *et al.* 2014).
- Fasting (Abdelmegeed *et al.* 2017).
- Omega 3 fatty acids (Maksymchuk *et al.* 2015).

Practical advice

- Check intake of acrylamides, cigarettes and coffee and advise on removing.
- Check medications and refer to GP for medication review if indicated.
- Check nutritional intake (ketone bodies and fasting) and address with patient.
- Advise re foods to enhance or reduce enzyme activity as appropriate.

Cytochrome P450 3A4: CYP3A4

CYP3A4 is highly expressed in the liver and small intestinal enterocytes and is tasked with metabolizing 45–60% of medications (Kandel & Lampe 2014). It is involved in the biotransformation of bile acids (Chen *et al.* 2014) with a therapeutic implication towards cholestasis. Regulation of this gene is complicated and highly variable (Martínez-Jiménez *et al.* 2007). The rsid 35539367 allele is down-regulated (Wang & Sadee 2016) and found in 4–8% of the population (Werk & Cascorbi 2014). Those taking simvastatin, for example, are said to need a 40% lower dose as a result (Kitzmiller *et al.* 2014).

Up-regulation of CYP3A4 has been associated heavily with a tenfold incidence of aggressive prostate cancer in African American males (Keshava *et al.* 2004) as this gene instructs the enzyme to oxidize oestrogen, testosterone, xenobiotics, aflotoxins and food mutagens. When CYP3A4 is expressing, this may lead to a reduced potential for oxidizing testosterone. Ultimately, this may leave more bioavailable testosterone for intracellular conversion to biologically active dihydroestosterone, the principal androgenic hormone regulating prostate growth (Basheer &

Kerem 2015). CYP3A4 can become down-regulated in the presence of the inflammatory signalling molecule interleukin 6 (Jover *et al.* 2002).

If CYP3A4 is over-expressed, it can be a huge factor in the pathophysiology of oestrogen-related cancers (Bai *et al.* 2017), as it plays a role in the 4 and 16α hydroxylation of oestrone in menopausal women. CYP1A2 may also play a role, as this enzyme catalyzes the formation of 2-hydroxyestrone, thereby negatively balancing the ratio of 2-hydroxyestrone: 16α-hydroxyestrone, associated with breast carcinogenesis (Basheer & Kerem 2015; Keshava *et al.* 2004). In fact, numerous studies have concluded expression of CYP3A4 in inflammatory and infectious diseases and liver cancer, leading to failure of treatment or harmful drug reactions (Taneja *et al.* 2019).

CYP3A4 is also noted for its ability to adapt structurally to many inhibitors and substrates that can precipitate many food/drug interactions. Perhaps one of the best-known interactions is that of grapefruit with over 85 prescription medications, including cyclosporine and felodipine (Basheer & Kerem 2015). However this mechanism can be inhibited by quercetin (Basheer & Kerem 2015) and thymoquinone from black seed oil (Elbarbry *et al.* 2018).

CYP3A4 expression due to caffeine ingestion appears controversial with more emphasis being placed on CYP1A2. Although Bailey *et al.* (2017) and others may have found notably elevated felodipine levels in subjects following two servings of coffee, Dresser *et al.* (2017) found no such correlation. Nor did they find a grapefruit-like effect of inhibition. However, all of these studies were really only pilot study size, so it would not be possible to infer a correlation.

**Possible interventions and considerations
based on CYP3A4 gene expression**
Nutrient cofactors that support CYP3A4 enzyme activity
Haem (Pai *et al.* 2007).

Inducers (activates CYP3A4 gene expression) and
substrates (substances on which the CYP3A4 enzyme
acts) that increase activity of the enzyme
Macrolide antibiotics (clarithromycin, erythromycin), antiarrhythmics, benzodiazepines, immune modulators (cyclosporine, tacrolimus,

sirolimus), HIV antivirals, prokinetics, antihistamines, calcium channel blockers, HMG-CoA reductase inhibitors, PDE-5 inhibitors, paracetamol, carbamazepine, garlic, glucocorticoids, phenytoin, St John's Wort.

- Vitamin D and ultraviolet exposure (Wang *et al.* 2013).
- Fatty acids (Hu *et al.* 2014).
- Being female (Zanger & Schwab 2013).

Unhelpful inhibitors that reduce CYP3A4 enzyme activity

- Polyphenols (black cohosh, ginger, ginseng), flavones (grapefruit), flavonols (quercetin), isoflavones, flavonoids (milk thistle), anthocyanin, stilbenoids (resveratrol), tannins (Basheer & Kerem 2015).
- H2 receptor antagonist cimetidine (Busty 2015).
- Antibiotics (clarithromycin, metronidazole), immunosuppressants (cyclosporine), corticosteroids (prednisone), lignans, SSRIs (sertraline).

Drug data accessed from www.drugbank.ca (Wishart *et al.* 2017, Law *et al.* 2014, Knox *et al.* 2011, Wishart *et al.* 2008, Wishart *et al.* 2006).

- Aloe vera juice (Djuv & Nilsen 2012).
- Mixed vegetable juice (Tsujimoto *et al.* 2016).
- Kale (Yamasaki *et al.* 2012).
- Garden cress (Al-Jenoobi *et al.* 2014).
- Fennel (Langhammer & Nilsen 2014).
- Green tea polyphenols (Basheer & Kerem 2015).

Practical advice

- Check mode of regulation with rsid and supportive evidence so you can advise effective management.
- Check medications and refer to GP for medication review if indicated.
- Advise patient on nutritional approach suitable for rsid identified.
- Support gastrointestinal health.

Cytochrome P450 3A5: CYP3A5

This is very similar to CYP3A4 except many people vary considerably with the expression of this one. It can be up- or down-regulated and many individuals don't have a functioning CYP3A5 enzyme (Diczfalusy *et al.* 2011). This gene (rs28365083, rs776746) is expressed in the liver and prostate predominantly, with lesser amounts in the epithelium of the small and large intestines. Small amounts are also evident in the bile duct, nasal mucosa, adrenal cortex, kidneys, gallbladder, pancreatic ducts and the parathyroid and ovaries. CYP3A5 also has a role in the oxidization of steroid hormones, fatty acids and xenobiotics in the NADPH-dependent electron transport chain. It also metabolizes medications such as cyclosporine, olanzapine, nifedipine, tacrolimus, testosterone, progesterone and androstenedione. Low levels of CYP3A5 have been associated with liver cancer and with reoccurrence after treatment (Jiang *et al.* 2015). There are two non-functional variants of CYP3A5: rs776746 occurs in 14% of Saharan Africans and over 95% of Europeans, while rs10264272 is frequent in Africans and rare or absent in Europeans (Suarez-Kurtz *et al.* 2014).

Tacrolimus is an interesting medication used to prevent organ rejection. Nephrotoxicity is a known side effect, with a large number of patients being affected by adverse effects. In vitro to in vivo scaling studies demonstrated a higher metabolic clearance of tacrolimus in those with the CYP3A5 –/– or wild-type allele (Dai *et al.* 2006). Those who have expressing mutations will require 1.5 to 2 times the regular tacrolimus dosage to reach therapeutic levels (Chen & Prasad 2018). There is evidence to suggest CYP3A enzymes may be responsible for interracial variations in the metabolism of many medications (Umamaheswaran *et al.* 2014). These medications include antipsychotics, antioestrogen, anticancer, antimalarial, immunomodulators, antihistamines, antiplatelets, antihypertensives, antivirals, HMG-CoA reductase inhibitors and steroids.

There is no definitive list of inhibitors and inducers for CYP3A5; they are assumed at this point to be the same as those for CYP3A4. Practitioners should consult the CYP3A4 section for recommendations until further evidence emerges.

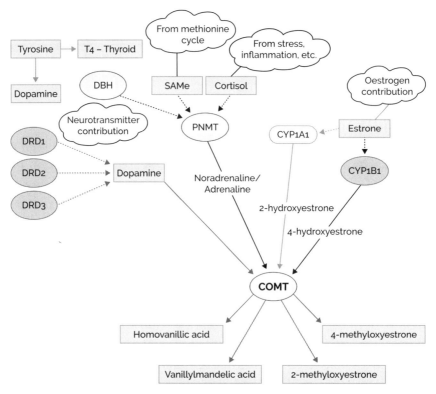

Figure 4.3: Ella's hormone/neurotransmitter SNPs
CYP1A2 +/+, CYP1B1 +/+, CYP2B6 +/−, CYP2C9
+/−, CYP2D6 +/+, and CYP3A4 +/+.
Key: CYP1B1 – up-regulated; DBH, PNMT, COMT all
down-regulated; DRD 1, 2 & 3 down-regulated.

As can be seen from Figure 4.3, Ella had a number of polymorphisms
corresponding with potential oestrogen dysregulation when expressing.
Also pyroluria is a haem-processing disorder, so CYP enzymes would all
likely express in her case. Although there were no laboratory results for
hormone testing, Ella's early history indicates earlier possible up-regulation of phase 1, creating fast oestrogen metabolism at CYP1B1 and in
phase 2 she has a down-regulated slow COMT in the form of irregular
menses with dysmenorrhoea and menorrhagia. Later, following years
of contraceptive use, she was also diagnosed with severe fibrocystic
breast disease. Thankfully for Ella, she was able to support much of this
herself by discontinuing oral contraceptive use at the time (Brkić *et al.*

2018), removing all dairy products from her nutritional intake (McCann *et al.* 2017), removing caffeine and supplementing with evening primrose oil (Jahdi *et al.* 2019; Murshid 2011) and supplementing B vitamins (Jahdi *et al.* 2019; Shobeiri *et al.* 2015) at fairly high dosages at the time of diagnosis. Ella also had low levels of homovanillic acid and vanillylmandelic acid on her urine organic acid test, indicating possible low levels of dopamine. This will be discussed in more detail in the section on neurotransmitters.

Polymorphisms associated with bile flow

As we are discussing detoxification, the gallbladder is a very important organ. It would therefore be remiss not to include polymorphisms associated with gallbladder and biliary function. These polymorphisms include BHMT, PEMT, MAT1, SULT2A1, PPARG and NRF2. With the exception of NRF2, these polymorphisms are all discussed within the methylation cycles.

Nuclear factor (erythroid-derived 2)-like 2: NFE2L2 (NRF2)

NRF2 is a key transcription factor in detoxification and antioxidant defence, regulating gene expression of many cytoprotective and detoxifying enzymes (Sova & Saso 2018). It governs many pathways such as glutathione synthesis, reactive oxygen species scavenging, drug excretion and detoxification, and NADP synthesis (Cai *et al.* 2019). NRF2 rs6726395 has being identified as a possible prognostic marker of cholangiocarcinoma (CCA) (Khunluck *et al.* 2014), offering a longer survival period in those affected by CCA (Prawan *et al.* 2014). CCA is a malignancy of the biliary tree with very poor prognosis, with liver fluke infection being identified as the most likely underlying aetiology (Prueksapanich *et al.* 2018).

Due to the NRF2 pathway being identified as the master regulator of antioxidant, detoxification and cell defence gene expression, it has been studied extensively. A number of brain-degenerating disorders have been linked to a down-regulation of the NRF2 pathway. Autism, Parkinson's disease, Alzheimer's disease and multiple sclerosis are some of the most common conditions studied, and in fact some studies have shown significant improvement in symptoms of autistic children with the addition of sulphoraphane, an extract of broccoli and a potent NRF2 pathway activator (Lynch *et al.* 2017).

NRF2 activation has also been widely accepted as useful for chemoprevention, thereby slowing the development of cancers. However, once neoplastic growth is established, it may be detrimental (Kensler & Wakabayashi 2010). NRF2 activation has been thought to interfere with chemotherapy and radiotherapy, thereby offering additional growth and survival opportunities for pre-established cancers (Gao, Doan & Hybertson 2014). Down-regulation of NRF2 conversely has indicated positive responses in cases of CCA (Sompakdee *et al.* 2018).

Possible interventions based on NRF2 genetic expression
Nutrient cofactors to support NRF2 enzyme activity

- Sulphoraphane such as diindolylmethane, broccoli seed extract (Kensler *et al.* 2013).
- Exercise (Pall & Levine 2015).
- Vitamin D (Jiménez-Osorio *et al.* 2015).
- Butyrate (Yaku *et al.* 2012).
- Garlic (Pall & Levine 2015).
- Curcumin (Macciò & Madeddu 2012).
- Luteolin (Zhang *et al.* 2013). Luteolin is a really good choice as it also inhibits NRF2 in many cancer cells (Chian *et al.* 2014).

Unhelpful inhibitors that reduce NRF2 enzyme activity

- Retinoic acid, 6-hydroxy-1-methylindole-3-acetonitrile (6-HMA), bleomycin (a type of antibiotic that binds to the DNA of cancer cells inhibiting cell division and growth), brusatol (quassinoid herbal product for amoebiasis treatment) (Gao, Doan & Hybertson 2014).

- N-acetylcysteine (Li *et al.* 2004); however, NAC is a strong antioxidant so do consider within the context of the case.

Drug data accessed from www.drugbank.ca (Wishart *et al.* 2017, Law *et al.* 2014, Knox *et al.* 2011, Wishart *et al.* 2008, Wishart *et al.* 2006).

ELLA'S BILE FLOW GENE PATTERN

Ella's genes included BHMT, PEMT, MAT1, PPARG and NRF2, which are all discussed in depth in their respective chapters. They are all relevant to Ella as they have a negative impact on bile flow when expressing. Ultrasound investigation and serum levels of alkaline phosphatase, bilirubin and liver enzymes showed a sluggish flow without stones. Ella's plan was already supporting bile flow so this was continued as in phase 1.

Foods to include encouraging bile flow

- Beetroot (Spiridonov 2012).
- Linseed tea (Goyal *et al.* 2014).
- High-fibre foods such as pulses caused bloating, so kitchari remained a good alternative (Naumann *et al.* 2019).
- Healthy fats – omega 3 (Jun *et al.* 2016).
- Tulsi ginger tea and broccoli (cruciferous vegetables with caution) – to support CYP1B1.

Supplements

- Beetroot complex and taurine (Ash 2008).
- Beetroot complex and ox bile when steatorrhoea was present (Ash 2008).
- Ensuring betaine levels were adequate to encourage CCK feedback loop triggering and also to gain haem from proteins to support CYP 450 enzymes.
- PC liquid (Wan *et al.* 2019).

- Zinc to support BHMT enzyme (Evans *et al.* 2002) and HCL production.

Lifestyle interventions

- Epsom salts baths (magnesium sulphate) for sulphation and for MAT1 and COMT.
- Stress-relieving techniques and tools (see Appendix).

Other polymorphisms associated with phase 1 detoxification

Human haemochromatosis protein: HFE

This gene encodes a membrane protein that is responsible for the regulation and storage of iron. Defects in this gene can result in the autosomal recessive or single-gene disorder known as hereditary haemochromatosis. This is an iron storage condition where excess iron cannot be effectively removed from the blood. Males are more affected due to the female menstruation cycle, and regular blood donors are unlikely to be affected. In serious cases, the excess iron can lead to iron overload that, if untreated, can cause heart disease, cardiogenic shock (Hughes *et al.* 2009), fatigue, depression, diabetes, hyperpigmentation of the skin and liver cirrhosis. Those with homozygous presentation of alleles are likely to have some difficulties processing iron, but unless blood levels exceed certain parameters (NICE 2010), they are unlikely to reach a formal diagnosis. Alcohol consumption, nutritional supplementation and dietary intervention can all affect blood iron levels. Roughly 1 in 200 with the homozygous mutation C282Y who are northern Europeans are at risk of haemochromatosis with two copies of this gene variant. Roughly 1 in 700 have the disease without any HFE gene. Having one C287Y and one H63D abnormal gene (compound heterozygous) usually leads to a milder form of haemochromatosis. A heterozygous presentation of either C287Y or H63D would render a person more likely a carrier of the disease (Haemochromatosis Australia 2021).

PRACTITIONER NOTES

Tests to consider if iron overload is suspected include:

- serum ferretin
- serum iron
- total iron-binding capacity
- serum transferrin saturation.

It is crucial to refer a patient with this presentation to an experi-enced medically qualified professional as iron mismanagement resulting in overload can accelerate neurodegenerative diseases such as Alzheimer's, Parkinson's, epilepsy and multiple sclerosis. Other combinations of SNPs to consider with HFE include SOD2 A16V. SOD2 is also iron binding and therefore could exacerbate the risk of heart disease tenfold if iron overload led to reduced function (Fargion *et al.* 2010; Valenti *et al.* 2004).

Other polymorphisms to consider in light of phase 1 detoxifica-tion include PON1 and SOD3 (discussed in the section on methyla-tion in Chapter 5).

Recap of phase 1 detoxification and biotransformation

In this chapter, phase 1 included CYP450 enzymes and their individual responsibilities within the terrain of metabolic toxin regulation. Recall that most CYP enzymes become up-regulated or work faster in the presence of certain endogenous or exogenous toxins, generally termed substrates. When the enzymes in phase 2 pathways are down-regulated or running slowly, the often toxic intermediary metabolites increase. This can result in higher levels of reactive oxygen species, resulting in cell danger response. Recall the example of oestrogen dysregulation in Ella resulting from this scenario. This will be reviewed again in the sec-tion on neurotransmitters in Chapter 5, with regard to dopamine and serotonin. Ella's case demonstrated one way to help detoxify the body in order to reduce the toxic load on the liver.

References

Abass K, Turpeinen M, Pelkonen O (2009) An evaluation of the cytochrome P450 inhibition potential of selected pesticides in human hepatic microsomes. *Journal of Environmental Science and Health B 44*, 6, 553–563. doi:10.1080/03601230902997766

Abass K, Lämsä V, Reponen P *et al.* (2012) Characterization of human cytochrome P450 induction by pesticides. *Toxicology 294*, 17–26.

Abdelmegeed MA, Ha SK, Choi Y *et al.* (2017) Role of CYP2E1 in mitochondrial dysfunction and hepatic injury by alcohol and non-alcoholic substances. *Current Molecular Pharmacology 10*, 3, 207–225. doi: 10.2174/1874467208666150817111114

Aitbali Y, Ba-M'hamed S, Elhidar N *et al.* (2018) Glyphosate based- herbicide exposure affects gut microbiota, anxiety and depression-like behaviors in mice. *Neurotoxicology and Teratology 67*, 44–49. doi:10.1016/j. ntt.2018.04.002

Akasaka T, Hokimoto S, Sueta D *et al.* (2016) Sex differences in the impact of CYP2C19 polymorphisms and low-grade inflammation on coronary microvascular disorder. *American Journal of Physiology – Heart and Circulatory Physiology 310*, 11, H1494–H1500. doi:10.1152/ajpheart.00911.2015

Al-Jenoobi FI, Al-Thukair AA, Alam MA *et al.* (2015) Effect of *Curcuma longa* on CYP2D6- and CYP3A4-mediated metabolism of dextromethorphan in human liver microsomes and healthy human subjects. *European Journal of Drug Metabolism and Pharmacokineti*cs 40, 1, 61–66. http:// dx.doi.org/10.1007/s13318-014-0180-2

Al-Jenoobi FI, Al-Thukair AA, Alam MA *et al.* (2014) Modulation of CYP2D6 and CYP3A4 metabolic activities by Ferula asafetida resin. *Saudi Pharmaceutical Journal 22*, 6, 564–569. doi:10.1016/j.jsps.2014.03.004

Amadasi A, Mozzarelli A, Meda C *et al.* (2009) Identification of xenoestrogens in food additives by an integrated in silico and in vitro approach. *Chemical Research in Toxicology 22*, 1, 52–63. doi:10.1021/ tx800048m

Amunugama HT, Zhang H, Hollenberg PF (2012) Mechanism-based inactivation of cytochrome P450 2B6 by methadone through destruction of prosthetic heme. *Drug Metabolism and Disposition 40*, 9, 1765–1770. doi:10.1124/dmd.112.045971

Androutsopoulos VP, Tsatsakis AM, Spandidos DA (2009) Cytochrome P450 CYP1A1: Wider roles in cancer progression and prevention. *BMC Cancer 9*, 187. doi:10.1186/1471-2407-9-187

Arellano AL, Martin-Subero M, Monerris M *et al.* (2017) Multiple adverse drug reactions and genetic polymorphism testing. *Medicine 96*, 45, e8505. doi:10.1097/ MD.0000000000008505

Arici M, Özhan G (2017) CYP2C9, CYPC19 and CYP2D6 gene profiles and gene susceptibility to drug response and toxicity in Turkish population. *Saudi Pharmaceutical Journal 25*, 3, 376–380. doi:10.1016/j. jsps.2016.09.003

Ash M (2008) Bile acids make you live longer: A new understanding. White Paper. https:// www.clinicaleducation.org/wp-content/ uploads/BileAcidsMakeYouLiveLonger.pdf

Bai X, Xie J, Sun S *et al.* D. (2017) The associations of genetic polymorphisms in CYP1A2 and CYP3A4 with clinical outcomes of breast cancer patients in northern China. *Oncotarget 8*, 24, 38367–38377.

Bailey DG, Dresser GK, Urquhart BL *et al.* (2016) Coffee-antihypertensive drug interaction: A hemodynamic and pharmacokinetic study with felodipine. *Am. J. Hypertens 29*, 1386–1393.

Basheer L, Kerem Z (2015) Interactions between CYP3A4 and dietary polyphenols, *Oxidative Medicine and Cellular Longevity 2015*, 854015. doi:10.1155/2015/854015

Bedada SK, Neerati P (2016) Resveratrol pretreatment affects CYP2E1 activity of chlorzoxazone in healthy human volunteers. *Phytotherapy Research 30*, 3, 463–468. doi:10.1002/ptr.5549

Bedada SK, Boga PK (2017) Effect of piperine on CYP2E1 enzyme activity of chlorzoxazone in healthy volunteers. *Xenobiotica 47*, 12, 1035–1041. doi:10.1080/00498254.2016.1241450

Bertilsson L, Dahl ML, Dalén P et al. (2002) Molecular genetics of CYP2D6: Clinical relevance with focus on psychotropic drugs. *British Journal of Clinical Pharmacology 53*, 2, 111–122.

Brkić M, Vujović S, Ivović M et al. (2018) The role of E2/P ratio in the etiology of fibrocystic breast disease, mastalgia and mastodynia. *Acta Clinica Croatica 57*, 4, 756–761. doi:10.20471/acc.2018.57.04.18

Busty AJ (2015) Are there any known drug interactions between histamine-2 receptor antagonists (H2RA) and clopidogrel (Plavix) that could compromise the efficacy on platelet inhibition? *Evidence Based Medical Consult.* www.ebmconsult.com/articles/histamine-receptor-antagonists-h2ra-plavix-clopidogrel-interaction-platelet

Cai SJ, Liu Y, Han S et al. (2019) Brusatol, an NRF2 inhibitor for future cancer therapeutic. *Cell and Bioscience 9*, 45. doi:10.1186/s13578-019-0309-8

Cederbaum AI (2003) Iron and CYP2E1-dependent oxidative stress and toxicity. *Alcohol 30*, 2, 115–120. doi:10.1016/S0741-8329(03)00104-6

Cederbaum AI (2010) Role of CYP2E1 in ethanol-induced oxidant stress, fatty liver and hepatotoxicity. *Digestive Diseases 28*, 6, 802–811. http://doi.org/10.1159/000324289

Cederbaum AI (2014) Methodology to assay CYP2E1 mixed function oxidase catalytic activity and its induction. *Redox Biology 2*, 1048–1054. doi:10.1016/j.redox.2014.09.007

Cerliani MB, Pavicic W, Gili JA et al. (2016) Cigarette smoking, dietary habits and genetic polymorphisms in *GSTT1*, *GSTM1* and *CYP1A1* metabolic genes: A case-control study in oncohematological diseases. *World Journal of Clinical Oncology 7*, 5, 395–405. doi:10.5306/wjco.v7.i5.395

Chen HW, Tsai CW, Yang JJ et al. (2003) The combined effects of garlic oil and fish oil on the hepatic antioxidant and drug-metabolizing enzymes of rats. *British Journal of Nutrition 89*, 2, 189–200. doi:10.1079/BJN2002766

Chen J, Zhao KN, Chen C (2014) The role of CYP3A4 in the biotransformation of bile acids and therapeutic implication for cholestasis. *Annals of Translational Medicine 2*, 1, 7. doi:10.3978/j.issn.2305-5839.2013.03.02

Chen L, Prasad G (2018) CYP3A5 polymorphisms in renal transplant recipients: Influence on tacrolimus treatment. *Pharmacogenomics and Personalized Medicine 11*, 23–33. doi:10.3978/j.issn.2305-5839.2013.03.02

Cheng J, Zhen Y, Miksys S et al. (2013) Potential role of CYP2D6 in the central nervous system. *Xenobiotica 43*, 11, 973–984. doi:10.3109/00498254.2013.791410

Chenoweth MJ, Sylvestre MP, Contreras G et al. (2016) Variation in CYP2A6 and tobacco dependence throughout adolescence and in young adult smokers. *Drug and Alcohol Dependence 158*, 139–146. doi:10.1016/j.drugalcdep.2015.11.017

Chian S, Thapa R, Chi Z et al. (2014) Luteolin inhibits the Nrf2 signalling pathway and tumor growth in vivo. *Biochemical and Biophysical Research Communications 447*, 4, 602–608. doi:10.1016/j.bbrc.2014.04.039

Choi EJ, Kim T, Kim GH (2012) Quercetin acts as an antioxidant and downregulates CYP1A1 and CYP1B1 against DMBA-induced oxidative stress in mice. *Oncology Reports 28*, 1, 291–296. doi:10.3892/or.2012.1753

Cohen S (2015) Medication-induced SNPs. Available from https://shop.suzycohen.com/products/medication-induced-snps-video

Dai Y, Hebert MF, Isoherranen N et al. (2006) Effect of CYP3A5 polymorphism on tacrolimus metabolic clearance in vitro. *Drug Metabolism and Disposition 34*, 5, 836–847. doi:10.1124/dmd.105.008680

Daly AK, Rettie AE, Fowler DM et al. (2017) Pharmacogenomics of CYP2C9: Functional and clinical considerations. *Journal of Personalized Medicine 8*, 1, 1. doi:10.3390/jpm8010001

Diczfalusy U, Nylén H, Elander P *et al.*
(2011) 4β-Hydroxycholesterol, an
endogenous marker of CYP3A4/5
activity in humans. *British Journal of
Clinical Pharmacology 71*, 2, 183–189.
doi:10.1111/j.1365-2125.2010.03773.x

Djuv A, Nilsen OG (2012) Aloe vera juice: IC$_{50}$
and dual mechanistic inhibition of CYP3A4
and CYP2D6. *Phytotherapy Research 26*, 3,
445–451. doi:10.1002/ptr.3564

Dresser GK, Urquhart BL, Proniuk J *et al.* (2017)
Coffee inhibition of CYP3A4 in vitro
was not translated to a grapefruit-like
pharmacokinetic interaction clinically.
Pharmacology Research and Perspectives 5, 5,
e00346. doi:10.1002/prp2.346

Ehrlich M (2019) DNA hypermethylation in
disease: Mechanisms and clinical relevance.
Epigenetics 14, 12, 1141–1163. doi:10.1080/15
592294.2019.1638701

Elbarbry F, Ung A, Abdelkawy K (2018) Studying
the inhibitory effect of quercetin and
thymoquinone on human cytochrome
P450 enzyme activities. *Pharmacognosy
Magazine 13*, Suppl 4, S895–S899.
doi:10.4103/0973-1296.224342

Evans JC, Huddler DP, Jiracek J *et al.* (2002)
Betaine-homocysteine methyltransferase: Zinc in a distorted barrel.
Structure 10, 9, 1159–1171. doi:10.1016/
s0969-2126(02)00796-7

Fargion S, Valenti L, Fracanzani AL (2010)
Hemochromatosis gene (HFE) mutations
and cancer risk: Expanding the clinical
manifestations of hereditary iron overload.
Hepatology 51, 4, 1119–1121. doi:10.1002/
hep.23541

Figueiras A, Estany-Gestal A, Aguirre C *et al.*
(2016) CYP2C9 variants as a risk modifier
of NSAID-related gastrointestinal bleeding:
A case-control study. *Pharmacogenetics
and Genomics 26, 2, 66–73.* doi:10.1097/
FPC.0000000000000186

Forsyth CB, Voigt RM, Keshavarzian A (2014)
Intestinal CYP2E1: A mediator of alcohol-induced gut leakiness. *Redox Biology 3*,
40–46. doi:10.1016/j.redox.2014.10.002

García-Suástegui WA, Ramos-Chávez LA,
Rubio-Osornio M *et al.* (2017) The role
of CYP2E1 in the drug metabolism or
bioactivation in the brain. *Oxidative Medicine and Cellular Longevity 2017* 4680732.
doi:10.1155/2017/4680732

Gao B, Doan A, Hybertson BM (2014) The
clinical potential of influencing Nrf2 signaling in degenerative and immunological
disorders. *Clinical Pharmacology: Advances
and Applications 6*, 19–34. doi:10.2147/
CPAA.S35078

Goh LL, Lim CW, Sim WC *et al.* (2017) Analysis
of genetic variation in CYP450 genes
for clinical implementation. *PLOS ONE
12*, 1, e0169233. doi:10.1371/journal.
pone.0169233

Goyal A, Sharma V, Upadhyay N *et al.*
(2014) Flax and flaxseed oil: An ancient
medicine and modern functional food.
Journal of Food Science and Technology 51, 9,
1633–1653. doi:10.1007/s13197-013-1247-9

Guengerich FP (2021) A history of the roles of
cytochrome P450 enzymes in the toxicity
of drugs. *Toxicological Research 37*, 1, 1–23.
doi:10.1007/s43188-020-00056-z

Haemochromatosis Australia (2021) Genetics of
haemochromatosis. https://haemochroma-
tosis.org.au/genetics

Han F, Tan Y, Cui W *et al.* (2013) Novel insights
into etiologies of leukemia: A HuGE review
and meta-analysis of CYP1A1 polymorphisms and leukemia risk. *American
Journal of Epidemiology 178*, 4, 493–507.
doi:10.1093/aje/kwt016

He XF, Wei W, Liu ZZ *et al.* (2014) Association
between the CYP1A1 T3801C polymor-
phism and risk of cancer: Evidence from
268 case-control studies. *Gene 534*, 2,
324–344.

He W, Wu JJ, Ning J *et al.* (2015) Inhibition
of human cytochrome P450 enzymes by
licochalcone A, a naturally occurring constituent of licorice. *Toxicology in Vitro 29*,
7, 1569–1576. http://dx.doi.org/10.1016/j.
tiv.2015.06.014

Heit C, Dong H, Chen Y *et al.* (2013) The role
of CYP2E1 in alcohol metabolism and
sensitivity in the central nervous system.
Subcellular Biochemistry 67, 235–247. doi:10.
1007%2F978-94-007-5881-0_8

Hicks JK, Swen JJ, Thorn CF *et al.* (2013) Clinical Pharmacogenetics Implementation Consortium guideline for CYP2D6 and CYP2C19 genotypes and dosing of tricyclic antidepressants. *Clinical Pharmacology and Therapeutics 93*, 5, 402–408. doi:10.1038/clpt.2013.2

Hodges RE, Minich DM (2015) Modulation of metabolic detoxification pathways using foods and food-derived components: A scientific review with clinical application. *Journal of Nutrition and Metabolism 2015*, 760689. doi:10.1155/2015/760689

Hu N, Hu M, Duan R *et al.* (2014) Increased levels of fatty acids contributed to induction of hepatic CYP3A4 activity induced by diabetes – in vitro evidence from HepG2 cell and Fa2N-4 cell lines. *Journal of Pharmacological Sciences 124*, 4, 433–444. doi:10.1254/jphs.13212FP

Hughes CG, Waldman JM, Barrios J *et al.* (2009) Postshunt hemochromatosis leading to cardiogenic shock in a patient presenting for orthotopic liver transplant: A case report. *Transplantation Proceedings 41*, 5, 2000–2002. http://dx.doi.org/10.1016/j.transproceed.2009.02.082

Hwang PH, Lian L, Zavras AI (2012) Alcohol intake and folate antagonism via CYP2E1 and ALDH1: Effects on oral carcinogenesis. *Medical Hypotheses 78*, 2, 197–202. doi:10.1016/j.mehy.2011.10.023

Ichikawa H, Sugimoto M, Sugimoto K *et al.* (2016) Rapid metabolizer genotype of CYP2C19 is a risk factor of being refractory to proton pump inhibitor therapy for reflux esophagitis. *Journal of Gastroenterology and Hepatology 31*, 4, 716–726. doi:10.1111/jgh.13233

Indiana University School of Medicine (2018) Drug Interactions Flockhart Table™. https://drug-interactions.medicine.iu.edu/MainTable.aspx

Iwuoha E, Ngece R, Klink M, Baker P (2007) Amperometric responses of CYP2D6 drug metabolism nanobiosensor for sertraline: A selective serotonin reuptake inhibitor. *IET Nanobiotechnology 1*, 4, 62–67. doi:10.1049/iet-nbt:20070005

Jahdi F, Tolouei R, Samani LN *et al.* (2019) Effect of evening primrose oil and vitamin B6 on pain control of cyclic mastalgia associated with fibrocystic breast changes: A triple-blind randomized controlled trial. *Shiraz E-Medical Journal 20*, 5, e81243. doi:10.5812/semj.81243

Jacob A, Hartz AM, Potin S *et al.* (2011) Aryl hydrocarbon receptor-dependent upregulation of Cyp1b1 by TCDD and diesel exhaust particles in rat brain microvessels. *Fluids and Barriers of the CNS 8*, 23. doi:10.1186/2045-8118-8-23

Jiang F, Chen L, Yang YC *et al.* (2015) CYP3A5 functions as a tumor suppressor in hepatocellular carcinoma by regulating mTORC2/Akt signaling. *Cancer Research 75*, 7, 1470–1481. doi:10.1158/0008-5472.CAN-14-1589

Jiménez-Osorio AS, González-Reyes S, Pedraza-Chaverri J (2015) Natural Nrf2 activators in diabetes. *Clinica Chimica Acta 448*, 182–192. doi:10.1016/j.cca.2015.07.009

Jin YY, Singh P, Chung HJ *et al.* (2018) Blood ammonia as a possible etiological agent for Alzheimer's disease. *Nutrients 10*, 5, 564. doi:10.3390/nu10050564

Jover R, Bort R, Gómez-Lechón M *et al.* (2002) Down-regulation of human CYP3A4 by the inflammatory signal interleukin 6: Molecular mechanism and transcription factors involved. *FASEB Journal 16*, 1799–1801. doi:10.1096/fj.02-0195fje

Jun WY, Cho MJ, Han HS *et al.* (2016) Use of omega-3 polyunsaturated fatty acids to treat inspissated bile syndrome: A case report. *Pediatric Gastroenterology, Hepatology and Nutrition 19*, 4, 286–290. doi:10.5223/pghn.2016.19.4.286

Kandel SE, Lampe JN (2014) Role of protein–protein interactions in cytochrome P450-mediated drug metabolism and toxicity. *Chemical Research in Toxicology 27*, 9, 1474–1486. doi:10.1021/tx500203s

Kane E (2017) Life on a membrane. Paper presented during the Membrane Medicine Seminar on 18 November.

Kensler TW, Wakabayashi N (2010) Nrf2: friend or foe for chemoprevention? *Carcinogenesis 31*, 1, 90–99.

Kensler TW, Egner PA, Agyeman AS *et al.* (2013) Keap1-nrf2 signaling: A target for cancer prevention by sulforaphane. *Topics in Current Chemistry* 329, 163–177. doi:10.1007/128_2012_339

Keshava C, McCanlies EC, Weston A (2004) CYP3A4 polymorphisms – Potential risk factors for breast and prostate cancer: A HuGE review. *American Journal of Epidemiology* 160, 9, 825–841.

Kharasch ED (2017) Current concepts in methadone metabolism and transport. *Clinical Pharmacology in Drug Development* 6, 2, 125–134. doi:10.1002/cpdd.326

Khunluck T, Kukongviriyapan V, Puapairoj A *et al.* (2014) Association of NRF2 polymorphism with cholangiocarcinoma prognosis in Thai patients. *Asian Pacific Journal of Cancer Prevention* 15, 1, 299–304. doi:10.7314/apjcp.2014.15.1.299

Kim HG, Lee HS, Jeon JS *et al.* (2020) Quasi-irreversible inhibition of CYP2D6 by berberine. *Pharmaceutics* 12, 10, 916. doi:10.3390/pharmaceutics12100916

Kitzmiller JP, Luzum JA, Baldassarre D *et al.* (2014) CYP3A4*22 and CYP3A5*3 are associated with increased levels of plasma simvastatin concentrations in the cholesterol and pharmacogenetics study cohort. *Pharmacogenetics and Genomics* 24, 10, 486–491. doi:10.1097/FPC.0000000000000079

Klein MD, Lee CR, Stouffer GA (2018) Clinical outcomes of CYP2C19 genotype-guided antiplatelet therapy: Existing evidence and future directions. *Pharmacogenomics* 19, 13, 1039–1046. doi:10.2217/pgs-2018-0072

Knox C, Law V, Jewison T *et al.* (2011) DrugBank 3.0: A comprehensive resource for 'omics' research on drugs. *Nucleic Acids Research* 39, D1035–1041. doi:10.1093/nar/gkq1126

Langhammer AJ, Nilsen OG (2014) In vitro inhibition of human CYP1A2, CYP2D6, and CYP3A4 by six herbs commonly used in pregnancy. *Phytotherapy Research* 28, 4, 603–610. doi:10.1002/ptr.5037

Law V, Knox C, Djoumbou Y *et al.* (2014) DrugBank 4.0: Shedding new light on drug metabolism. *Nucleic Acids Research* 42, 1, D1091–1097. doi:10.1093%2Fnar%2Fgkt1068

Lee HI, McGregor RA, Choi MS *et al.* (2013) Low doses of curcumin protect alcohol-induced liver damage by modulation of the alcohol metabolic pathway, CYP2E1 and AMPK. *Life Sciences* 93, 18–19, 693–699. doi:10.1016/j.lfs.2013.09.014

Lilja JJ, Kivistö KT, Neuvonen PJ (2000) Duration of effect of grapefruit juice on the pharmacokinetics of the CYP3A4 substrate simvastatin. *Clinical Pharmacology and Therapeutics* 68, 4, 384–390. doi:10.1067/mcp.2000.110216

Li R, Shugart YY, Zhou W *et al.* (2009) Common genetic variations of the cytochrome P450 1A1 gene and risk of hepatocellular carcinoma in a Chinese population. *European Journal of Cancer* 45, 7, 1239–1247. doi:10.1016/j.ejca.2008.11.007

Li N, Alam J, Venkatesan MI *et al.* (2004) Nrf2 is a key transcription factor that regulates antioxidant defense in macrophages and epithelial cells: Protecting against the proinflammatory and oxidizing effects of diesel exhaust chemicals. *Journal of Immunology* 173, 5, 3467–3481. doi:10.4049/jimmunol.173.5.3467

Lim YP, Cheng CH, Chen WC *et al.* (2015) Allyl isothiocyanate (AITC) inhibits pregnane X receptor (PXR) and constitutive androstane receptor (CAR) activation and protects against acetaminophen- and amiodarone-induced cytotoxicity. *Archives of Toxicology* 89, 1, 57–72. doi:10.1007/s00204-014-1230-x

Livezey M, Nagy LD, Diffenderfer LE *et al.* (2012) Molecular analysis and modeling of inactivation of human CYP2D6 by four mechanism based inactivators. *Drug Metabolism Letters* 6, 1, 7–14. doi:10.2174/187231212800229318

Liu HX, Li J, Ye BG (2016) Correlation between gene polymorphisms of CYP1A1, GSTP1, ERCC2, XRCC1, and XRCC3 and susceptibility to lung cancer. *Genetics and Molecular Research* 15, 4. doi:10.4238/gmr15048813

López-García MA, Feria-Romero IA, Serrano H *et al.* (2017) Influence of genetic variants of CYP2D6, CYP2C9, CYP2C19 and CYP3A4 on antiepileptic drug metabolism in pediatric patients with refractory epilepsy. *Pharmacological Reports* 69, 3, 504–511. doi:10.1016/j.pharep.2017.01.007

Lynch B (2017) SHEICON 2017 Conference Proceedings And Pathway Planner v5. Seattle.

Lynch R, Diggins EL, Connors SL et al. (2017) Sulforaphane from broccoli reduces symptoms of autism: A follow-up case series from a randomized double-blind study. Global Advances in Health and Medicine 6, 2164957X17735826. doi:10.1177/2164957X17735826

Macciò A, Madeddu C (2012) Management of anemia of inflammation in the elderly. Anemia, 563251. doi:10.1155/2012/563251

Maksymchuk O, Shysh A, Chashchyn M et al. (2015) Dietary omega-3 polyunsaturated fatty acids alter fatty acid composition of lipids and CYP2E1 expression in rat liver tissue. International Journal for Vitamin and Nutrition Research 85, 5–6, 322–328. doi:10.1024/0300-9831/a000296

Mann A, Miksys SL, Gaedigk A et al. (2012) The neuroprotective enzyme CYP2D6 increases in the brain with age and is lower in Parkinson's disease patients. Neurobiology of Aging 33, 9, 2160–2171. doi:10.1016/j.neurobiolaging

Marshall TM (2015) Lithium as a nutrient. Journal of American Physicians and Surgeons 20, 4, 104–109.

McCann SE, Hays J, Baumgart CW et al. (2017) Usual consumption of specific dairy foods is associated with breast cancer in the Roswell Park Cancer Institute Databank and BioRepository. Current Developments in Nutrition 1, 3, 2017. doi:10.3945/cdn.117.000422

Martínez-Jiménez CP, Jover R, Donato MT et al. (2007) Transcriptional regulation and expression of CYP3A4 in hepatocytes. Current Drug Metabolism 8, 2, 185–194. doi:10.2174/138920007779815986

Mohebati A, Guttenplan JB, Kochhar A et al. (2012) Carnosol, a constituent of Zyflamend, inhibits aryl hydrocarbon receptor-mediated activation of CYP1A1 and CYP1B1 transcription and mutagenesis. Cancer Prevention Research 5, 4, 593–602. doi:10.1158/1940-6207

Murshid KR (2011) A review of mastalgia in patients with fibrocystic breast changes and the non-surgical treatment options. Journal of Taibah University Medical Sciences 6, 1, 1–18. doi:10.1016/S1658-3612(11)70151-2

Naumann S, Schweiggert-Weisz U, Eglmeier J et al. (2019) In vitro interactions of dietary fibre enriched food ingredients with primary and secondary bile acids. Nutrients 11, 6, 1424. doi:10.3390/nu11061424

NICE Guidelines Hemachromatosis. www.nice.org.uk/guidance/gid-tag423/documents/chronic-iron-over-load in people with-thalassaemia-des-ferrioxamine-deferiprone-and-defera-sirox-draft-scope-for-consultation-december-2010-2

Niu RJ, Zheng QC, Zhang JL (2011) Analysis of clinically relevant substrates of CYP2B6 enzyme by computational methods. Journal of Molecular Modeling 17, 11, 2839–2846. doi:10.1007/s00894-011-0970-2

Ohno M, Darwish WS, Ikenaka Y et al. (2011) Astaxanthin can alter CYP1A-dependent activities via two different mechanisms: induction of protein expression and inhibition of NADPH P450 reductase dependent electron transfer. Food and Chemical Toxicology 49, 6, 1285–1291. doi:10.1016/j.fct.2011.03.009

Pai AB, Norenberg J, Boyd A et al. (2007) Effect of intravenous iron supplementation on hepatic cytochrome P450 3A4 activity in hemodialysis patients: A prospective, open-label study. Clinical Therapeutics 29, 12, 2699–2705. doi:10.1016/j.clinthera.2007.12.024

Pall ML, Levine S (2015) Nrf2, a master regulator of detoxification and also antioxidant, anti-inflammatory and other cytoprotective mechanisms, is raised by health promoting factors. Sheng Li Xue Bao 67, 1, 1–18.

Park CM, Cha YS, Youn HJ et al. (2010) Amelioration of oxidative stress by dandelion extract through CYP2E1 suppression against acute liver injury induced by carbon tetrachloride in Sprague-Dawley rats. Phytotherapy Research 24, 9, 1347–1353. doi:10.1002/ptr.3121

Park Y, Kim H, Choi JY et al. (2019) Star allele-based haplotyping versus gene-wise variant burden scoring for predicting 6-mercaptopurine intolerance in pediatric acute lymphoblastic leukemia patients. Frontiers in Pharmacology 10, 654. doi:10.3389/fphar.2019.00654

Peñas-Lledó EM, Llerena A (2014) CYP2D6 variation, behaviour and psychopathology: Implications for pharmacogenomics-guided clinical trials. *British Journal of Clinical Pharmacology 7*, 4, 673–683. doi:10.1111/bcp.12227

Pesticide Action Network UK (2019) Pesticides in our food. www.pan-uk.org/site/wp-content/uploads/Pesticides-in-our-food-multiple-residues-June-2019-1.pdf

Poon CH, Wong TY, Wang Y *et al.* (2013) The citrus flavanone naringenin suppresses CYP1B1 transactivation through antagonising xenobiotic-responsive element binding. *British Journal of Nutrition 109*, 9, 1598–1605. doi:10.1017/S0007114512003595

Prawan A, Khuntikeo N, Senggunprai L *et al.* (2014) Association of NRF2 polymorphism with cholangiocarcinoma prognosis in Thai patients. *Asian Pacific Journal of Cancer Prevention 15*, 1, 299–304.

Prueksapanich P, Piyachaturawat P, Aumpansub P *et al.* (2018) Liver fluke-associated biliary tract cancer. *Gut and Liver 12*, 3, 236–245. doi:10.5009/gnl17102

Rastogi H, Jana S (2014) Evaluation of inhibitory effects of caffeic acid and quercetin on human liver cytochrome p450 activities. *Phytotherapy Research 28*, 12, 1873–1878. doi:10.1002/ptr.5220

Reding KW, Chen C, Lowe K *et al.* (2012) Estrogen-related genes and their contribution to racial differences in breast cancer risk. *Cancer Causes and Control 23*, 5, 671–681. doi:10.1007/s10552-012-9925-x

Reis LM, Tyler RC, Weh E *et al.* (2016) Analysis of *CYP1B1* in pediatric and adult glaucoma and other ocular phenotypes. *Molecular Vision 22*, 1229–1238.

Reynolds KK, McNally BA, Linder MW (2016) Clinical utility and economic impact of CYP2D6 genotyping. *Clinics in Laboratory Medicine 36*, 3, 525–542. doi:10.1016/j.cll.2016.05.008

Rodriguez-Melendez R, Griffin JB, Zempleni J (2004) Biotin supplementation increases expression of the cytochrome P450 1B1 gene in Jurkat cells, increasing the occurrence of single-stranded DNA breaks. *Journal of Nutrition 134*, 9, 2222–2228. doi:10.1093/jn/134.9.2222

Röhrich CR, Drögemöller BI, Ikediobi O *et al.* (2016) CYP2B6*6 and CYP2B6*18 predict long-term efavirenz exposure measured in hair samples in HIV-positive South African women. *AIDS Research and Human Retroviruses 32*, 6, 529–538. doi:10.1089/AID.2015.0048

Rosemary J, Adithan C, Gene TC (2007) The pharmacogenetics of CYP2C9 and CYP2C19: Ethnic variation and clinical significance. *Current Clinical Pharmacology 2*, 1, 93–109.

Samavat H, Kurzer MS (2015) Estrogen metabolism and breast cancer. *Cancer Letters 356*, 2 Pt A, 231–243. doi:10.1016/j.canlet.2014.04.018

Samsel A, Seneff S (2013) Glyphosate, pathways to modern diseases II: Celiac sprue and gluten intolerance. *Interdisciplinary Toxicology 6*, 4, 159–184. doi:10.2478/intox-2013-0026

Samsel A, Seneff S (2015) Glyphosate, pathways to modern diseases III: Manganese, neurological diseases, and associated pathologies. *Surgical Neurology International 6*, 45. doi:10.4103/2152-7806.153876

Santes-Palacios R, Romo-Mancillas A, Camacho-Carranza R *et al.* (2016) Inhibition of human and rat CYP1A1 enzyme by grapefruit juice compounds. *Toxicology Letters 258*, 267–275. doi:10.1016/j.toxlet.2016.07.023

Seneff S, Davidson R, Mascitelli L (2012) Might cholesterol sulfate deficiency contribute to the development of autistic spectrum disorder? *Med Hypotheses 78*, 2, 213–217.

Shahabi HN, Westberg L, Melke J *et al.* (2009) Cytochrome P450 2E1 gene polymorphisms/haplotypes and Parkinson's disease in a Swedish population. *Journal of Neural Transmission 116*, 567–573. doi:10.1007/s00702-009-0221-1

Shankar E, Goel A, Gupta K *et al.* (2017) Plant flavone apigenin: An emerging anticancer agent. *Current Pharmacology Reports 3*, 6, 423–446. doi:10.1007/s40495-017-0113-2

Shobeiri F, Oshvandi K, Nazari M (2015) Clinical effectiveness of vitamin E and vitamin B6 for improving pain severity in cyclic mastalgia. *Iranian Journal of Nursing and Midwifery Research 20*, 6, 723–727. doi:10.4103/1735-9066.170003

Šmerdová L, Svobodová J, Kabátková M et al. (2014) Upregulation of CYP1B1 expression by inflammatory cytokines is mediated by the p38 MAP kinase signal transduction pathway. *Carcinogenesis 35*, 11, 2534–2543. doi:10.1093/carcin/bgu190

Smith C (2015) *SNPBit Compendium*. Chicago, IL: Life Zone Wellness.

Sova M, Saso L (2018) Design and development of Nrf2 modulators for cancer chemoprevention and therapy: A review. *Drug Design, Development and Therapy 12*, 3181–3197. doi:10.2147/DDDT.S172612

Sompakdee V, Prawan A, Senggunprai L et al. (2018) Suppression of Nrf2 confers chemosensitizing effect through enhanced oxidant-mediated mitochondrial dysfunction. *Biomedicine and Pharmacotherapy 101*, 627–634. doi:10.1016/j.biopha.2018.02.112

Spink DC, Wu SJ, Spink BC et al. (2008) Induction of CYP1A1 and CYP1B1 by benzo(k)fluoranthene and benzo(a)pyrene in T-47D human breast cancer cells: Roles of PAH interactions and PAH metabolites. *Toxicology and Applied Pharmacology 226*, 3, 213–224. doi:10.1016/j.taap.2007.08.024

Spiridonov NA (2012) Mechanisms of action of herbal cholagogues. *Medicinal and Aromatic Plants 1*, 5. doi:10.4172/2167-0412.1000107

Suarez-Kurtz G, Vargens DD, Santoro AB et al. (2014) Global pharmacogenomics: Distribution of CYP3A5 polymorphisms and phenotypes in the Brazilian population. *PLOS ONE 9*, 1, e83472. doi:10.1371/journal.pone.0083472

Surapaneni KM, Priya VV, Mallika J (2014) Pioglitazone, quercetin and hydroxy citric acid effect on cytochrome P450 2E1 (CYP2E1) enzyme levels in experimentally induced non alcoholic steatohepatitis (NASH). *European Review for Medical and Pharmacological Sciences 18*, 18, 2736–2741.

Sutti S, Rigamonti C, Vidali M et al. (2014) CYP2E1 autoantibodies in liver diseases. *Redox Biology 3*, 72–78. doi:10.1016/j.redox.2014.11.004

Taneja G, Maity S, Jiang W et al. (2019) Transcriptomic profiling identifies novel mechanisms of transcriptional regulation of the cytochrome P450 (*Cyp)3a11* gene. *Scientific Reports 9*, 6663 doi:10.1038/s41598-019-43248-w

Tsujimoto M, Uchida T, Kozakai H et al. (2016) Inhibitory effects of vegetable juices on CYP3A4 activity in recombinant CYP3A4 and LS180 cells. *Biological and Pharmaceutical Bulletin 39*, 9, 1482–1487. doi:10.1248/bpb.b16-00263

Turpeinen M, Raunio H, Pelkonen O (2006) The functional role of CYP2B6 in human drug metabolism: substrates and inhibitors in vitro, in vivo and in silico. *Current Drug Metabolism 7*, 7, 705–714.

Umamaheswaran G, Krishna Kumar D, Adithan C (2014) Distribution of genetic polymorphisms of genes encoding drug metabolizing enzymes and drug transporters – A review with Indian perspective. *Indian Journal of Medical Research 139*, 1, 27–65.

Valenti L, Conte D, Piperno A et al. (2004) The mitochondrial superoxide dismutase A16V polymorphism in the cardiomyopathy associated with hereditary haemochromatosis. *Journal of Medical Genetics 41*, 12, 946–950.

Van Booven D, Marsh S, McLeod H et al. (2010) Cytochrome P450 2C9–CYP2C9. *Pharmacogenet Genomics 20*, 4, 277–281. doi:10.1097/FPC.0b013e3283349e84

Villard PH, Sampol E, Elkaim JL et al. (2002) Increase of CYP1B1 transcription in human keratinocytes and HaCaT cells after UV-B exposure. *Toxicology and Applied Pharmacology 178*, 3, 137–143. doi:10.1006/taap.2001.9335

Wan S, Kuipers F, Havinga R et al. (2019) Impaired hepatic phosphatidylcholine synthesis leads to cholestasis in mice challenged with a high-fat diet. *Hepatology Communications 3*, 2, 262–276. doi:10.1002/hep4.1302

Wang D, Sadee W (2016) CYP3A4 intronic SNP rs35599367 (CYP3A4*22) alters RNA splicing. *Pharmacogenetics and Genomics 26*, 1, 40–43. doi:10.1097/FPC.0000000000000183

Wang F, Zou YF, Sun GP et al. (2011) Association of CYP1B1 gene polymorphisms with susceptibility to endometrial cancer: A meta-analysis. *European Journal of Cancer Prevention 20*, 2, 112–120. doi:10.1097/CEJ.0b013e3283410193

Wang H, Leung LK (2010) The carotenoid lycopene differentially regulates phase I and II enzymes in dimethylbenz[a]anthracene-induced MCF-7 cells. *Nutrition 26*, 11–12, 1181–1187. doi:10.1016/j.nut.2009.11.013

Wang H, Zhang Z, Han S *et al.* (2012) CYP1A2 rs762551 polymorphism contributes to cancer susceptibility: A meta-analysis from 19 case-control studies. *BMC Cancer 12*, 528. doi:10.1186/1471-2407-12-528

Wang SC, Ho IK, Tsou HH *et al.* (2011) CYP2B6 polymorphisms influence the plasma concentration and clearance of the methadone S-enantiomer. *Journal of Clinical Psychopharmacology 31*, 4, 463–469. doi:10.1097/JCP.0b013e318222b5dd

Wang Z, Gong Y, Zeng DL *et al.* (2016) Inhibitory effect of apigenin on losartan metabolism and CYP2C9 activity in vitro. *Pharmacology 98*, 3–4, 183–189. doi:10.1159/000446808

Wang Z, Schuetz EG, Xu Y *et al.* (2013) Interplay between vitamin D and the drug metabolizing enzyme CYP3A4. *Journal of Steroid Biochemistry and Molecular Biology 136*, 54–58. doi:10.1016/j.jsbmb.2012.09.012

Wei D-Q Wang J-F, Chen C *et al.* (2008) Molecular modeling of two CYP2C19 SNPs and its implications for personalized drug design. *Protein and Peptide Letters 15*, 1, 27. doi:10.2174/092986608783330305

Werk AN, Cascorbi I (2014) Functional gene variants of CYP3A4. *Clinical Pharmacology and Therapeutics 96*, 3, 340–348. doi:10.1038/clpt.2014.129

Williams SN, Shih H, Guenette DK *et al.* (2000) Comparative studies on the effects of green tea extracts and individual tea catechins on human CYP1A gene expression. *Chemico-Biological Interactions 128*, 3, 211–229. doi:10.1016/s0009-2797(00)00204-0

Wishart DS, Feunang YD, Guo AC *et al.* (2017) DrugBank 5.0: A major update to the DrugBank database for 2018. *Nucleic Acids Research 46*, D1, D1074–D1082. doi:10.1093/nar/gkx1037

Wishart DS, Knox C, Guo AC *et al.* (2006) DrugBank: A comprehensive resource for in silico drug discovery and exploration. *Nucleic Acids Research 34*, D668–D672.

Wishart DS, Knox C, Guo AC *et al.* (2008) DrugBank: A knowledgebase for drugs, drug actions and drug targets. *Nucleic Acids Research*, D901–D906. doi: 10.1093/nar/gkm958

Xu JY, Wu L, Shi Z *et al.* (2011) Upregulation of human CYP2C9 expression by bisphenol A via estrogen receptor alpha (ERα) and Med25. *Environmental Toxicology 32*, 3, 970–978. doi:10.1002/tox.22297

Yaku K, Enami Y, Kurajyo C *et al.* (2012) The enhancement of phase 2 enzyme activities by sodium butyrate in normal intestinal epithelial cells is associated with Nrf2 and p53. *Molecular and Cellular Biochemistry 370*, 1–2, 7–14. doi:10.1007/s11010-012-1392-x

Yamasaki I, Yamada M, Uotsu N *et al.* (2012) Inhibitory effects of kale ingestion on metabolism by cytochrome P450 enzymes in rats. *Biomedical Research 33*, 4, 235–242. doi:10.2220/biomedres.33.235

Yang F, Zhuang S, Zhang C *et al.* (2013) Sulforaphane inhibits CYP1A1 activity and promotes genotoxicity induced by 2,3,7,8-tetrachlorodibenzo-p-dioxin in vitro. *Toxicology and Applied Pharmacology 269*, 3, 226–232. doi:10.1016/j.taap.2013.03.024

Yang Y, Lewis JP, Hulot JS *et al.* (2015) The pharmacogenetic control of antiplatelet response: Candidate genes and CYP2C19. *Expert Opinion on Drug Metabolism and Toxicology 11*, 10, 1599–1617. doi:10.1517/17425255.2015.1068757

Yao HT, Hsu YR, Lii CK *et al.* (2014) Effect of commercially available green and black tea beverages on drug-metabolizing enzymes and oxidative stress in Wistar rats. *Food and Chemical Toxicology 70*, 120–127. doi:10.1016/j.fct.2014.04.043

Zabalza A, Orcaray L, Fernández-Escalada M *et al.* (2017) The pattern of shikimate pathway and phenylpropanoids after inhibition by glyphosate or quinate feeding in pea roots. *Pesticide Biochemistry and Physiology 141*, 96–102. doi:10.1016/j.pestbp.2016.12.005

Zanger UM, Schwab M (2013) Cytochrome P450 enzymes in drug metabolism: Regulation of gene expression, enzyme activities, and impact of genetic variation. *Pharmacology and Therapeutics 138*, 1, 103–141.

Zhang L, Miao XJ, Wang X *et al.* (2016) Antiproliferation of berberine is mediated by epigenetic modification of constitutive androstane receptor (CAR) metabolic pathway in hepatoma cells. *Scientific Reports 6*, 28116. doi:10.1038/srep28116

Zhang JW, Liu Y, Cheng J *et al.* (2007) Inhibition of human liver cytochrome P450 by star fruit juice. *Journal of Pharmacy and Pharmaceutical Sciences 10*, 4, 496–503. doi:10.18433/j30593

Zhang YC, Gan FF, Shelar SB *et al.* (2013) Antioxidant and Nrf2 inducing activities of luteolin, a flavonoid constituent in *Ixeris sonchifolia* Hance, provide neuroprotective effects against ischemia-induced cellular injury. *Food and Chemical Toxicology 59*, 272–280. doi:10.1016/j.fct.2013.05.058

Zhou Q, Wang Y, Chen A *et al.* (2015) Association between the COMT Val158Met polymorphism and risk of cancer: evidence from 99 case-control studies. *Onco Targets and Therapy*, 2791–2803. doi:10.2147/OTT. S90883

5
Biotransformation and Elimination Phase 2

Methylation

To some of us, methylation is somewhat of a mystery. It is taught in biochemistry sessions but often forgotten or purely associated with homocysteine. Methylation is far more than this and in this chapter the whole concept of methylation will be explored in light of the biochemical pathways and SNPs associated with the process. The practitioner will be guided through the individual pathways and SNPs, and instructed how to assess gene expression and how to support the pathways in the safest possible way.

What is the importance of methylation?

Methylation is the most widely known epigenetic modification. It occurs mostly on a cytosine preceding guanine base (CpG dinucleotide). There are two components to this, namely methyl CpG binding proteins and DNA methyltransferase (DNMT) (He *et al.* 2018). The joint actions of these in recognizing methylation-related marks and in maintaining methylation patterns respectively maintain the dynamic changes of DNA methylation over time. Without methylation, there is no life. It commences before conception; 70–80% of CpG sites are methylated in human somatic cells. This happens billions of times daily, until death. It determines us in terms of appearance and behaviour, but also how we feel mentally, emotionally and physically.

In technical terms, methylation starts with the creation of methyl groups. These methyl groups contain a carbon atom and three hydrogen atoms. These are added and removed to and from other molecules that may be DNA or protein, so these molecules are then methylated. A worthy note here is that methylation is a homeostatic mechanism. It works hard to keep the body in equilibrium, very like the pH of the blood that needs to remain at 7.35–7.45 in order to maintain life. Homocysteine can be one measure highlighting the loss of equilibrium in the methylation system and this has been correlated with a number of disease processes. Methylation helps to regulate gene expression so some conditions associated with poor methylation include birth defects (Imbard *et al.* 2013), cancer (Klutstein *et al.* 2016; Board *et al.* 2007), autoimmune disease (Strickland *et al.* 2013), heart disease (Zhong *et al.* 2016), learning disability (Iwase *et al.* 2017) and dementia (Fransquet *et al.* 2018). Methylation dysfunction has also been linked to emotional conditions such as depression (Iwase *et al.* 2017) due to methylation helping to create and assimilate neurotransmitters, which in turn are linked to the immune system.

Due to this need for equilibrium, there are times and situations when one aspect of the methylation pathway may be running fast or slow, or, as some would determine, under- or over-expressed, and another pathway may compensate. Over- and undermethylation are arbitrary terms rather than a black-and-white situation. This is why it can be dangerous to SNP treat. One example of this is the blind recommendation of 5-methylfolate on the basis of a MTHFR polymorphism. Although this practice may be safe for about half of the population, the other half may be temporarily harmed if they have what we call slow (underactive) SNPs in the dopamine pathway, for example. Trapping dopamine can be a serious issue, resulting in severe anxiety, psychosis or suicidal ideology (Carballo *et al.* 2008). This is because folate drives methylation and is taken into the biopterin pathway via the DHFR enzyme to create dopamine and other neurotransmitters. If these cannot be assimilated due to a slow COMT, dopamine will get trapped. It is of the utmost importance that practitioners understand this mechanism and practise safely. There will be an example of catecholamine trapping in the section on neurotransmitters in Chapter 5.

Methylation also plays a central role in the regulation of fat metabolism as it plays a role in the regulation of lipid levels (Mittelstraß & Waldenberger 2018; He *et al.* 2018). It produces melatonin, which is required for circadian rhythm regulation, and it is one of the major ways the body clears histamine as discussed in Chapter 3. Hormones are also assimilated within the methylation pathways; this will be discussed further under 'Dopamine pathway'.

Probably the first and most important function of methylation is that of maintaining and protecting DNA. This is hugely important in order to keep cells healthy. When DNA methylation is dysfunctional due to expressing SNPs or dysfunctional enzymes, cells can become cancerous, turn into an autoimmune response or begin to age prematurely. Methylation also instructs the cells in defining their role in the body, be that as lung, liver or other organs of the body. Really important cells such as myelin basic protein that are part of the myelin sheath are also methylated. Myelin sheath acts as nerve insulation, ensuring nerve impulses reach their target tissue. If methylation is underperforming, the proteins can fall into a state of disrepair, opening up the opportunity for conditions associated with severe nervous system disease; however, these appear to be epigenetically regulated and therefore can be reversed (Weng *et al.* 2013). The second function of methylation is an epigenetic process. This process alters the expression of other genes. These may or may not be methylation genes.

Cell membrane integrity

It would be remiss to write this chapter without considering cell membranes. Methylation makes the membranes that surround every cell in the body. For a full understanding of the cell membrane, the reader would be advised to consult books such as Mary Luckey's *Membrane Structural Biology* (2012) as it is beyond the scope of this book to cover anatomy and physiology.

The cell membrane has been quite rightly identified as the brain of the cell, with 50% of the membrane being phospholipid (Lipton 2015). In the late 1960s, Lipton's work was focused on cell biology, in particular cloning of stem cells. While under the guidance of Dr Irv Konigsberg, Lipton experimented on genetically identical cells and their environment, and how changing the growth medium could encourage a cell to grow into either bone, adipose or muscle tissue. The nucleus of the cell is what most of us would see as the brain, but Lipton never believed this. He started to look at the cell membrane and learned that through the action of the cell membrane genes and biology can be controlled. Using computer analogy, Lipton identifies the cell membrane as a chip and the nucleus as a hard drive. The genes he sees as the programmes.

Cell membranes are a phospholipid bilayer containing channels and gates that allow the exchange of life-supporting minerals and electrolytes such as sodium and potassium to enter and leave the cell as necessary. Methylation maintains membrane fluidity of the cell. Drs Ed and Patricia Kane of the Neurolipid Research Foundation have spent the best part of their lives researching cell membranes. Dr Patricia Kane has a long-standing interest in the challenging area of severe and refractory neurological disease. This has culminated in the production of a world-renowned version of the PK protocol or PLX therapy (discussed in Chapter 3) to restabilize cell membranes.

Essential fatty acids and non-essential fats make up the cell membrane (Rong *et al.* 2013). In humans, the cell must be continually fed with the correct combination of lipids in order to function to the greatest effect. Although there have been a number of theories around the specific ratio of omega 6 and omega 3 lipids required for cell membrane stability, Dr's Kane research has identified that the 4:1 balance of omega 6:3 as their raw sources of linoleic acid and alpha linolenic acid respectively is the key to cell membrane stability. This balance was originally theorized by Udo Erasmus (1993) in his book *Fats that Heal, Fats that Kill.*

Lipton (2015) from his own studies described the relationship between the DNA and cell membrane. Lipton states that a cell can exist for months without its DNA if left in a petri dish with cell nourishment. If a cell membrane becomes ruptured, the cell dies instantaneously. DNA holds the programme for the production of all the proteins the body requires – the intelligence in effect (Kane 2017). Phospholipids, cholesterol, cerebrosides, gangliosides and sulphatides are the lipids within the bilayers in the brain (Bazan & Scott 1990). The fatty acid tails of the phospholipids provide secondary messaging and signal mediation (Schachter *et al.* 1983). They are also vital for cell signalling within the neuron (Rapoport 2007). Phospholipids also surround neurotransmitters, allowing release at the appropriate time, and this is dependent on a high concentration of DHA (Kane 2017). Remodelling of the phospholipids may be accomplished by providing a balance of 80% omega 6 to 20% omega 3 (Yehuda *et al.* 2005). This is provided via intravenous and/ or oral routes within the PK protocol.

Folate cycle

Before reading further here, it would be really useful for practitioners to download and print a copy of a full-sized pathway planner. Printing this in A3-size or larger will allow the reader to follow the SNPs within their respective pathways as they read.

While the folate and methionine cycles may be within the central core of methylation, it needs to be appreciated that these will likely be the last cycle in which to commence nutritional support in many cases. This is because the practitioner will need to assess detoxification via transsulphuration and to assess assimilation of neurotransmitters. To increase methylation before addressing the other two pathways could make a patient more toxic or anxious. The folate cycle is the first area to attract our attention. It is responsible for the conversion of synthetic folic acid and natural plant-based folates into 5-methyltetrahydrofolate. It is also responsible for urine nucleotide synthesis, histidine and serine metabolism.

The cycle is familiar to most practitioners, and defects in it have been identified as a factor in the pathogenesis of renal disease and hyperhomocysteinemia (HHCY) (Fowler 2001).

Possible SNPs within the folate cycle are FOLR1 and 2, SLC19A1, DHFR, MTHFD1, MTHFR, MTHFS, SHMT1, TYMS and MTR (see Figure 5.1). Practitioners are advised to follow the corresponding diagram in this book in order to understand the sequence of enzymatic activity.

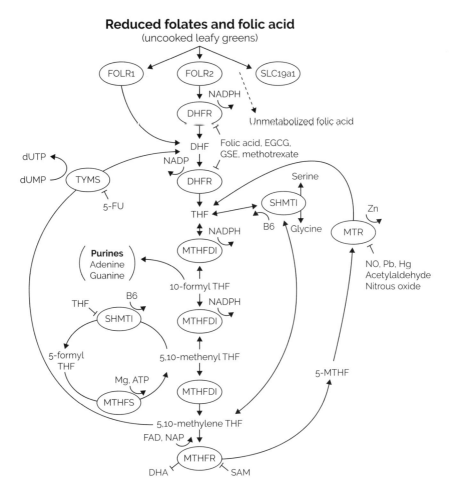

Reduced folates and folic acid
(uncooked leafy greens)

Figure 5.1: Folate cycle
Source: Methylation Planner by Dr Ben Lynch (author
of Dirty Genes and creator of StrateGene)

Prior to discussion of the relevant SNPs in this pathway, it would be beneficial for the reader to follow the chart above in the direction of the arrows. Where there are opposing arrows on a section (MTHFR to SHMT), the reaction is bidirectional. Commence with FOLR1 and 2 and SCL19A1, tracing down. All potential SNPs will be discussed in the order they are read on the pathway.

The purpose of this pathway is to create methylfolate (5-MTHF). Folate from food (or synthetic folic acid) is converted to 5-MTHF via the pathway down the centre. On reaching the MTHFR enzyme, some 5-MTHF is sent to the DHFR enzyme for the biopterin cycle and neurotransmitter production. The rest is recycled via SHMT back to tetrahydrofolate. Some also is sent to the MTR enzyme to meet B12 before entering the methionine cycle.

FOLR1–3 and SLC19A1

At the top of the folate pathway, the FOLR genes encode the protein for the folate receptor family. Commencing at the top of the folate cycle and following the arrows down, there are three folate receptors. FRα, FRβ and FRγ are cysteine-rich cell surface glycoprotein folate receptors. Practitioners will see these presented as FOLR1, FOLR2 and FOLR3 on genetic profiles. These receptors bind to folate and synthetic folic acid, having a higher binding affinity at a neutral pH. While SNPs in these are generally expressed in very low numbers in most tissues, studies have shown them to be expressed at high levels in a number of cancers. Rapidly dividing cells may be a sign of folate deficiency (Kelemen 2006).

The expression of FOLR1 SNP (rs2071010) is one gene related to cerebral folate deficiency (Al-Baradie & Chaudhary 2014), and synthetic folic acid has been shown to prevent or block the transport of L-methylfolate across the blood–brain barrier in cerebral folate deficiency. Also, many of the general population do not metabolize folic acid well so can become vulnerable to folic acid toxicity (Bailey *et al.* 2010; Ramaekers *et al.* 2002). FOLR2 (rs651933) was originally thought to be specific to the placenta but is now known to exist within many organs, predominantly focusing on gallbladder, urinary bladder, adrenal glands and lymph nodes. It may also play a role in the transport of methotrexate in synovial macrophages in subjects with rheumatoid arthritis. Activated macrophages are isolated in the synovial joints of those with inflamed arthritis (Wong & Choi 2015) and as a result the FOLRs are considered appropriate targets for cancer and inflammation intervention.

FOLR3 is generally not measured; instead, practitioners will find SLC19A1 (rs1888530, rs3788200) as evidence has demonstrated that this particular gene carries folates and antifolates such as methotrexate into the cell. Methotrexate is a cytotoxic drug used in childhood acute myeloid leukaemia (AML) and as a gold-standard disease-modifying antirheumatic (DMARD) in rheumatoid arthritis and other autoimmune conditions. In a small study (n=88), Kotnik *et al.* (2017) explored methotrexate toxicity in children and teenagers with AML and found that while SLC19A1 rs1051266 expression conferred an increase in methotrexate toxicity, SLC19A1 rs1131956 was significantly associated with protection.

Dihydrofolate reductase: DHFR

The DHFT gene encodes for the enzyme dihydrofolate reductase. This converts dihydrofolate into tetrahydrofolate using nicotinamide adenine dinucleotide phosphate hydrogen (NADPH) as a cofactor. Tetrahydrofolate is a methyl group shuttle needed for the novel synthesis of purines, thymidylic acid (a thiamine nucleotide also known as thymidine monophosphate) and some amino acids. Homozygous DHFR expression or down-regulation which slows the enzyme (Fei *et al.* 2016) has been linked to megaloblastic anaemia and cerebral folate deficiency (Cario *et al.* 2011) and also tentatively to moderately severe mental health disorders and epilepsy.

Some drugs and natural food state products have been identified as inhibitors of DHFR; these include antimalarial, folate inhibitors (such as methotrexate), antibiotics (trimethoprim) and thiazide loop diuretics (triamterene), antimicrobial chemotherapeutic agents (such as vancomycin, rifamycin, metronidazole) and anti-toxoplasma medications (sulfadiazine, pyrimethamine).

Possible interventions based on DHFR genetic expression
Nutrient cofactors to support DHFR enzyme activity
NADPH (Lynch 2017).

Unhelpful inhibitors that reduce DHFR enzyme activity

- Green tea catechins (EGCG) (Navarro-Perán *et al.* 2005). Patients should abstain or limit their green tea intake to one or two cups daily.
- Grapefruit seed extract (Kao *et al.* 2010).

Askari and Krajinovik (2010) would advocate that inhibiting DHFR expression with EGCG in fast-cell proliferative diseases such as cancer would be advantageous. However, in a potential folate-dependent condition such as risk of spina bifida, this might warrant abstinence from EGCG.

Practical advice

- Advise to reduce green tea or eliminate (Navarro-Perán *et al.* 2005).
- Avoid grapefruit seed extract (Kao *et al.* 2010).
- Check medications and serum folate or formiminoglutamic acid (FiGlu) or uracil on organic acid test.
- Refer to GP for a medication review if indicated.
- Check gastrointestinal health and absorption and rebalance microbiome.
- Support enzyme with NADPH.

Methylenetetrahydrofolate reductase: MTHFD1

This particular gene (rs1076991 and 2236225) encodes a protein that converts tetrahydrofolate to 10-formyltetrahydrofolate to 5,10-methenyltetrahydrofolate to 5,10-methylenetetrahydrofolate in three consecutive steps. This gene/enzyme requires nicotinamide adenine dinucleotide phosphate (NADP) as a cofactor. Homozygous +/+ expression of this gene is down-regulation and has been associated with neural tube defects and, in those with colorectal cancer, a progression from adenoma to advanced adenocarcinoma.

Possible interventions based on MTHFD1 genetic expression
Nutrient cofactors to support MTHFD1 enzyme activity
NADP/NADPH (Lynch 2017).

Unhelpful inhibitors that reduce MTHFD1 enzyme activity
Corticosteroids (hydrocortisone, prednisolone, beclometasone), antibiotics, HRT, sulphonamides (co-trimoxasole, bactrim, trimethoprim),
stimulants (methylphenidate) (Cohen 2015).

Practical advice

- Increase foods rich in niacin (beef, fish, poultry and pulses).
- Check all other SNPs in this pathway to assess overall picture of
  folate conversion.
- Check medications and refer to GP for review if necessary.
- If the patient is taking long-term steroids, check the overall
  impact (gastrointestinal, endocrine) and address those. Consider
  medications that may reduce niacin.
- Consider nutrient cofactor NADP alongside cofactors for other
  expressing genes in the pathway.

Methylenetetrahydrofolate synthase: MTHFS

This gene encodes the instruction for the initial intracellular conversion
of 5-formyltetrahyrofolate to other reduced folates. An increased activity
of the enzyme may result in increased folate turnover rate and associated
folate depletion. 10-formyltetrahydrofolate (10-formylTHF) is required
to synthesize the purine bases of guanine and adenine. High levels of
10-formylTHF may reduce the activity of this enzyme; practitioners are
therefore advised to ensure MTHFD1 (Figure 5.1) is functioning well.
Those with a deficiency in this enzyme may have difficulties metabolizing
folinic acid; the drug equivalent is leucovorin, which can often be found
in prenatal multivitamin products and some vitamin B complex products
(Ogwang *et al.* 2011). MTHFS uses magnesium as a cofactor.

Serine hydroxymethyltransferase: SHMT

SHMT encodes for the cytosolic form of the enzyme serine hydroxymethyltransferase. This enzyme plays two simultaneous roles. SHMT1 (rs9909104 and 1979277) catalyzes the reversible conversion of L-serine to glycine followed by the conversion of tetrahydrofolate to 5,10-MTHF. The latter conversion requires SAM as a cofactor (Rao *et al.* 2003). Reduced SHMT enzyme activity or a SNP down-regulation when expressing may result in lower levels of glycine. Pyridoxal-5-phosphate is the cofactor for this enzyme. Factors that may inhibit the action of the enzyme include B6 antagonists, sulfasalazine, zinc chelators, vitamin A. The practitioner may also need to consider medications that are known to deplete B2/riboflavin/FAD, niacin/NADPH, magnesium and B12. It can be considered an easy solution to support this enzyme with high levels of B6 but, as will be demonstrated in the section on transsulphuration later in this chapter, this can be detrimental if transsulphuration enzymes, particularly cystathionine beta-synthase (CBS), are over-expressing at the time.

Possible interventions based on SHMT genetic expression
Nutrient cofactors to support SHMT enzyme activity
Magnesium, ATP (Lynch 2017), pyridoxine-5-phosphate (Perry *et al.* 2007).

Unhelpful inhibitors that reduce SHMT enzyme activity
Antimalarials (Nonaka *et al.* 2019), antifolates (Ducker *et al.* 2017), pyridoxine antagonists, penicillamine (aids copper elimination), contraceptive steroids, antihypertensives (hydralazine), sulfasalazine (anti-inflammatory) (Cohen 2015), zinc chelators (copper, iron, azole medications) (Hatcher *et al.* 2009).

Practical advice

- Check medications for interactions with enzymes of SNPs and nutrient depletion of pyridoxine.

- Check other SNPs and particularly their expression in the folate and biopterin pathway.
- Check gastrointestinal health and address as appropriate.
- Increase foods high in pyridoxine and magnesium (salmon, tuna, halibut, turkey, chicken, duck, hazelnuts, walnuts) and magnesium (green leafy vegetables, brown rice, hazelnuts, cashews) (Linus Pauling Institute n.d.).

Thymidylate synthetase: TYMS

TYMS is a protein-coding gene that encodes for the thymidylate synthetase enzyme. High expression of TYMS has been identified in colon cancer (Castro-Rojas *et al.* 2017) and HER2 negative breast cancer (Chao & Anders 2018) as down-regulation or slowing of enzyme activity can lead to poor cell growth and DNA damage. Due to high expression of TYMS in most cases, it has become an important target for chemotherapy agents in cancers of the colorectal, ovarian, pancreatic, breast and gastric organs. Jiang *et al.* (2019) reported that TYMS expression could be a useful marker for efficacy of chemotherapy agents. Burdelski *et al.* (2015) also found high expression of TYMS in those with aggressive tumour features and early rise in prostate specific antigen (PSA) on testing. The interest has arisen due to inhibition of the TYMS enzyme because it catalyzes the conversion of deoxyuridine monophosphate (dUMP) to deoxythymidine monophosphate (dTMP), one of the three nucleotides that form thymine. The other important step here is that the 5,10-MTHF produced in the three stages of MTHFD1 activity is used partly by TYMS to generate dihydrofolate (DHF) in a loop and partly to generate 5-methylenetetrahydrofolate (5-MTHF) via the well-known methylenetetrahydrofolate reductase (MTHFR) enzyme. Dihydrofolate deficiency may lead to cerebral folate deficiency and megaloblastic anaemia (Cario *et al.* 2011).

Possible interventions based on TYMS genetic expression
Nutrient cofactors that support the TYMS enzyme
5-methylfolate.

Helpful inducers that increase TYMS enzyme activity

- Oestrogen (Chen *et al.* 2001).
- Disease-modifying antirheumatic medications (DMARDs) such as methotrexate and sulfasalazine (James *et al.* 2008).
- Infection (Schober *et al.* 2019).
- Rapid cell division (Bazzocco *et al.* 2015).

Unhelpful inhibitors that reduce TYMS enzyme activity
Antitumour medications (fluorouracil) (Kim *et al.* 2008), cisplatin (Ko *et al.* 2011), methotrexate (Blits *et al.* 2013), leucovorin (prescription folinic acid) (Ardalan *et al.* 2010), organophosphates (Hreljac & Filipic 2009).

Practical advice

- Advice on avoidance and removal of the following: airborne pollutants, food toxins, household toxins, industrial/workplace toxins, natural toxins, pollutants.
- Advice to patient on avoidance of oestrogen-disrupting chemicals from herbicides, plastics, skin care, antiperspirants and make-up.
- Ensure good levels of folate-containing foods (dark green leafy vegetables, peas, beans and lentils) (Linus Pauling Institute n.d.).
- Check medications and refer to GP for medicine review if appropriate.
- Test for possible infections and support immunity to reduce infection, support gut microbiome and gut-barrier integrity.
- Requires effective conversion of folate to 5-10 methylene tetrahydrofolate to be able to take this to DHFR for the biopterin cycle, so do check other SNPs and their expression.
- Check serum folate, urine FiGlu or Uracil.

Methylenetetrahydrofolate reductase (MTHFR)

The MTHFR gene encodes the protein for the enzyme methylenetetrahydrofolate reductase. There are a number of alleles of MTHFR but the two with the most robust research are C677T (rs1801133) and A1298C (rs2274976). MTHFR is the rate-limiting enzyme at the end of the folate pathway that converts 5,10-MTHF to 5-MTHF before it joins cobalamin in the methionine cycle. It is here that it is a crucial enzyme for the conversion of homocysteine to methionine (De Mattia & Toffoli 2009). This means that with expressing SNPs in the MTHFR gene, the enzyme activity is reduced, leading to poor folate conversion from food or synthetic folic acid to 5-methylenetetrahydrofolate (5-MTHF). This is required to drive methylation. Having homozygous C677T +/+ and a raised homocysteine would appear to increase the risk of blood agglutination or clotting disorders (Hickey *et al.* 2013). However, having two variants or being compound heterozygous +/– of MTHFR means the individual has one of each C677T +/– and A1298C +/– and is equivocal in terms of risk (Dean 2016). This situation can have serious ramifications to health generally. MTHFR is also a key enzyme in the formation of folate to S-adenosylhomocysteine, the universal methyl donor in cells affecting DNA status.

MTHFR C677T SNPs have been associated with various forms of cancer (Izmirli 2013), cerebrovascular accident (strokes) (Gao *et al.* 2012), heart disease where serum folate levels are low (Klerk *et al.* 2002), autism spectrum disorders (Rai 2016), Parkinson's disease (Hua *et al.* 2011), dementia (Mansoori *et al.* 2012), rheumatoid arthritis (Shahvali *et al.* 2015) and many others. MTHFR A1288C also has a negative impact on health when expressing; however, it seems to have much less impact than the C677T allele.

The important takeaway is that SNPs in the MTHFR gene are not by themselves a threat to life. We do currently live in a zeitgeist of fear around the MTHFR enzyme, so the practitioner does need to be mindful of all the other SNPs in the pathways in and around methylation and how these also may be impacting the MTHFR. As stated previously, methylation is a homeostatic mechanism, so there are likely to be compensatory mechanisms occurring to offset any slow conversions at this juncture. This is why SNP treating can be detrimental to the patient's health. An example of this might be when giving nutrients to increase folate cycle activity when the ability to break down and eliminate hormones and neurotransmitters is reduced. There is a case example of this in the section on neurotransmitters later in this chapter.

Folic acid vs methylfolate

This is quite a controversial view but there are studies now considering the effects of supplementation with folic acid versus 5-methylfolate (5-MTHF). Higher risk of cancer has been identified with the fortification of foods with folic acid and supplementation (Tomita 2016). One reason for this may be that unmetabolized folic acid is responsible for reduced levels of natural killer cell cytotoxicity in postmenopausal women according to Troen *et al.* (2006). A randomized control trial also found a higher rate of prostate cancer in those supplementing 1mg of synthetic folic acid daily (Figueiredo *et al.* 2009). Morris *et al.* (2007) found a higher incidence of anaemia and cognitive decline in those with low B12 who were supplementing folic acid. Folate from natural sources is highly recommended.

How can we provide support for MTHFR?

The nutrient cofactors to support this enzyme are FAD and NADPH. However, we need to be mindful of the conditions that may encourage expression of the gene. Dihydrofolate (DHF), S-adenosylmethionine (SAM), high levels of T4, folic acid and/or anything that would initiate the cell danger response (Naviaux 2013) (see the sections on cell membrane integrity in Chapter 5, and PLX in Chapter 4) might impede the action of MTHFR, so these should all be considered (dysbiosis, heavy metals, reactive oxygen species, sulfasalazine) before recommending 5-MTHF as these toxins are all inhibitors of MTHFR. There are also a host of medications that are known to reduce the action of this enzyme. These include hormone replacement therapy (HRT), diuretics, antidepressants, cholestyramine, non-steroidal anti-inflammatory drugs (NSAIDs), rifampin, and selective oestrogen receptor modulators (Cohen 2015). Practitioners may need to work around the medications, ensuring that FAD and NADPH are optimal and that any other potential deficiencies as a result of prescription medications are addressed. There are many avenues to explore and support when considering the cell danger response, and as the cell membrane has been identified as the brain of the cell, this is paramount.

Possible interventions based on MTHFR genetic expression
Nutrient cofactors to support MTHFR enzyme activity
FAD, NADPH (Lynch 2017).

Unhelpful inhibitors that reduce MTHFR enzyme activity
Thyroxin, dihydrofolate, S-adenosylmethionine, cell danger response, folic acid (Lynch 2017), HRT, diuretics, antidepressants, cholestyramine, NSAIDs, rifampin (Cohen 2015).

Practical advice

- Encourage an organic diet where possible or at least follow the dirty dozen/clean fifteen lists.
- Assess the potential impact of all genes in the pathway for a clear picture of the impact.
- Reduce environmental toxin exposure.
- Test for heavy metals and rebalance with minerals/use binders as appropriate (Joneidi *et al.* 2019).
- Test for dysbiosis and re-establish microbiome diversity as appropriate (Sharma *et al.* 2020).
- Include foods high in riboflavin and niacin such as dairy, chicken, beef, fish, eggs, peas, beans, lentils (Linus Pauling Institute n.d.).
- Supplement riboflavin or riboflavin-5-phosphate as tolerated and nicotinamide riboside or niacin. Nicotinamide riboside increases NAD by 60% in studies, whereas there are no studies on the clinical use of niacinamide (Martens *et al.* 2018).

PRACTITIONER NOTES

In the unfortunate scenario that a patient takes too much 5-MTHF and becomes extremely anxious, this generally means there is a temporary overproduction of methyl donors. Please do not use niacin as a 'methyl group rescue'. Niacin does neutralize excess methyl donors and it does that because niacin needs methylating and supraphysiological doses are being used. The methylated niacin is then passed out in the urine, so effectively we are using niacin in the same way we would use a drug. Methyl groups are reduced because there is too much niacin in the body, not because there are too many methyl groups. In effect, the body will create more methyl groups to be able to methylate the niacin. This is an unstable situation that lends itself to the uncomfortable biochemical rollercoaster between hyper- and hypo-methylation. Glycine is a much better solution because glycine is methylated when there are too many methyl groups, not because there is too much glycine. Also glycine is part of the methylation system, so a regular dose of glycine is all that is required as a methyl group rescue (Locasale 2013).

Methionine cycle

The function of the methionine cycle is to convert and recycle homocysteine from methionine. It also creates S-adenosylmethionine (SAM), which in turn produces and regulates hormones and many other proteins in the body. See Figure 5.2 – SAM is a methyl donor. Cell membranes are produced in the methyltransferase part of the cycle – top right.

SNPs associated with the methionine cycle include MTR, MTRR, MAT1a, DMGDH, GNMT, PEMT, GAMT, PON1, MARS, AHCY and CBS. Then to the right, creating uric acid and hydrogen peroxide, are AHCY, ADA, SOD2, SOD3, MPO, CAT, GPX (see Figure 5.2).

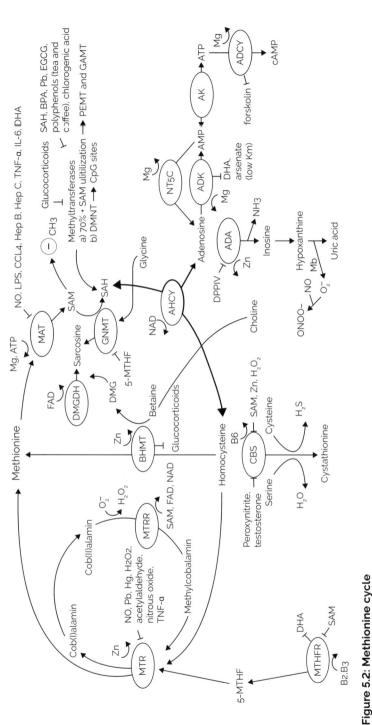

Figure 5.2: Methionine cycle

Source: Methylation Planner by Dr Ben Lynch (author of Dirty Genes and creator of StrateGene)

Key: MTR = methionine synthase, MTRR = methionine synthase reductase, MAT = methionine adenosyltransferase, SAM = S-adenosylmethionine, SAH = S-adenosylhomocysteine, AHCY = adenosylhomocysteinase, ADA = adenosine deaminase, BHMT = beta homocysteine methyltransferase, CBS = cystathionine beta-synthase, DMGDH – dimethylglycine dehydrogenase, GNMT = glycine N-methyltransferase.

How to read the methionine pathway

Reading from left to right, 5-MTHF from the MTHFR enzyme meets with methylcobalamin at the MTR enzyme where cobalamin has been methylated from MTRR. Through the addition and subtraction of methyl groups, methionine is converted to S-adenosyl methionine, then up into methyltransferase, transferring a methyl group to DNA, using S-adenosylmethionine as a methyl donor. The S-adenosylmethionine/S-adenosyl homocysteine (SAM/SAH) ratio with homocysteine can tell the practitioner how successful methylation is and is a marker for atherosclerosis (Zhang *et al.* 2021). Coming down the right-hand side of the cycle, SAH becomes homocysteine as it donates methyl groups. Homocysteine is the toxic by-product of methylation which, when raised, is a marker of inflammation and a signal of poor methylation. Reference ranges for homocysteine are 0–15umol/L.

Three routes can dispose of homocysteine:

- via MTR back to methionine
- via BHMT (short route to methionine)
- via CBS into the transsulphuration pathway for sulphur detoxification and conversion to glutathione.

Methionine synthase: MTR

MTR encodes the protein for 5-methyltetrahydrofolate-homocysteine methyltransferase. This is the final step in methionine biosynthesis. SNPs in the MTR gene have been identified as one cause of methylcobalamin deficiency as cobalamin is methylated to methylcobalamin via MTR/MTRR. There are again a number of MTR alleles that practitioners may see on reporting, but the A66G (rs1801394) and the A2765G (rs1805087) appear to be those most researched and applied to health. Sterling Hill Erdei (Hill Erdei & Ledowski 2015) is one of the founding members of MTHFR support and author of the original SNPbit compendium 1. In her analyses on Sterling's app, she considers a further 18 MTRs at this time, although evidence for their inclusion is sparse. As can be seen from Figure 5.2, 5-MTHF meets methylcobalamin at the MTR enzyme where they both drive the methylation of methionine into subsequent compounds that will be discussed in this section. MTR also regenerates methionine from homocysteine. The enzyme is zinc- and methylcobalamin-dependent and many medications are known to reduce the function. These include ACE inhibitors, diuretics, oral contraceptives, HRT, psychiatric medications and proton pump inhibitors (PPIs). Cadmium and casein are also culprits (Cohen 2015). Diseases associated with MTR deficiency include homocystineuria-megaloblastic anaemia. Neural tube defects are also known to be folate-sensitive, the most common being open spina bifida.

Possible interventions based on MTR genetic expression
Nutrient cofactors to support MTR enzyme activity
Zinc (Lynch 2017; Cohen 2015).

Unhelpful inhibitors that reduce MTR enzyme activity
Aluminium, cadmium, mercury, lead, reactive oxygen species, hydrogen peroxide, TNFα, thyroxin (Lynch 2017), antacids, ACE inhibitors, diuretics, oral contraceptives, HRT, psychiatric medications, casein (Cohen 2015).

Practical advice

- Check levels of active B12 and folate in serum or urine organic acids and address if indicated (Palmer *et al.* 2017).
- Check heavy metals in blood, hair and/or urine and address imbalances.
- Encourage foods high in zinc such as oysters, crab, beef, dark meat, pork, chickpeas, black beans and pumpkin seeds (Linus Pauling Institute n.d.).
- Support digestion (may be the root cause of potential B12 deficiency).
- Supplement zinc if indicated.

Methionine synthase reductase: MTRR

MTRR encodes the protein for the 5-Methyltetrahydrofolate-Homo-cysteine Methyltransferase Reductase enzymes. Two alleles of MTRR appear to be important for genome analysis, A66G (rs18001394) and C524T (rs1532268). MTRR regenerates cobalamin in order to maintain MTR in a functional state via reductive methylation. This is necessary in order to utilize methyl groups from the folate pathway. SNPs on the MTRR gene are generally associated with decreased enzyme activity and therefore possible reduction in methylation capacity due to a limited amount of active methylcobalamin being available. MTRR is one of the most widely researched SNPs and as such has been associated with a variety of conditions such as cancers (Wang *et al.* 2017), birth defects (Guo *et al.* 2017), mood disorders (Wan *et al.* 2018) and metabolic syndrome (Kim & Hong 2019).

Nutrient cofactors for MTRR include FAD, NAD and SAM. MTRR can be negatively affected by reactive oxygen species and medications such as antibiotics, antacids, PPIs, cholestyramine, colestipol, diabetes drugs such as metformin and Parkinson's medications. Medications that deplete B12 should also be considered, such as hydrocortisone, prednisolone, quinolones, phenobarbital, potassium chloride, colchicine and ulcer medications such as cimetidine and ranitidine. This is a very long list of medications so perhaps this is one reason why practitioners are observing a higher incidence of B12 deficiency currently.

Possible interventions based on MTRR genetic expression
Nutrient cofactors to support MTRR enzyme activity
SAM, FAD, NAD (Lynch 2017), riboflavin (García-Minguillán *et al.* 2014).

Inhibitors that reduce MTRR enzyme activity (may be helpful or unhelpful depending on dopamine pathway status)
Reactive oxygen species (Lynch 2017), antibiotics, antacids, PPIs, cholestyramine/colestipol, diabetes medications, Parkinson's medications (Cohen 2015).

Practical advice

- Check levels of active B12 and folate in serum or urine organic acids and address if indicated (Horita *et al.* 2016).
- Check heavy metals in blood, hair and/or urine and address imbalances.
- Encourage foods high in riboflavin such as dairy, chicken, beef, fish and egg, and those high in niacin such as beef, fish, poultry, beans, peas and lentils (Linus Pauling Institute n.d.).
- SAM is produced though methylation so support as necessary.
- Support digestion (may be the root cause of potential B12 deficiency).
- Supplement zinc if needed.

Methionine adenosyltransferase: MAT1a

MAT1 encodes the protein that produces the enzyme methionine adenosyltransferase. If expressing, it is generally down-regulated. This is a very important enzyme (rs72558181) because it starts the conversion of methionine to adenosylmethionine (AdoMet) or SAMe. AdoMet/SAMe is a major methyl donor. Lai *et al.* (2010) identified eight alleles of this gene associated with a high risk of hypertension, DNA damage and cerebrovascular accident or stroke. During the first pass through the liver, 50% of available methionine is converted to SAM, which in turn creates DNA, RNA, protein and phospholipids. SAM also methylates many drugs, xenobiotics, hormones and neurotransmitters. An expressing mutation in MAT1a may result in hypermethioninemia due to MAT deficiency or slowing down of the enzyme. The practitioner may not observe clinical symptomology associated with this. However, studies have linked severe MAT1 deficiency with neurological disorders (Furujo *et al.* 2012).

Possible interventions based on MAT1 genetic expression
Nutrient cofactors to support MAT1 enzyme activity

- Magnesium, potassium (Lynch 2017) and ATP.

- Fasting (Lynch 2017).

Unhelpful inhibitors that reduce MAT1 enzyme activity

- Oxidative stress leading to inflammation, in particular raised TNFα and interleukin 6.
- Glutathione depletion (check for transsulphuration defects and conditions known to deplete glutathione such as neurodegenerative disease, cancer, cystic fibrosis, cardiovascular, inflammatory and/or immune) (Ballatori *et al.* 2009).
- Poor tyrosine metabolism (check biopterin), endotoxins from disturbed microbiome.
- Hepatitis B and C and cirrhosis of the liver.

Medications such as folate antagonists (e.g. methotrexate and trimethoprim), corticosteroids (such as hydrocortisone and prednisolone), HRT, sulphonamides (such as sulfadiazine), methylphenidate and antibiotics may also reduce enzyme activity (Cohen 2015).

It would be prudent to discuss methionine levels generally at this point. Methionine can be low or high for a variety of reasons, so excluding some of them helps inform clinical practice. High methionine can occur due to:

- methionine or SAM supplementation
- magnesium deficiency
- impaired liver function
- enzyme defects (MAT or AHCY).

Low methionine levels may be due to:

- diet – poor protein or unbalanced protein intake
- gastrointestinal dysfunction
- methylation defects
- environmental exposure to heavy metals such as thimerosol or aluminium (Waly *et al.* 2004)
- infection.

It is worth noting that fasting and starvation may increase activity of MAT1.

Practical advice

- Check SAM/SAH ratio and homocysteine to assess expression of MAT1 and correct if necessary.
- Encourage intermittent fasting (Sakata *et al.* 2005).
- Ensure good mitochondrial production of ATP (consider OAT testing for mitochondrial nutrients). For a more in-depth understanding please consult the sister book in this series *Mitochondria in Health and Disease* (Griffiths 2018) and/or *Diagnosis and Treatment of Chronic Fatigue Syndrome and Myalgic Encephalitis* (Myhill 2018).
- Check glutathione levels in serum or urine organic acids and correct if necessary. The two most absorbable forms available to nutrition practitioners include liposomal glutathione and S-acetyl glutathione (Ash 2011).
- Epsom salts baths with the addition of electrolytes to provide magnesium and potassium for MAT1 enzyme support and sulphate for the transsulphuration system (discussed in the section on transsulphuration below).
- Supplement magnesium and or electrolytes according to red cell magnesium and serum or hair mineral electrolytes.
- Encourage food high in magnesium and electrolyte minerals (whole grains, green leafy vegetables, nuts and seeds) (Linus Pauling Institute n.d.).

Adenosylhomocysteinase: AHCY

This gene encodes for the production of the S-adenosylhomocysteine hydrolase enzyme. This enzyme breaks down methionine in a multi-step process. It regulates the intracellular S-adenosylhomocysteine (SAH) levels thought to be important for transmethylation reactions. This reaction regulates the addition of methyl groups. AHCY converts

SAH to adenosine, which is then converted to ATP and cyclic adenosine monophosphate (cAMP) or to inosine for conversion to uric acid. True AHCY deficiency is a rare autosomal recessive condition resulting in psychomotor delay, delayed myelination and myopathy (absent tendon reflex from birth). It is associated with hypermethioninemia, elevated serum creatinine kinase and increased genome-wide DNA methylation. However, this does not appear to be a consistent feature (Motzek *et al.* 2016). This is a reflection of the tri-directional pathway of AHCY between SAH, homocysteine and adenosine. Belužić *et al.* (2018) have highlighted that reduced AHCY activity has resulted in decreased proliferation of cells, DNA damage, depletion of adenosine and cell cycle arrest. These authors purport that ACHY could be used as a tumour marker.

Possible interventions based on AHCY genetic expression

Nutrient cofactors to support AHCY enzyme activity

- Magnesium and manganese (Lynch 2017).
- NAD (Hill Erdei & Ledowski 2015).
- Fasting and starvation (Lynch 2017).

Unhelpful inhibitors that reduce AHCY enzyme activity
Copper, green tea catechins, NADH+ (Lynch 2017).

Practical advice

- Check SAM/SAH ratio and homocysteine to assess gene expression.
- Check digestion and absorption/dysbiosis and rebalance as necessary.
- Encourage intermittent fasting as appropriate to the client (Aksungar *et al.* 2005).
- Encourage magnesium-rich foods such as whole grains, green leafy vegetables, nuts and seeds; manganese-rich foods such as brown rice, pecans, almonds and pineapple; and niacin-rich

foods such as beef, fish, poultry, beans, peas and lentils (Linus Pauling Institute n.d.).

Dimethylglycine dehydrogenase: DMGDH and glycine N-methyltransferase: GNMT

These genes instruct the enzymes involved in the catabolism of choline. Dimethylglycine is demethylated to form sarcosine. Four alleles have been identified in the DMGDH gene: rs479405, rs2255262, rs402701 and rs532964. Mutations result in enzyme deficiency, so slow enzyme activity has resulted in fish-like body odour, chronic muscle fatigue and elevated levels of muscle creatine kinase in serum (Magnusson *et al.* 2015). Magnusson's genome-wide association study (GWAS) also identified the possibility of DMGDH enzyme deficiency being a factor on the development of diabetes.

Possible interventions based on DMGDH genetic expression
Nutrient cofactors to support DMGDH enzyme activity
FAD (Lynch 2017; Barile *et al.* 2016).

Nutrient cofactors to support GNMT enzyme activity
SAM (Lynch 2017), so optimizing methylation is key.

Helpful enhancers that increase DMGDH and GNMT enzyme activity
Cortisol, methionine, glucocorticoids (Lynch 2017).

Unhelpful inhibitors that reduce DMGDH and GNMT enzyme activity
These include elevated levels of dimethylglycine and hypotonic dehydration (Lynch 2017). Test serum urea and electrolytes as high levels of sodium and/or potassium could indicate dehydration or possible poor kidney function.

Practical advice

- Encourage choline from foods as much as possible (eggs, poultry, beef, shellfish) and glycine (beans, nuts, seeds and bone broth). Egg yolks are the greatest source (Linus Pauling Institute n.d.).
- Reduce stress and check for exogenous delivery of glucocorticoids.
- Manage blood glucose regulation to help balance glucocorticoids by reducing the strain on the HPA axis and reducing the stress response (Tanaka *et al.* 2020).
- Encourage beetroot for the betaine; use small amounts due to possible negative effects on blood glucose regulation (Lee *et al.* 2014).
- Encourage creative activities and relaxation/meditation to support cortisol production (Drexel University 2016).
- Ensure adequate methylation to produce SAM for GNMT enzyme.
- Encourage niacin-containing foods such as beef, fish, poultry, beans, peas and lentils (Linus Pauling Institute n.d.).

Phosphatidylethanolamine methyltransferase: PEMT

This oestrogen-responsive gene encodes the transferase enzyme that converts phosphatidylethanolamine (PE) to phosphatidylcholine (PC) in the liver (Vance 2013). Down-regulation or slowing down of enzyme activity may lead to lower levels of PC being made available for cell membrane repair and this can have negative effects body-wide. The allele rs7946 seems to be prominent in the evidence base to date, although rs4646406 and rs4244593 are reported on some genetic reports. PC is the key component of cell membrane structure, making this one of the most important enzymes to be supporting. PC is derived from the B vitamin choline. The enzyme uses three molecules of SAM as a nutrient cofactor to make this conversion in three sequential steps. Although the CDP–choline pathway is the predominant one for the biosynthesis of PC, the PEMT pathway was identified as being crucial in times of starvation (Vance 2014) as it can produce PC from methylation in the absence of food sources of choline. Oestrogen (Resseguie *et al.* 2007) and histamine (Hirata & Axelrod 1978) have been identified as two possible activators of PEMT when the body lacks dietary choline. The two pathways operate differently in that the CDC–choline pathway uses choline from dietary sources such as eggs, whereas the PEMT pathway makes PC via the conversion of phosphatidylethanolamine. PC is utilized in hepatocyte membrane structures, choline synthesis, bile secretion and VLDL secretion (Pm24184426). The PEMT enzyme is found in endoplasmic reticulum (Gao *et al.* 2015) and mitochondria associated membranes and the PC it creates accounts for more than 50% of cell membrane phospholipids and 30% of cellular lipid content, and is therefore of paramount importance for the stabilization of cell membranes.

PC plays a crucial role in cell membrane fluidity, permeability and signal transduction. It is required for cell growth and maturation, brain and neurotransmitter function (as a precursor to acetylcholine) and for liver function and detoxification (Van der Veen *et al.* 2017).

Oestrogen has also been identified as a positive regulator of hepatocyte PEMT transcription, particularly on the allele rs12325817. This determines a possible advantageous clinical use of PC in menopausal women with expressing PEMT SNPs, unless contraindicated by antiphospholipid antibodies (Resseguie *et al.* 2007). PC is predominantly utilized via bile secretion into the intestine, retarded release of which has been linked to acute exacerbations of ulcerative colitis (Stremmel *et al.* 2005). PC is abundant in the mucin layer of the gastrointestinal tract (Stremmel *et al.* 2016), suggesting clinical application for inflammatory bowel disorders.

Recent evidence has highlighted the need for dietary choline in females who present with low oestrogen at menopause (Fischer *et al.* 2010). The Fischer study also confirmed that 82% of those postmenopausal women who were given oestrogen when deficient did not develop choline deficiency-induced organ dysfunction. However, 72% receiving placebo did. Males do not seem to be influenced by the oestrogen promoter region (Kohlmeier 2013).

When methyl donors are required due to compromised methylation (e.g. low folate and/or B12 or other cofactors) cell membranes will donate methyl groups to the detriment of bile production and the cell membrane itself (Hill Erdei & Ledowski 2015). PEMT can also partially modulate levels of homocysteine by producing trimethylglycine (TMG), which BHMT uses to reduce homocysteine back to methionine.

The nutrient cofactor for PEMT is SAM, but this needs to be balanced as too much or too little can be detrimental to enzyme function.

Dietary choline per 100g portion

- Beef liver (cooked, braised or pan fried) 330–420mg.
- Lamb, veal, game liver 310–410mg.
- Chicken liver (pan fried) 330mg.
- Raw egg yolk 147mg.
- Whole eggs hard-boiled (two whole eggs, medium-sized) 230mg.
- Seafood – scallop 94mg.
- Meat, fish, pork and poultry 80–100mg.

(Linus Pauling Institute n.d.)

Vegetarian sources of choline per 100g

Vegans and vegetarians are at a higher risk of choline deficiency as plant foods contain significantly less choline than animal foods. Raw soybean seeds contain 120mg of choline per 100g so one portion would provide only 25% of the daily requirement. Antinutrients such as lectins, phytates, proteinase inhibitors, urease, trypsin and chymotrypsin inhibitors might reduce that further. Fermenting and/or cooking may reduce the antinutrient load. However, a vegan is unlikely to meet the daily requirements for PC. This will be more obvious if they are low oestrogen and or PEMT is expressing.

- Raw soybeans 116mg.
- Tofu fried 106mg.
- Flax seeds 79mg.
- Pistachio nuts 71mg.
- Quinoa 70mg.
- Pine nuts and sunflower seeds 55–56mg.

- Almonds 52mg.
- Brassicas 40mg.
- Legumes, cooked 30–40mg.

NutritionData (2018)

Practical advice

- Encourage a choline-rich diet.
- Manage histamine as necessary – refer to the histamine section in Chapter 3 for a full review. However, optimizing methylation and a low-histamine diet until dysbiosis has been rebalanced might be useful.
- The Snellen visual acuity test can be used to assess the requirement for supplemental PC (Hirsch 2015, p.46). This test refers to the ability to see shapes and details in things we see. There are a number of online testing companies where visual acuity can be self-tested for a small fee.

PRACTITIONER NOTES

While some would advocate the use of lecithin to support the need for more PC, there appears to be a contraindication to this. Hazen and colleagues (Wilson *et al.* 2013) in their research found that lecithin actually feeds some microbes in the gut that create trimethylamine N-oxide (TMAO). Interestingly, TMAO has been linked to cardiac events (heart attacks), cerebrovascular events (stroke) and death even where there was no evidence of risk (Yang *et al.* 2019).

Betaine homocysteine methyltransferase: BHMT

BHMT encodes the cytosolic enzyme betaine homocysteine methyltransferase/betaine homocysteine S-methyltransferase.

There are three alleles for BHMT rs6875201, BHMT-02 (rs567754) and BHMT-08 (rs651852). The BHMT enzyme converts betaine (TMG) to dimethylglycine and methionine. Irreversible oxidation of choline also results from this reaction. Practitioners will often see this referred to as the short route or shortcut pathway. BHMT SNPs are generally down-regulated, meaning less conversion occurs, resulting in higher glycine levels. In addition, a higher level of homocysteine with lower methionine and SAM in the liver occurs. CBS down-regulates to counter the loss of methionine (Strakova *et al.* 2011).

BHMT expression appears to increase the level of noradrenaline relative to dopamine, so the practitioner may see internalization of stress and possible ADHD (Saha *et al.* 2018).

The nutrient cofactor for BHMT is zinc, although PC and phosphatidylserine are also important.

Possible interventions based on BHMT genetic expression
Nutrient cofactors to support BHMT enzyme activity
Zinc, betaine, PC (Lynch 2017; Obeid 2013).

Unhelpful inhibitors that reduce BHMT enzyme activity

- S-adenosylmethionine and PPIs.
- ACE inhibitors (lisinporil, perindopril).
- Diuretics (furosemide, bendroflumethiazide, spironolactone).
- Cadmium (cigarettes, metal plating, batteries).
- Oral contraceptives and HRT.
- Psychiatric medications.
- Casein.

Note that these are the same inhibitors as for MTR.

Practical advice

- Check medications for nutrient depletions and effect on the BHMT enzyme.
- Refer to GP for medicine review as appropriate.

- Check methionine levels as low levels increase BHMT activity (Pérez-Miguelsanz *et al.* 2017).
- Encourage zinc-rich foods such as seafood, oysters, crab, beef, dark meat, pork, chickpeas and black beans (Linus Pauling Institute n.d.).
- Test zinc levels in serum, creatinine kinase, creatinine kinase MB or troponin levels as these are inversely correlated with low zinc (Huang *et al.* 2017) or urine (OAT) and correct if necessary.
- Check stomach acid levels for optimal absorption, as zinc is required to optimize stomach acid production. Question how the patient feels after heavy proteins or a mixed meal of protein and grain. If they feel excessively tired after eating, they may require digestive support or assistance with food combining.

Guanidinoacetate N-methyltransferase: GAMT

The GAMT gene (rs17851582 and rs55776826) encodes for the enzyme guanidinoacetate N-methyltransferase, which is expressed mainly in the liver. The enzyme potentiates the second step of a two-stepped synthesis of creatine from glycine, arginine and methionine. In the second step, creatine is produced from guanidinoacetate. Creatine provides the energy for muscle contraction and muscle building. Down-regulation of GAMT has been identified in ovarian cancers (Alur *et al.* 2019). Where there are also expressing SNPs in catechol-O-methyltransferase and/or MAT, it may be prudent to supplement with creatine, depending on the case, in order to free up SAM. Guanidinoacetate N-methyltransferase is also thought to activate fatty acid oxidation (Hill Erdei & Ledwoski 2015). This process mobilizes fatty acids for energy during times of stress such as when glucose is scarce. Guanidinoacetate N-methyltransferase deficiency is an inherited disorder consistent with severe intellectual disability, speech delay, epilepsy, autism and tics. Weak muscle tone gives rise to poor motor development (Barić *et al.* 2017).

Possible interventions based on GAMT genetic expression
Nutrient cofactors to support GAMT enzyme activity
S-adenosylmethionine (SAMe). Note that SAM and 5-MTHF modulate
GNMT enzyme function (Joo *et al.* 2011).

Unhelpful inhibitors that reduce GAMT enzyme activity

- High levels of SAM.
- Selective oestrogen receptor modulator (tamoxifen).
- Heavy alcohol intake (Lynch 2017).
- 5-MTHF (Lynch 2017).
- Growth hormones (Lynch 2017).

Practical advice

- Optimize methylation in order to create SAMe. Please note that European law prevents nutrition practitioners from recommending SAMe as a supplement because this is a prescription drug in Europe.
- Reduce alcohol intake.
- Optimize digestion and microbiome diversity with a high percentage of foods from plant sources, to reduce aldehydes created via digestion.
- Check medications and nutrient depletions. Refer for medical review if warranted.

Paraoxonase 1: PON1

PON1 encodes for the enzyme paraoxonase 1. PON1 hydrolyzes the toxic metabolites of a variety of organophosphorus insecticides and nerve gases. Although generally a SNP will be down-regulated, the developmental process also regulates the expression of PON1. Newborns have very low levels of PON1, leaving them very susceptible to toxicity if living on farms where organophosphates are sprayed readily. The author has experienced two small children of farmers with this exposure, resulting in conditions akin to amyotrophic lateral sclerosis. This is a devastating condition characterized by progressive muscle weakness due to the loss of motor neurons. Sporadic amyotrophic lateral sclerosis has been associated with this type of exposure (Sánchez-Santed *et al.* 2016).

There is also a growing interest in this enzyme's association with prevention of lipid oxidation, making it a possible target for intervention in cardiovascular disease. PON1 is capable of hydrolyzing homocysteine thiolactone, which can impair protein function, leading to endothelial dysfunction and vascular damage (Esin *et al.* 2013).

Possible interventions based on PON1 genetic expression
Nutrient cofactors to support PON1 enzyme activity
Calcium (Harel *et al.* 2004).

Unhelpful inhibitors that reduce PON1 enzyme activity
Antibiotics, thyroid medications (levothyroxine), aspirin, oral contraceptives, HRT, calcium channel blockers (amlodipine, nifedipine), naringenin (Mahrooz *et al.* 2011).

Practical advice

- Advise organic diet for gene expression. If this is not possible, recommend following the dirty dozen/clean fifteen lists and eat organic as much as possible.
- Check living situation for crop-spraying exposure. Lymphocyte sensitivity testing may be useful or urine organophosphates profile.
- Check medications for interactions and nutrient depletions and correct with the help of testing in serum or urine. Refer to GP for a medication review if necessary.
- Encourage a good intake of high-calcium foods such as yogurt, milk, cheese, sardines and green leafy vegetables (Linus Pauling Institute n.d.).

Key points for the folate and methionine pathways

For the practitioner, this pathway may need addressing, of course. However, to blindly recommend B12 and folate without fully appreciating the effects of this on neurotransmission and transsulphuration may initiate undesirable effects.

Tests to consider

- Methylation profile.
- Red cell magnesium.
- Red blood cells (RBC) glutathione.
- Serum urea and electrolytes.
- Organic acids.

ELLA'S CASE: METHYLATION

As can be seen in Figure 5.3, Ella has many polymorphisms, both heterozygous (grey) and homozygous (black), within the folate and methionine cycles. These SNPs could potentially limit her ability to methylate. She may have a propensity towards poor cell membrane repair due to the PEMT gene, but MAT1 may also be slowing the conversion of methionine into methyltransferase towards PEMT. Ella also has possible poor conversion of folate to methylfolate, which drives methylation and biopterin via the DHFR enzyme.

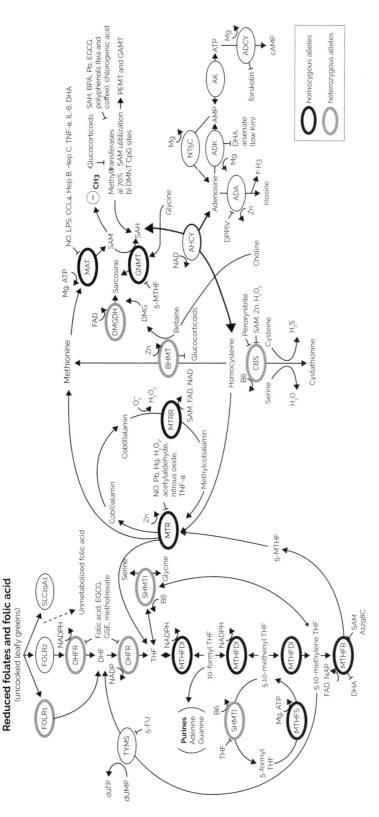

Figure 5.3: Ella's folate and methionine cycle SNPs

Source: Methylation Planner by Dr Ben Lynch (author of Dirty Genes and creator of StrateGene)

Homozygous polymorphisms are defined by thick black outlines. Heterozygous polymorphisms are defined by thick grey outlines.

Ella's folate cycle demonstrated a potential problem with folate metabolism (FOLR1, DHFR, MTHFD1, MTHFR, SHMT1, MTHFS) in the form of possible poor conversion of natural folate from food to methylfolate or 5-MTHF and also recycling of 5,10-methylene THF. This was confirmed with very high levels of formiminoglutamic acid (FiGlu) and moderately high levels of methylmalonic acid (MMA).

Ella's ability to add a methyl group to her cobalamin to create methylcobalamin may be compromised given her MTR and MTRR polymorphisms. This may have had an impact on her levels of MMA in urine. However, she may also have a suppressed ability to carry B12 into the cells due to TCN2 polymorphisms, and, of course, her gut health and her pyroluria may be compromising her ability to absorb and assimilate B12 from food.

As methylation is a homeostatic mechanism, as discussed earlier, Ella's methylation may have down-regulated more than usual, due to her near-death experience with the pneumonia. In this instance, although methylation may need to be addressed, if this is increased while Ella is still unwell, the body may make more sick cells (Pfeifer 2018) although there is still no firm conclusion in the evidence. Cole *et al.* (2007) report folate as being beneficial in the reduction of pre-cancerous cell formation but detrimental once cancer cells have established. This, according to Cole *et al.*, is due to the increased need for folate in cancer cells and the associated increase in folate receptors in cancer cells. This scenario, of course, appears to be tumour-promoting.

Another factor to consider is that once methylation is driven by folate, Ella's neurotransmitter production will increase, but at this time anxiety was still a fairly major issue without the full knowledge of the aetiology. To increase dopamine production if Ella was unable to assimilate it fully may lead to dopamine trapping and symptoms such as increased levels of anxiety, obsessive behaviours or even suicide ideology and/or psychosis. After some work supporting transsulphuration, Ella was able to use folinic acid effectively on days when she needed more brainpower.

At this point, it was decided to consider causes for genetic expression of Ella's methylation pathway and address those first. Recall her timeline of almost constant stress and autoimmunity, and, of course, she has the BHMT polymorphism which, when expressing, seems to clinically correspond with the internalization of stress. This was very clear from Ella's demeanour and the way she appeared to disassociate from highly stressful life events. MAT1 was also homozygous and this is the gene that precedes the gateway to the methyltransferase system and where SAMe and PC for cell membranes are produced.

Ella's previous near-death experience was quite profound. She reported a very significant emotional shock a few weeks prior to the onset of the pneumonia in which she immediately handed in her notice at work. She was then resident in a hotel with a mould issue and was unable to remove herself from the exposure. Ella was not overly concerned about the exposure as she was aware of her mould intolerance; this manifested as extreme fatigue and a barking cough with no evidence of infection otherwise. She would normally feel much better on arrival home and, if necessary, consider a short-term antifungal. This time was no exception. However, on the flight home Ella inadvertently was exposed to high-fructose corn syrup on her in-flight meal. Immediately, she suffered a quite severe asthmatic-type reaction as the mould from the exposure had created expression of her histamine genes (DAO, HNMT, MAO, ALDH), rendering her unable to break down the histamine from the high-fructose corn syrup. Recall these SNPs from Figure 3.3.

Luckily, a doctor on board the plane dealt with this, and following a full examination in Accident and Emergency on landing, she was discharged from the hospital. Ella continued to work after her arrival home and five days later collapsed; at this point the pneumonia was diagnosed and she was treated with antibiotics. After four rounds of antibiotics, Ella was not improving. Intravenous phospholipid exchange (PLX) was therefore initiated, in order to rebuild her cell membranes (see Chapter 3).

Day 1:

- 10 ampules intravenous phospholipid in 25ml dextrose 5% over one hour

Day 2:

- 10 ampules intravenous phospholipid in 250ml dextrose 5% over one hour
- 5ml intravenous phenylbutyrate in 250ml dextrose 5% over one hour

Day 3

- 5 ampules intravenous phospholipid in 100ml dextrose 5% over 30 minutes
- intravenous vitamin C: 10g in 250ml dextrose over 90 minutes.

This was in addition to oral PC, fatty acids and electrolytes as dictated by fatty acid analysis. Fatty acids included a range of flax, safflower, fish oil and evening primrose oil with PC liquid and PC capsules. Ella was initially very apprehensive at the need to consume 40ml of oils twice daily but reported that her body just cried out for the oils as soon as she put them to her lips. The environmental cause of genetic expression would seem to be the mould, yeast and bacterial overgrowth and the potentially sluggish cholecystokinin feedback loop. Low to moderate levels of mercury and arsenic were also evident on Ella's toxicology profile. Ella's metabolic markers of ethanolamine, phosphoethanolamine and phosphoserine were extremely low on the organic acids, as was glycine. These gave clear indication for the need to support cell membranes with a direct infusion of oils in the 4:1 balance of omega 6:3 as reported by Erasmus (1993) and Assies *et al.* (2010). Cell membrane modulation is now a recognized adjuvant therapy in naturopathic cancer (Zalba & Ten Hagen 2016), neurotoxic syndromes, depression (de Groot & Burgas 2015) and psychiatric disease (Haag 2003) treatments.

This approach helped Ella markedly. Her mobility and flexibility had improved with the gentle exercises. She was able to stand long enough to make a very quick, simple meal of steamed vegetables and protein. Her lower digestive symptoms had improved (wind, bloating) but she was still struggling with the gastroparesis symptoms of feeling heavy after tiny meals despite taking betaine HCL to support protein digestion, severe pain in the gastric region radiating through to lower thoracic spine, and sluggish bowels. She continued to make progress with the chiropractic NSA care. She found the sessions made her feeling amazing and so relaxed immediately afterwards, but she couldn't maintain the feeling between sessions. Her organic acid results had indicated possible small intestinal bacterial overgrowth (SIBO) (hydroxyphenylacetic acid, hydroxybenzoic acid and hydroxyhippuric acid) and this was consistent with her symptomology.

There was no SIBO-specific test undertaken at this time as it was felt to be counterproductive given Ella's anxiety and the inability to be able to recommend antimicrobials at this time due to her reactions to any new products or foods. She was doing well with the kitchari at lunchtime and the introduction of more vegetables and chicken in the evening. Her digestive system was showing small signs of improvement. Stool quality was improving, heaviness after eating was less and the open feeling Ella reported at the last consultation continued to improve and sustain for longer after the NSA appointments. To this end, a small number of organic herbs and spices were added to the kitchari on a daily basis. These included oregano, cinnamon, clove bud, cumin (seed and powder), coriander, rosemary, turmeric and black pepper. These offered anti-inflammatory (turmeric) and antimicrobial effects for Ella. The addition of vegetables and a switch from white rice to brown (soaked for 2–4 hours before cooking) gave Ella more variety. When Ella felt her blood glucose levels were a little unbalanced, she was advised to add a tiny portion of organic chicken to the meal.

Ella's supplementation 3

- Betaine HCL + pepsin 700mg caps x 3 per meal to support protein digestion in the stomach (Guilliams & Drake 2020).
- Digestive enzymes x 1 per meal to support digestion in the small intestine (Ianiro *et al.* 2016).
- Bifidobacteria x 2 daily to support detoxification, immunity, antihistamine and rebalancing of gut flora in the large intestine (O'Callaghan & van Sinderen 2016).

- *Lactobacillus plantarum, L. rhamnosus, L. salivaricus* x 1 daily to support immunity in the small intestine and reduce histamine (Krzyściak *et al.* 2017; Sasikumar *et al.* 2017; Segers & Lebeer 2014).
- Liposomal glutathione x 4 sprays daily due to elevated levels of pyroglutamic acid and 2-hydroxybutyric acids on the organic acid result and to poor transsulphuration (see the section on transsulphuration later in the chapter).
- Broccoli seed extract x 1 tsp twice daily in water to support microbiome diversity, reduce gut inflammation, antihistamine and detoxification of oestrogen (Heber *et al.* 2014).
- Phosphatidylcholine 10ml daily to support cell membranes and mucin (Van der Veen *et al.* 2017).
- 4:1 balance of omega 6:3 oils 10ml daily mixed with PC for cell membrane repair and stability.
- KPU multimineral was changed to a methylated multivitamin and mineral.
- B6, zinc and magnesium combination (to ensure pyroluria was still supported) alongside methylation.
- Methyl and adenosyl cobalamin (active B12) with 5-MTHF as a lozenge due to high urinary MMA and uracil (1. Bailey, 2. Sun).

Lifestyle interventions

Ella wanted to continue with trampet rebounding and add in beginners Pilates once weekly.

Ella was to continue with her weekly walking group and gradually extend the walk distance if possible.

Ella particularly enjoyed the HeartMath techniques and found she was able to incorporate them into her chiropractic care to enhance the effects.

Ella also reported that the breathing techniques were helping her to meditate, too. She was managing around a half-hour daily. As her breathing and meditation improved, her digestive function also improved. This was presumably because all the therapies Ella was combining to combat her anxiety were affecting her vagal tone (Gerritsen & Band 2018). This in turn may be modulating the gut–brain axis (Breit *et al.* 2018). Ella had also noticed that specific traumas she was holding from childhood were surfacing gently due to the NSA practice. As the traumas surfaced, Ella also reported great insight that helped her to process them quickly. This was an unexpected bonus.

Transsulphuration cycle

The transsulphuration cycle is primarily focused on the regulation of cysteine levels and the production of glutathione. Homocysteine provides the cysteine substrate for the formation of glutathione, taurine, sulphate, hydrogen sulphide and some TCA cycle intermediaries such as pyruvate. Those practitioners who have been supporting patients with autism spectrum conditions may be more familiar with transsulphuration as researchers such as Rosemary Waring of the University of Birmingham wrote extensively on the topic prior to her retirement. Stephanie Seneff is a world-leading authority on sulphation for practitioners who would like more information. Many practitioners know of the virtues of the Epsom salts (magnesium sulphate) bath to provide much-needed sulphate when the transsulphuration cycle fails to deliver (Adams *et al.* 2018). Magnesium is a very useful (Ismail & Ismail 2016) and much-needed by-product of the therapy but not usually the main therapeutic aim.

Why do we need sulphate?
The main findings of Dr Waring's research (Waring n.d.; Waring & Klovrza 2000) highlighted higher plasma levels of sulphites concurrent with higher protein excretion and lower levels of sulphate in autism. This would suggest a poor conversion from sulphite to sulphate at the end of the transsulphuration cycle, resulting in many aberrant functions within digestion and assimilation and, of course, in the biopterin cycle. Inorganic sulphate is essential for cell growth and other physiological mechanisms that are critical for the life of the organism. Being so crucial to life, sulphate is the fourth most abundant ion in plasma (Markovich & Aronson 2007).

Sulphation helps the body to neutralize and eliminate used neurotransmitters (Cook *et al.* 2017), maintains gut integrity (Tobisawa *et al.* 2010) via sulphated glycoproteins, helps release various digestive enzymes (Pomin 2017) and metabolizes a number of drugs (Levy 1986). In fact, poor sulphation can also lead to salicylate and/or phenol sensitivity, encouraging sensitivity to many foods of salicylate or phenol nature and therefore a very restricted diet in many cases. Sulphate is vastly underappreciated. It protects the blood from coagulation (Na *et al.* 2012), detoxifies food additives and environmental toxins such as aluminium and mercury. Sulphate is an essential component of extracellular matrix proteins throughout all body tissues. Cerebrosides sulphate is a major component of myelin sheath. Sulphated glycosaminoglycans (GAGs) are crucial for maintaining the negative charge of cells and for protecting from infection (Seneff 2014). This makes it one of the most crucial biochemical processes in the body and yet the research is not fully adopted into mainstream or natural medicine. Interestingly, recent advances in the evidence are pointing towards SIBO as being an adaptive mechanism to provide sulphation (Nigh 2019).

Glutathione

Glutathione is the body's major antioxidant, being present in all tissues. Some functions of glutathione include epigenetic mechanisms (García-Giménez *et al.* 2017), xenobiotic metabolism (Wu *et al.* 2004), immune system support (Fraternale *et al.* 2017), cell proliferation and apoptosis (Circu & Aw 2012) and phase 2-biotransformation conjugation (Jancova *et al.* 2010).

Deficiency or dysregulation of glutathione has been associated with a number of diseases such as cancer (Traverso *et al.* 2013), liver disease (Lu 2020), cognitive impairment (Rae & Williams 2017), cystic fibrosis (Kettle *et al.* 2014), neurodegenerative disorders (Aoyama & Nakaki 2013), Parkinson's disease (Coles *et al.* 2017) and ulcerative colitis (Loguercio *et al.* 2003) to name a few.

In situations of high oxidative stress, the glutathione-S-transferase genes are up-regulated. However, 20–50% of the population are said to have an absence of the GSTM1 gene, which decreases the ability of the host to detoxify effectively. When excessively exposed to environmental triggers such as pollution, smoking and/or heavy metals, conditions such as asthma, cancer, cardiovascular disease, hypertension and autism may be more likely.

Low levels of the amino acid substrates (glycine, cysteine and glutamic acid) may contribute to poor production of glutathione, and this is why lots of studies on NAC supplementation have been undertaken. While some studies have shown promise in the use of NAC in a variety of disorders, other studies have shown that polymorphisms in the GST gene may determine the efficacy of this as a therapeutic intervention (Rushworth & Megson 2014).

Hypochlorhydria is another consideration as low levels of stomach acid or digestive enzymes limit the host ability to break down food proteins into amino acids. Stress, ageing and nutrient deficiencies such as pyridoxine and zinc may all contribute, as does poor sulphation of the cholecystokinin feedback loop (Nigh 2019).

Inflammation anywhere in the body will use up vital glutathione stores readily, so ensuring an anti-inflammatory nutritional and lifestyle approach can be very useful. Finally, glutathione is continually recycled from oxidized to reduced glutathione in the lower part of the transsulphuration pathway. Too much oxidized glutathione increases inflammation for some who choose to supplement with glutathione. If they oxidize it and can't recycle it back due to low levels of riboflavin, then supplementing can be counterproductive. Recycling from reduced glutathione requires selenium, but again too much may increase the inflammatory response (Ashoori & Saedisomeolia 2014).

Polymorphisms associated with transsulphuration

CBS, CTH, GCL, GSS, GGT, GSR, GST; CDO1, CSAD, SUOX, PAPSS; AHCY, ADA, SOD, MPO, CAT, GPX, G6PD.

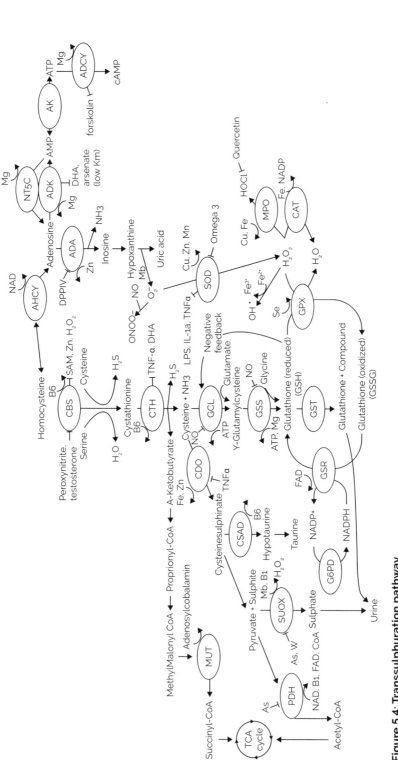

Figure 5.4: Transsulphuration pathway

Source: Methylation Planner by Dr Ben Lynch (author of Dirty Genes and creator of StrateGene)

When following the pathway planner, four routes can be identified within the transsulphuration pathway. The vertical axis converts homocysteine to glutathione; to the right, S-adenosyl homocysteine takes the route down to uric acid and eventually to hydrogen peroxide. To the left, cysteine becomes pyruvate for the TCA cycle, taurine and sulphate. Alpha-ketobutyrate becomes succinyl coA for the TCA cycle. The genes and enzymes will be traced in this order for ease.

Cystathione beta-synthase:
CBS – glutathione production

The CBS enzyme (C699T, A360A, N212N) is the first step in the conversion of homocysteine to glutathione. It converts homocysteine to cystathionine by condensing homocysteine with serine. CBS pathway up-regulations mean a faster clearance of homocysteine but not necessarily higher levels of glutathione, so a slow enzyme further down may result in higher levels of ammonia production alongside urinary sulphites, in addition to lower levels of glutathione synthesis and/or possible imbalances in glutathione redox reactions. A major catastrophe that could also occur is a high loss of methyl groups because these may be drawn down the up-regulated CBS pathway. CBS is like a leaking sump drain where the fluid contents eternally drip rather than collect. The primary antioxidant in every cell is glutathione. Methyl groups are required to create to synthesize phosphatidylcholine; and in reactions involving neurotransmitters, creatine, carnitine and antioxidants (such as glutathione and taurine). So the loss of methyl groups can be catastrophic and lead the body into a cell danger response (Naviaux 2013). A functional vitamin D receptor (VDR) is also necessary for CBS to function effectively (Kriebitzsch *et al.* 2011).

There is no simple way to discern if the CBS enzyme is up-regulating, although there does appear to be a decrease in toxic metal release in hair, stool and urine samples. When practitioners are considering the symptomology of a potential CBS up-regulation, they may also need to consider a BHMT down-regulation, as this would likely predispose to similar effects – recall this was discussed under the BHMT gene.

The CBS enzyme can also be down-regulated. GABA/glutamate balance is also relevant with the CBS enzyme as an up-regulation may also cause increase alpha-ketoglutarate that in turn converts to glutamate, which is excitatory to the brain (Yudkoff 2012).

Sulphur metabolism may also be altered with expression of this gene and subsequent up-regulation of its respective enzyme. High levels of sulphur dioxide (Bai & Meng 2010) and sulphites (Berry *et al.* 2020) may be evident, which can be toxic. During highly toxic states, the body attempts to create more cysteine in order for the conversion of thiol-containing antioxidants metallothionein and glutathione. However, cysteine has a high degree of reactivity so it is likely to oxidize to sulphur dioxide and hydrogen sulphide. Down-regulation of genes and enzymes below CBS in the transsulphuration cycle may lead to an accumulation of these toxic substances. However, hydrogen sulphide neutralizes methyl mercury so an increase may also be an adaptive mechanism to neutralize this (Yoshida *et al.* 2011).

In Down's syndrome, an up-regulated CBS enzyme is well known for being causal in the increased amount of cystathione and cysteine (Pogribna *et al.* 2011). The debate continues as to whether this happens in others. It is now widely accepted that CBS is a rate-limiting enzyme (Maclean 2002).

Possible interventions based on CBS genetic expression
Cofactors to support CBS enzyme activity
B6, serine, haem (Lynch 2017), zinc (Cohen 2015).

Helpful or unhelpful (dependent on expression)
inhibitors that reduce CBS enzyme activity
Nitric oxide and hyperhomocysteinemia (Lynch 2017), antacids (Gaviscon, Alka-Seltzer, Milk of Magnesia, Pepto-Bismol), ACE inhibitors (enalopril, lisinopril, ramipril), casein (dairy), diuretics (furosemide, bendroflumethiazide, spironolactone), HRT, cadmium (cigarettes, metal plating, plastics) (Cohen 2015).

Inducers that increase CBS enzyme activity
Hydrogen sulphide (Hellmich *et al.* 2015) thought to be the third gas produced by small intestinal bacterial overgrowth (Banik *et al.* 2016).

Practical advice
CBS up-regulations can cause increased levels of ammonia and taurine, especially when conversion of homocysteine to glutathione is poor. When analyzing CBS up-regulations, the following may be considered:

- Elevated urinary sulphites above 800. If these are consistently above 1000, then CBS up-regulation is likely (Jethva 2019).
- Elevated ammonia (orotate, citrate, isocitrate) on organic acids.
- Elevated taurine (taurine is synthesized by cysteine) on organic acids.
- Blood urea nitrogen (BUN) above 20.
- Elevated serum alanine aminotransferase ALT.
- Decreased homocysteine.
- Cravings or aversions to sulphur foods (may also be reflective of SIBO).
- Sleepy after glutamine ingestion.
- Elevated orotate, citrate and isocitrate on organic acids may indicate elevated ammonia.

When assessing for CBS down-regulations, please consider the following:

- Low ammonia (organic acids (OAT)).
- Low taurine (OAT).
- High homocysteine (OAT/serum).
- Low B6 (OAT).
- Low RBC glutathione.
- Sulphite to sulphate conversion poor.
- Check for symptoms of CBS up-regulation such as cravings, aversions or sensitivity to sulphur-rich foods (onions, garlic, brassicas and eggs). Also check for aggressive or sedated behaviour after consuming glutamine.

- Check CBS up-regulation with down-regulation of enzymes further down the pathway.
- Check medication nutrient depletions and refer to the GP for a medication review if necessary.
- Check for heavy metals and address as necessary.
- Consider butyrate to sequester ammonia (Bedford & Gong 2018) and check kidney function in serum (urea, creatinine, eGFR).
- May need to encourage low-sulphur diet initially until pathway has been supported and dysbiosis has been brought under control.
- Check B6 and zinc levels in serum and recommend as necessary.

PRACTITIONER NOTES

Plasma homocysteine is a gross average rather than a tissue-specific measure. Recall there are three possible routes for the metabolism of homocysteine. Much of homocysteine is metabolized by the long route (MTR/MTRR) and short route (BHMT). Roughly 50% is eliminated via the CBS enzyme as the only elimination route. The CBS enzyme has been discussed in this section as part of the methionine cycle for completeness. Questions to ask clients below are related to this.

- MTR/MTRR – requires B12 and MTHF (Lynch 2017).
- BHMT – requires trimethylglycine (TMG), dimethylglycine (DMG) and zinc. TMG contains more methyl donors (Lynch 2017; Cohen 2015).
- CBS – requires B6 (P-5-P) (Lynch 2017; Cohen 2015).

Questions to ask clients:

- Is there a family history of cardiovascular disease, dementia, cancer, non-insulin dependent diabetes (type 2), autism spectrum disorders and/or rheumatoid arthritis?
- Are there symptoms of generalized inflammation?

- Are there any fertility issues, especially recurrent miscarriages?
- Are hormonal imbalances prominent (PMT/menopause)?
- Is there excessive fatigue?

With overexpression of CBS and/or reduced activity in the lower part of this cycle, there is a strong likelihood of producing too much ammonia and/or cysteine/taurine/sulphites, so do pay close attention to this. This can also occur if too much pyridoxine is recommended to support CBS. It is really important, particularly here, to commence with low doses, slowly increasing with nutrient support.

Cystathione gamma-lyase: CTH

This enzyme encodes the cytosolic protein cystathionine gamma-lyase, which converts cystathionine to cysteine and has one common single allele G1364T. Studies have associated this enzyme with elevated levels of homocysteine (Wang *et al.* 2004) via down-regulation and pre-eclampsia (Mrozikiewicz *et al.* 2015) so it has been included for completeness. However, many genetic companies are not measuring CTH.

PRACTITIONER NOTES

Consult the section on CBS expression.

Glutamate cysteine ligase: GCLC

GCLC encodes the protein for the enzyme glutamate cysteine ligase. This enzyme is responsible for the conversion of cysteine to glutamyl-cysteine. Expression as a down-regulation on the rs17883901 allele has been linked to sulfamethoxazole sensitivity (Wang *et al.* 2012) and glutathione deficiency in mycotoxin illness (Guilford & Hope 2014). Dr Ben Lynch is the first to account for the action of this enzyme in his genetic analysis. It may become a prominent gene/enzyme to observe for the future. GCLC levels increase with cysteine depletion (Lee *et al.* 2006).

Possible interventions based on GCLC genetic expression
Nutrient cofactors to support GCLC enzyme activity
ATP, manganese, magnesium and glutamate.

Unhelpful inhibitors that reduce GCLC enzyme activity
Myctoxin and TGF-β1. The latter is known to be regulate cell maturation and growth and is frequently up-regulated in tumour growth (www.ncbi.nlm.nih.gov/gene/7040).

Practical advice

- Consider options as included in CBS enzyme practitioner advice above.
- Encourage foods high in manganese (brown rice, peanuts, pecan, almonds and pineapple) and magnesium (whole grains if tolerated, green leafy vegetables, nuts and seeds – especially hazelnuts and cashews) (Linus Pauling Institute n.d.).
- Check for mould exposure and signs of mycotoxin illness and address as appropriate.
- Check glutathione levels in serum or urine organic acids and correct as appropriate.

Glutathione Synthetase: GSS

The GSS gene encodes the enzyme glutathione synthase, which in turn participates in the gamma-glutamyl cycle to create glutathione in all cells. In addition to the antioxidant capacity of glutathione, medications and cancer-causing compounds are also processed. It also helps to build DNA and proteins. This gene can be down-regulated or deleted (Chattopadhyay *et al.* 2013).

More than 30 mutations have been found in glutathione synthase deficiency, related to abnormal destruction of blood cells. Neutropenia has also been identified in children with GSS deficiency (Humphreys *et al.* 2005), as has haemolytic anaemia. Long-term clinical outcome appears to offer some degree of amelioration with supplementation of vitamins C and E (Ristoff *et al.* 2001), depending on severity. The GSS enzyme is said to transfer glutathione into the mitochondria via NDUFS7. This gene seems to be crucial for the biogenesis of complex 1 in the electron transport chain (Lebon *et al.* 2007). It has not been included in the gene descriptors as it is a novel gene not measured on most genetic tests and the evidence is limited.

Possible interventions based on GSS genetic expression
Nutrient cofactors to support GSS enzyme activity
Magnesium, glycine and ATP (Lynch 2017).

Helpful inducers and substrates that stimulate GSS enzyme activity
Tumour necrosis factor (TNFα), nuclear factor kappa B (NF-kB) and nuclear factor (erythroid-derived 2) (NRF2), assuming all other factors are addressed (Lynch 2017).

Unhelpful inhibitors that reduce GSS enzyme function
Infection, human immunodeficiency virus, surgical trauma, heavy drinking (Lynch 2017), corticosteroids (prednisolone, hydrocortisone) HRT, antibiotics, sulphonamides (sulphadiazine), ADHD stimulants (methylphenidate) (Cohen 2015).

Practical advice

- Check underlying cause for inflammation and infection (gut health) and address as appropriate.
- Check for medicine interactions and depletions and refer to GP for medication review as appropriate.
- Check underlying viral load and address as appropriate.
- Encourage foods high in magnesium (whole grains if tolerated, green leafy vegetables, nuts and seeds, especially hazelnuts and cashews).

- Encourage foods high in glycine (bone broth, meat, gelatine, chicken, seafood).
- Support ATP production via an antioxidant-rich diet; balance blood glucose levels with good-quality protein and fats; eliminate extrinsic sugars (Chanseaume *et al.* 2006).

Glutathione reductase: GSR

This gene (rs2551755 and rs3594) encodes a homodimeric (composed of two polypeptide chains) flavoprotein that is central to reducing oxidized glutathione disulphide (GSSG) to the sulphydryl form (GSH), an important cellular antioxidant. This enzyme maintains optimal levels of glutathione in cytosol. The ratio of GSSG to GSH within the cell is the key factor controlling oxidative balance of the cell. Mutations or down-regulation due to SNPs in this gene may predispose to hereditary glutathione reductase deficiency, pyridoxine deficiency and haemolytic anaemia due to glutathione reductase deficiency. It has also been highly associated with systemic lupus erythematosus in African Americans (Ramos *et al.* 2013).

GSR works in tandem with the GST family and GPX, and it also recycles NADP + NADPH via G6PD, to be discussed further.

Possible interventions based on GSR genetic expression
Nutrient cofactors to support GSR enzyme activity
FAD (Lynch 2017).

Unhelpful inhibitors that reduce GSR enzyme activity
Arsenic and reactive nitrogen species (Lynch 2017).

Practical advice

- Test for arsenic in hair, lymphocytes or urine if suspected and rebalance.
- Avoid rice and groundwater (arsenic).
- Check levels of riboflavin in serum and address if needed.

- Check glutathione levels and address if needed.
- Ensure oxidized glutathione is being recycled back to reduced glutathione as too much oxidized glutathione can lead to anxiety.
- Support with foods high in riboflavin (milk, yogurt, cheese, chicken, beef, fish and egg) and supplement as necessary. Those with dairy intolerance may be more prone to riboflavin deficiency (Powers *et al.* 2011).

Glutathione peroxidase: GPX

This gene (rs8177412) encodes extracellular glutathione peroxidase, which detoxifies hydrogen peroxide, lipid peroxidation and oxygen hydroperoxide. In simple terms, GPX3 scavenges peroxides, thereby offering cellular protection by maintaining redox balance within cells. When expressing, there is a down-regulation or slow activity of this enzyme. The function of GPX is to oxidize reduced glutathione along with GST. It is generally expressed in the placenta, lung, breast and kidney. This gene is often down-regulated in a variety of cancer cases (Chen *et al.* 2011) and may be an important factor in cerebrovascular accident (Polonikov *et al.* 2012). It has, however, been shown to become positively regulated by 17β-estradiol in skeletal muscle (Baltgalvis *et al.* 2010). Selenium-methylselenocysteine has been shown to support enzyme activity. GPX3 has also been identified as having decreased activity in prostate cancer, thyroid, cervical, gastric and colon cancers, suggesting a possible role in carcinogenesis modulation (Sekine *et al.* 2011).

GPX also supports the breakdown of hydrogen peroxide with catalase (CAT). The production of hydrogen peroxide is a split-second reaction within cells, used by the cells to keep bacteria in check. However, if GPX and CAT are unable to reduce the hydrogen peroxide levels, this can become highly toxic, initiating the cell danger response. Other genes that manage hydrogen peroxide levels include MPO, SOD2 and SOD3.

Possible interventions based on GPX genetic expression
Nutrient cofactors to support GPX enzyme activity
Selenium (Lynch 2017).

Unhelpful inhibitors that reduce GPX enzyme function
High levels of mercury, copper, iron and zinc, low levels of selenium, dopamine quinone, heavy drinking (Lynch 2017), statins, co-careldopa, tricyclic antidepressants (amitriptyline, imipramine), antacids (Gaviscon, Rennie, Alka-Seltzer, Milk of Magnesia) (Cohen 2015).

Practical advice

- Check for heavy metals and address as appropriate.
- Check medication interactions and depletions and correct as appropriate; refer to GP for medication review if indicated.
- Encourage foods high in selenium (beef, chicken, pork, Brazil nuts, sunflower seeds, tuna, clams and shrimp).
- Testing for serum selenium is difficult to undertake. Hair and nail are more common for long-standing issues. Correct as appropriate.

Myeloperoxidase: MPO

This is a peroxidase enzyme encoded by the MPO gene. It is generally expressed in neutrophils, and the haem pigment it contains gives pus the green colour when the pus or mucous is rich in neutrophils. MPO creates hypochlorous acid from hydrogen peroxide. This too can create much free-radical damage if it becomes unregulated. Down-regulated expression of the rs2333227 allele has been linked to Alzheimer's disease (Ji & Zhang 2017), lung cancer, gastric cancer and lupus in much older studies; however, Yang *et al.* (2013) in a meta-analysis of 22 cases found no correlation with lung cancer.

Wang *et al.* (2011) later produced a further meta-analysis of 66 cases and concluded that the MPO-463G polymorphism may be a useful marker for producing a protective effect in gastric cancer. However, it may also provide a marker for risk of lung cancer but only in Asians.

Possible interventions based on MPO genetic expression
Nutrient cofactors to support MPO enzyme activity
Copper and iron (Lynch 2017).

Unhelpful inhibitors that reduce MPO enzyme activity
Sulphonamides (dapsone) and non-steroidal anti-inflammatory medicines (indomethacin) (Malle *et al.* 2007).

Practical advice

- Support digestion as appropriate.
- Check medication interactions and depletions and address as appropriate; refer to GP for medication review if indicated.
- Check copper and iron levels and correct if necessary.
- Encourage foods high in iron (haem iron – red meat; non-haem iron – lentils and vegetables especially the dark green leafy type).
- Encourage foods high in copper (oysters, clams, crab, hazelnuts, almonds, peas, beans, lentils and liver).
- Check for high zinc intake – zinc depletes copper, as does vitamin C.
- Consider chlorophyll drinks to support copper needs.

Superoxide dismutase: SOD

The SOD gene is a member of the iron/manganese superoxide dismutase family. It encodes a mitochondrial protein that forms a homotetramer (four identical sub-units, associated but not covalently bonded). Superoxide dismutase is an important antioxidant system which degrades superoxide radicals into oxygen and hydrogen peroxide. There are three forms of SOD, aptly named SOD1, 2 and 3. There is some tentative literature suggesting SOD1 mutations may be over-expressed or up-regulated, contributing to higher levels of hydrogen peroxide, but this gene is still poorly understood. Some studies (such as Banci *et al.* 2008) have linked mutations in SOD1 to amyotrophic lateral sclerosis. Xie *et al.* (2015) have proposed a mechanistic link via mediated impairment of late endosome transport to autophagy-lysosomal deficits and mitochondrial pathology. This is a zinc- and copper-dependent enzyme.

There is more literature supporting mutation effects in SOD2 and 3. SOD3 (rs2855262) is thought to protect the lungs and brain from oxidative stress. It protects the extracellular space from the toxic effects of superoxide free radicals. The risk allele rs1799895 has been associated with a higher cardiovascular and emphysema risk (Juul *et al.* 2004). SOD3 is also copper- and zinc-dependent.

SOD2 has a number of alternative names such as IPO-B, IPOB, MnSOD, Mn-SOD and MVCD6. These are all names the practitioner may see in the literature. SOD2 is the manganese-dependent form of the SODs enzymes. Mutations have been linked to prostate cancer (Li *et al.* 2016), especially in smokers (Woodson *et al.* 2003).

Possible interventions based on SOD genetic expression
Nutrient cofactors to support SOD enzyme activity
Manganese, copper and zinc (Lynch 2017).

Unhelpful inhibitors that reduce SOD enzyme activity
Aluminium, selenium, insulin-like growth factor 1, high-fat diet (SOD2) and aluminium, transforming growth factor 1, platelet-derived growth factor, fibroblast growth factor (SOD3) (Lynch 2017), antacids (Gaviscon, Rennie, Alka-Seltzer, Milk of Magnesia), resveratrol supplements, antivirals (oseltamivir, acyclovir), zinc, oral contraceptives (Cohen 2015).

Practical advice

- Balance blood glucose levels.
- Check for the use of antacids (reduce stomach acid capacity) and address digestive distress if this is an issue.
- Test for heavy metals via urine, serum or lymphocyte sensitivity and address as appropriate.
- Encourage foods high in manganese (brown rice, pecans, pineapple), copper (chlorophyll drinks, liver, oysters, cashew nuts, lentils) and zinc (oysters, crab, beef, dark meat, pork, black beans and chickpeas).

Glucose-6-phosphate dehydrogenase: G6PD

G6PD encodes the protein for the glucose-6-phosphate enzyme. This enzyme (rs2230037, rs722554664, rs1050829 and rs1050828) is involved in the pentose phosphate pathway. The major role of this pathway is to generate NADPH, which in turn protects the red blood cells from free-radical damage. It also generates ribulose-5-phosphate for the synthesis of nucleotides. G6PD deficiency is one of the most common human enzyme defects, occurring in more than 400 million people worldwide (Von Seidlein *et al.* 2013). G6PD deficiency has been identified in numerous types of tumour (Hu *et al.* 2013).

Another name for G6PD deficiency is favism due to the links with certain negative reactions to the fava bean, a cousin of the broad bean. The fava bean is dried on the plant and harvested much later than the broad bean. The x-linked genetic predisposition to favism may cause spontaneous haemolysis of red blood cells, resulting in jaundice, as a result of coming into contact with certain medications (aspirin, quinine, other antimalarials and sulphonamides) (Luzzatto & Seneca 2014), fava beans, moth balls (naphthalene) and stress from bacterial or viral infections. Not all individuals with G6PD deficiency will show symptoms of favism and the condition appears more prevalent in children and in Mediterranean and African communities. Some studies have demonstrated a correlation between iron overload and G6PD deficiency (Pigatto *et al.* 2016). These patients should be considered at risk due to increased bone marrow activity. Sterling Hill Erdei (2014) has also identified fluoroquinolones as risk factors for those with G6PD deficiency according to anecdotal research.

Possible interventions based on G6PD genetic expression
Nutrient cofactors to support G6PD enzyme activity
Magnesium (Burhanettin *et al.* 2012).

Unhelpful inhibitors that reduce G6PD enzyme function
Aluminium, DHEA, high levels of cAMP, quinolinic acid, TNFα, aldosterone, DHA, high levels of omega 6 fatty acids.

Practical advice

- Check heavy metals (aluminium) and advise removal of all cooking foils, anti-perspirants and cosmetics.
- Check HPA axis function (DHEA) and address as appropriate.
- Check red cell fatty acids and address if indicated.
- Check quinolinic acid on organic acids and correct if indicated. Evaluate kynurenine pathway SNPs and metabolic markers.
- Encourage foods high in magnesium (whole grains, green leafy vegetables, nuts and seeds, especially cashews and hazelnuts).
- Check red cell magnesium and supplement oral or transdermal as appropriate.

Glutathione S-transferase: GST

GST encodes the cytosolic and membrane forms of glutathione S-transferase.

The common alleles of GST include GSTM1 (specific to the brain), GSTT1 and GSTP1 (specific to the biliary tract). Roughly 50% of the general population have null genotype, or a homozygous deletion of GSTM1; 92% are said to have a heterozygous/null genotype. This enzyme is slower functioning. The wild type is the unchanged gene. As the enzyme is instructed to conjugate electrophilic xenobiotics with glutathione for excretion via urine and bile, this could predispose the person to a higher level of environmental toxicity than usual (Conklin & Bhatnagar 2011). As previously mentioned, this could be a risk factor for the development of acute myeloid leukaemia (Dunna *et al.* 2013). GSTP1 is also located in the brain, heart, lungs, testes, skin, kidney and pancreas (Bocedi *et al.* 2019).

Savukaitytė *et al.* (2015) studied 80 young breast cancer patients and identified women with GSTT1 null genotype and SULT1A1 G638A AA genotype. The women with GSTT1 null genotype had 3.5 times higher risk of cancer progression than those with wild-type presentation. Those who also had SULT1A1 G638A AA genotype were more likely to have HER2 breast cancer. The authors suggest these could be useful genetic markers for breast cancer prognosis.

Allocati *et al.* (2018) have identified polymorphisms in GST genes to be associated with a variety of diseases such as Alzheimer's, epilepsy, Parkinson's, spinocerebellar ataxia type 2 and amyotrophic lateral sclerosis. The GSTs also appear to be the main detoxification route of alatoxin B1 and some anticancer drugs (canfosfamide). Piperlongumin has been developed to inhibit the GST enzyme in order to maximize the effects of chemotherapy.

Possible interventions based on GST genetic expression
Helpful inducers of GST enzyme activity
Butyrate (Pool-Zobel *et al.* 2005), brassica and allium family of vegetables (Minich & Brown 2019), resveratrol (Chow *et al.* 2010).

Unhelpful inhibitors of GST enzyme activity
Synthetic and naturally occurring phenols, quinones, dopamine (Bolton & Dunlap 2017).

Practical advice

- Nutritional approach for GST enzyme dysfunction:
  - Increase cruciferous vegetables and alliums.
  - Increase antioxidant status with 80% plant-based nutrition.
  - Increase phytonutrients (Minich & Brown 2019).
  - Increase GSH precursors and cofactors including methionine-rich foods, N-acetyl cysteine, glutamine, glycine, pyridoxine and magnesium.
  - Limit glutathione depletion with alpha-lipoic acid (Minich & Brown 2019), milk thistle and taurine.
- Curcumin may shift the emphasis to glutathione rather than taurine (Biswas *et al.* 2005).
- Minimize exposure to xenobiotics including polycyclic aromatic hydrocarbons and toxic metals.

We head back up the pathway to the CBS gene again and this time track to the right-hand side.

Adenosylhomocysteinase: AHCY

AHCY (rs819147, rs41301825) is another important gene in the methionine cycle. It encodes for the enzyme S-adenosylhomocysteine hydrolase, which converts S-adenosylhomocysteine to either adenosine or homocysteine. This conversion is reversible to ensure the regulation of intracellular S-adenosylhomocysteine concentration and the production of methyl groups. If S-adenosylhomocysteine rises too high, the production of S-adenosylmethionine is impaired. Supplementing SAMe at this point could overload an already compromised pathway, so care needs to be taken. Although nutritional therapists are not permitted to recommend SAMe in the UK, some patients may be self-administering. Excessive intake of SAMe can induce free-radical damage and lipid peroxidation. Also an expressing down-regulation of AHCY may lead to hypermethioninemia. While many may not display symptomology associated with AHCY expression, others may suffer developmental delay or muscle weakness, and body excretions of sweat, breath and urine may have a distinctive smell resembling boiled cabbage. It is important for the practitioner to rule out homocysteineuria, tyrosinemia and galactosemia as other possible causes, in addition to excessive dietary intake of methionine-based foods. Adenosine is also vital for promoting healthy sleep (Landolt 2018).

Possible interventions based on AHCY genetic expression
Nutrient cofactors for to support AHCY enzyme activity
NAD (Hill Erdei & Ledowski 2015), magnesium and manganese (Lynch 2017).

Unhelpful inhibitors that reduce AHCY enzyme activity
Copper, NADH+, epigallocatechin gallate, methylthioadenosine and hypoxia or ischaemia (Lynch 2017).

Practical advice

- Check copper levels and possible zinc:copper ratios.
- Check predisposition towards hypoxia and ischaemia (comorbidities of the heart and lung such as chronic obstructive pulmonary disease). Also check for mouth breathing and refer for sleep studies as appropriate.
- Check green tea intake and reduce if necessary.
- Encourage foods high in niacin (beef, fish, poultry, beans, peas and lentils), manganese (whole grains, peanuts, almonds, pineapple) and magnesium (whole grains if tolerated, green leafy vegetables and nuts and seeds).

Adenosine deaminase: ADA

The ADA gene encodes for the adenosine deaminase enzyme and is present in all mammalian cells. It has a primary function of development and maintenance of the immune system, with ADA deficiency being a common cause of severe combined immunodeficiency (SCID) (Rubinstein 2016). This generally presents prior to the age of six months (Hershfield 2017) with diarrhoea, serious lung infection and failure to thrive. However, some individuals have partial ADA deficiency resulting in a more benign condition and fairly normal immunity.

ADA converts adenosine to inosine which then is also involved in purine metabolism and the production of cyclic adenosine monophosphate (cAMP). Purines are primarily synthesized as nucleotides and attached to ribose-5-phosphate.

Possible interventions based on ADA genetic expression
Nutrient cofactors to support ADA enzyme activity
Zinc (Hill Erdei & Ledowski 2015), magnesium (Lynch 2017).

Unhelpful inhibitors that reduce ADA enzyme activity

- Curcumin (Akinyemi *et al.* 2017).

- Nettle in prostate cancer cases (Durak *et al.* 2004).
- Mercury (Bellé *et al.* 2009).
- Progesterone in epilepsy cases (Pençe *et al.* 2009).

Practical advice

- Check heavy metals in hair, serum and/or urine and address as appropriate.
- Check for diabetes medications and possible berberine use.
- Check digestive health and function and address as appropriate.
- Serum zinc can be difficult to measure (Wieringa *et al.* 2015) so consider hair mineral testing.
- Encourage foods high in magnesium (green leafy vegetables, nuts and seeds) and zinc (oysters, crab, beef, dark meat and pork, chickpeas and black beans).
- Supplement with magnesium and zinc if indicated.

Having already discussed CBS and CTH above, it is now appropriate to venture across to the left of the transsulphuration pathway. This arm of transsulphuration converts cysteine to taurine, sulphate and TCA cycle intermediaries. Travelling from CTH again, the next gene is CDO1. This gene maintains hepatic concentration of intracellular free cysteine.

Cysteine dehydrogenase: CDO1

This gene encodes the enzyme cysteine dioxygenase type 1 to catalyze the first stage of cysteine oxidation to cysteine sulphate or sulphino-alanine which can be converted to taurine or pyruvate and sulphite. Inhibition of this enzyme may lead to cysteine excitotoxicty; the symptoms of this are anger and headaches. As many pathogens create sulphur by-products, it is very important to reduce pathogenic activity in order to stabilize gene expression of CDO. This should also include assessment for heavy metals due to them being a precursor to pathogenic activity. Interestingly, Adams and Shearer (2020) have written extensively about how yeast (in pathogenic form) and mould express CDO enzyme activity.

Possible interventions based on CDO1 genetic expression
Nutrient cofactors to support CDO1 enzyme activity
Iron and oxygen, in the absence of cysteine CDO, may become inactive (Dominy *et al.* 2008).

Unhelpful inhibitors that reduce CDO1 enzyme activity
Tumour necrosis factor alpha (Lynch 2017).

Practical advice

- Check for heavy metals and address as appropriate.
- Test and correct dysbiosis (urine and stool).
- Encourage anti-inflammatory diet such as Mediterranean (Sureda *et al.* 2018).
- Encourage foods high in cysteine (all protein, especially chicken, turkey, yogurt and cheese) and iron (red meat and dark green leafy vegetables).

Cysteine sulphinic acid decarboxylase: CSAD

This gene encodes the rate-limiting enzyme involved in taurine synthesis. The CSAD enzyme catalyzes the decarboxylation (removal of carbon) of cysteine sulphinate to hypotaurine. Expression of the gene appears to be up-regulated by bile acids and suppressed by cholestyramine (Kerr *et al.* 2014).

Possible interventions based on CSAD genetic expression
Nutrient cofactor to support CSAD enzyme activity
Pyridoxine (Lynch 2017).

Unhelpful inhibitors that reduce CSAD enzyme activity

Protein kinase inhibitors (Wu *et al.* 1998) are responsible for phosphorylation. This means they add the terminal phosphate group of ATP to serine, threonine or tyrosine residues. Phosphorylation regulates signalling pathways to change the function of the target protein or substrate. Two per cent of the human genome encodes for protein kinases (Kannaiyan & Mahadevan 2018). Protein kinase inhibitors have become a target as medicinal intervention for cancer. There are currently 66 clinically approved kinase inhibitors (these can be seen here: www.ppu.mrc.ac.uk/list-clinically-approved-kinase-inhibitors).

Practical advice

- Check medication interactions/depletions and address as appropriate. Refer to GP for medication review as necessary.
- Check taurine levels in urine and serum – high levels may be cardioprotective.
- May need to check gallbladder function if taurine is low as taurine is implicated in bile acid synthesis. Check for symptoms of cholestasis and refer or support gallbladder as necessary.
- Check digestive function and dysbiosis and address as appropriate.

Sulphite oxidase: SUOX

The SUOX gene encodes the mitochondrial enzyme sulphite oxidase. It has been extensively studied and found to be really important in autism spectrum disorders (Kou *et al.* 2012). This gene encodes sulphite oxidase, which in turn adds an oxygen molecule to sulphurs that the body no longer needs. This marks the conversion of sulphites to sulphates, which then become 3'-phosphoadenosine 5'-phosphosulphate (PAPS) (Günal *et al.* 2019). Expressive down-regulations in SUOX may lead to sulphite toxicity or sulphite sensitivity and the inability to sulphate hormones, neurotransmitters, metabolic toxins, cell membranes, vitamin D (Nair & Maseeh 2012) and the cholecystokinin feedback loop of digestion. It is also a common clinical feature to see down-regulation of the SUOX enzyme without obvious gene expression in cases of autism spectrum disorders and chronic fatigue syndrome. This could be because molybdenum deficiency is the root cause or that the evidence base has not yet identified the correct SNPs of the SUOX gene.

Sulphites are used extensively as preservatives in food manufacturing and will ultimately be found in delicatessen meats, processed meats such as bacon and sausage, dried fruits (usually non-organic), alcohols and wines particularly. Other products such as bottled citrus and grape juices, commercial sauerkraut, molasses, pickled cocktail onions, fruit toppings and dried foods such as potato also contain them. In fact, just about any food that has been through processing into a product that will keep is likely to contain sulphites. They are deemed necessary to keep the microbial population away from the food to increase shelf life.

Sulphites are usually labelled as:

- sodium sulphite
- sodium sulphate
- sodium thiosulphate
- sulphurous acid
- sulphur dioxide
- sodium metabisulphite
- potassium metabisulphite
- sodium bisulphite.

Sulphite sensitivity can manifest as any or all of the following from simple dermatitis, urticaria, flushing, hypotension, abdominal pain and diarrhoea, to life-threatening anaphylaxis and severe asthma attacks (Vally & Misso 2012). Reactions are variable but seem to be more extreme in individuals with already compromised lung capacity such as children with chronic asthma.

Sulphite oxidase deficiency can be due to an isolated defect in the SUOX enzyme or a secondary issue with cofactor defects of molybdenum (Claerhout *et al.* 2018). The molybdenum cofactor is also crucial for the xanthine oxidase and aldehyde oxidase enzymes, so SUOX presentation can be differentiated from molybdenum cofactor deficiency by the presence of normal levels of uric acid, hypoxanthine and xanthine in urine and plasma (Hobson *et al.* 2005; Tan *et al.* 2005).

Possible interventions based on SUOX genetic expression
Nutrient cofactors to support SUOX enzyme activity

- Molybdenum and thiamine (Lynch 2017).
- Molybdenum and riboflavin (Rudolph *et al.* 2003; Burton & Foster 1988; Rajagopalan 1988).

Unhelpful inhibitors that reduce SUOX enzyme activity
Arsenic and tungsten (Lynch 2017).

Practical advice

- Check for sulphite sensitivity to wines and non-organic dried fruit. Fermented foods are also high in histamine and some of the histamine reaction symptoms are similar. Check for hives and itching, diarrhoea and/or vomiting, flushing (often seen as red ears in children with autism), difficulty breathing or not being able to take a deep breath.
- Check for heavy metals and tungsten exposure and address as appropriate. Welders are more likely to be exposed to tungsten.
- Encourage a sulphite-free nutritional programme – natural foods only.
- Encourage foods high in molybdenum (legumes – beans, peas and lentils), thiamine (peas, beans, lentils, whole grains, pork) and riboflavin (milk, yogurt, cheese, beef, chicken, fish and egg).
- Test and supplement with molybdenum, thiamine and riboflavin as appropriate.
- Epsom salts baths three times weekly for 20–30 minutes (Mitchell & Waring 2016).

PRACTITIONER NOTES

Practitioners can – and do, of course – recommend Epsom salts baths to provide the sulphate at the end of this pathway where sulphite oxidase is suspected or known to be down-regulated. However, it is still necessary to remove excess sulphite from the body, thereby optimizing pathway function. In addition, the xanthine oxidase enzyme also uses up a lot of molybdenum. Sulphate is required by the body to detoxify various metabolic end products and crucial metabolic processes. Those to consider include the cholecystokinin (CCK) feedback loop, sulphation of vitamin D (Kurogi *et al.* 2017), sulphation of waste hormones and neurotransmitters. Interestingly, this is one area where enzyme activity can be clearly seen as poorly functioning when the SNP appears to remain intact (presenting as a wild card –/–). Mitchell and Waring (2016) found that soaking in a bath with 500–600g Epsom salts three times weekly increases levels of both magnesium and sulphate in blood and urine.

3'-phosphoadenine 5'-phosphosulphate synthase: PAPSS1

3'-phosphoadenosine 5'-phosphosulphate is the sulphate donor for all the SULT enzymes and the 3'-phosphoadenosine 5'-phosphosulphate synthase 1 and 2 genes encode the enzymes to ensure 3'-phosphoadenylylsulphate is produced from ATP and inorganic sulphate. This is a two-step process, the first being the addition of a sulphate group to ATP to yield adenosine 5'-phosphosulphate and the second stage to transfer a phosphate group to yield 3'-phospho-adenylylsulphate. Research has focused primarily on heart disease risk (Navab *et al.* 2011; Gaita *et al.* 2010).

Practical advice

- Check for heavy metals and address as appropriate.

- Check kidney (eGFR, albumin to creatinine ratio, urea and electrolytes in serum) and liver function (LFTs in serum).
- Encourage polyphenol-rich diet.
- Check calcium levels – support with high-calcium foods (yogurt, milk, cheese, sardines, green leafy vegetables). Supplement as appropriate and be mindful that calcium absorption requires good levels of stomach acid.
- Some of the key nutrients of the transsulphuration pathway are vitamin B6, molybdenum, taurine, NAC, glycine, selenium and riboflavin.

**Health challenges as an occurrence of expression
of SNPs within the transsulphuration pathway**
Sulphur is the eighth most important mineral to humans, and sulphur amino acids are the foundation of many enzymes including glutathione. However, when the body metabolizes sulphur, it produces ammonia. Mostly, we are able to excrete it through urine but occasionally, for a number of reasons, it reaches toxic levels.

This can lead to

- brain fog
- fatigue
- mood disturbances
- insomnia
- muscle weakness
- nausea and vomiting
- headaches
- diarrhoea
- clumsiness and loss of coordination
- growth retardation
- hypothermia
- ataxia, tremors and seizures
- shortness of breath.

Ammonia is produced during normal protein metabolism but factors such as stress, via gluconeogenesis, and/or dysbiosis can be responsible for an increase in ammonia (Kang *et al.* 2016).

Individuals with an up-regulated expression of the CBS C699T enzyme are more likely to suffer the effects of high ammonia levels. They may also have high levels of taurine, low cystathionine and homocysteine (Paré *et al.* 2009). If a NOS mutation is also expressing, this can exacerbate the elevated ammonia. Urea cycle metabolites of ammonia, citrulline, ornithine and urea may also indicate difficulties with the conversion of ammonia to urea for urinary excretion.

As the practitioner will appreciate, those with up-regulated CBS mutations may temporarily need to limit their intake of sulphur by removing garlic, onions, cruciferous vegetables, eggs, legumes, and/or protein-rich animal products with care to assess specific food reactions as this is not an exhaustive list. All sulphur-based amino acids and alpha-lipoic acid, chlorella, spirulina, glutathione, MSM, DMSO and N-acetyl-cysteine may need to be avoided until transsulphuration has been stabilized and ammonia levels reduced.

The nutrition plan should focus on high fat, low carbohydrate and low protein, working from ratios of around 70% fat, 20% carbohydrate and 10% protein of the daily allowance. Meat should be grass-fed and pasture-raised and kept below 50g per day, using the bones to create broth. Fat content in the form of grass-fed ghee and coconut products should feature highly. Avocado and low-sulphur vegetables such as romaine lettuce, parsley, celery and carrots, flax, pumpkin, chia and sunflower seeds, and macadamia nuts can be eaten in moderation. Ginger, rosemary, cinnamon, thyme, basil, oregano and turmeric can be used generously with copious amount of olive oil.

Glucoronidation, glutathione conjugation and sulphation are all sulphur-based processes that the liver depends upon and this can be a challenge for those with expressing CBS mutations. Vitamin C with bioflavonoids, parsley and dandelion are all low sulphur (Zhao *et al.* 2008) and can support the liver to recycle glutathione for detoxification. Chlorophyll can neutralize both ammonia and carbon monoxide (Wang *et al.* 2019), so liquid chlorophyll added to water can be a real bonus. Wheat grass and barley grass are more nutrient-dense, of course, and contain high levels of chlorophyll, so clean varieties can be used in foods and smoothies.

Celery juice appears to be currently making a name for itself as being a superfood to aid ammonia reduction by supporting electrolyte balance in the body. Kooti and Daraei (2017) have systematically reviewed a number of animal studies highlighting the beneficial properties of celery juice in many conditions. It appears to improve glutathione status. Celery juice is, of course, a good source of vitamin K, potassium and flavonoids, which all assist with blood glucose, blood pressure and management of inflammation. The health benefits are related to its compounds of caffeic acid, apigenin, tannins, saponins, luteolin, ferulic acid, p-coumaric acid and kaempferol. All of these compounds support mitochondrial health due to their powerful removal of reactive oxygen species. There are no human studies to support these health claims and maybe the anecdotal effects are purely due to adequate hydration. Although it can be so tempting to advocate food such as celery in this manner, caution should be advised in those with potential thyroid-related disease as it can interfere with iodine uptake (Felker *et al.* 2016) in addition to containing high levels of oxalates (Dolan *et al.* 2010) that are known to bind minerals such as calcium and potassium.

Down-regulation of CBS
There appears to be two differing perspectives on the action of CBS mutations. The opposing view offered by Kruger and Gupta (2015) is that some with CBS deficiency present with high homocysteine, decreased cysteine and increased methionine. These researchers compared the interventions of N-acetyl-cysteine (NAC), betaine supplemented diet (BSD), reduced methionine diet (MRD) and a regular diet (RD) in mice.

The diets were ranked from best to worst MRD, BSD, RD, NAC in terms of the reduction in methionine and homocysteine. They postulate that a reduced methionine diet, supplemented with betaine for those who are less compliant would be far more beneficial than supplementing with NAC.

Sulphate and sulphation

Rosemary Waring and Margaret Moss have studied sulphation issues in autism spectrum disorders (ASD) for decades. Sulphate is converted from sulphite in the penultimate conversion to 3'-phosphoadenosine-5'-phosphosulphate (PAPSS 1 and 2) at the end of the transsulphuration pathway. PAPSS are critical for the biopterin pathway. Low SULT1A1, 2 and/or 3 activities can determine less ability to sulphate dietary phenols and catecholamines in the gut. Such individuals might be more at risk of migraines resulting from the ingestion of cheese (tyramine), chocolate (phenylethylamine) and bananas (serotonin). Foods high in flavonoids may also inhibit these enzymes. According to Ghazali and Waring (1999), sulphate is needed for the following functions:

- formation of proteins in joints (low levels of sulphate are found in synovial fluid in rheumatoid arthritis)
- the commencement of CCK feedback loop activity, initiating bile flow and a cascade of digestive enzymes from the pancreas
- formation of mucin proteins that line the gut walls for protection from gastric juices and toxins (low plasma sulphate has been found in cases of IBS)
- formation of brain tissue (sulphated carbohydrate chains support brain neurons)
- major pathway to detoxify medications and environmental contaminants.

Sulphate is formed in the body via oxidation of cysteine and methionine, but this is suboptimal in a large percentage of the population and especially in the ASD population. Sulphate is not easily absorbed across the gut wall; transdermal delivery is far advanced and predominantly in the form of Epsom salts (Mitchell & Waring 2016). Sulphation increases the body's resistance to colonization of bacteria and viruses and, interestingly, *Helicobacter pylori*, a stomach colonizer, can only colonize once it has produced a sulphatase enzyme to de-sulphate gastric mucin (Slomiany *et al.* 1992). Gut hyperpermeability, of course, is a known side effect.

**What about small intestinal bacterial
overgrowth as a human adaptation?**

Nigh's (2019) paper is worth noting. He suggests that small intestinal bacterial overgrowth (SIBO) may be a human adaptation to poor sulphation. For many years, practitioners have steadfastly followed the outdated germ theory in delivering many 4R approaches to clients suffering with dysbiosis and intestinal hyperpermeability. There are situations that require this approach as a short-term solution. However, the approach has been vastly over-used and the pathogenic bacteria are now becoming resistant. Many patients attend clinic having undergone years of antifungal, antimicrobial approaches and diets with limited success. Nigh is suggesting these cases of long-term SIBO should be considered differently and he has a very valid point.

When the cell danger response is triggered, the cystathionine gamma-lyase enzyme moves from the cytosol to the outer mitochondrial membrane where it utilizes the high concentration of cysteine to produce hydrogen sulphide, the substrate for sulphate production. Sulphite may also be generated from hydrogen sulphide via endothelial nitric oxide synthase (eNOS) (Hildebrandt & Grieshaber 2008) and via activated neutrophils (Mitsuhashi *et al.* 2005).

Glyphosate may chelate molybdenum and iron while impeding haem synthesis, thereby leaving sulphate in short supply (Samsel & Seneff 2013). Sulphate is also produced in the skin on sunlight exposure (Seneff *et al.* 2012) so the use of ultraviolet-blocking sunscreens and reduction in daily sunlight quotient in some countries would have a great impact. The use of oral sulphated glycosaminoglycans such as chondroitin sulphate has shown extensive promise in the treatment of osteoarthritis and plaque psoriasis (Vergés *et al.* 2005). Vitamin D deficiency may therefore be better addressed with sulphated vitamin D via the use of a Sperti (FDA approved) vitamin D lamp (Dabai *et al.* 2012; Chandra *et al.* 2007).

Heavy metals such as tungsten, cadmium, arsenic and copper can all attach to the molybdenum cofactor within the SUOX enzyme (Neumann & Leimkühler 2008), rendering it inactive. Nigh purports that over a dozen sulphate-producing bacteria, including Helicobacter pylori, *Klebsiella* species, *Campylobacter jejuni*, *E. coli*, *Bilophilia wadsworthia, Desulfovibrio* and *Staphylococcus aureus* (Rees *et al.* 2008) can create hydrogen sulphide from many different sulphur substrates and these can then be converted to sulphate under conditions of good enzyme activity.

Studies are demonstrating a 44% recurrence of SIBO after successful treatment with rifaximin (Lauritano *et al.* 2008). In a further study, Waring (2010) identified that in 19 subjects who soaked in 400g (four cups) Epsom salts every night for seven nights in a row, sulphate levels in the blood improved to a steady state and with that a dramatic improvement in digestive symptoms in those with SIBO.

To conclude, Nigh is saying that providing the body with transdermal sulphate via Epsom salts baths is sulphating all hormones and neurotransmitters. As a result, sulphated cholecystokinin and secretin are stimulating the gallbladder and pancreas. Less stagnation and inflammation in the small intestine allows the bacterial overgrowth to naturally decrease.

ELLA'S CASE: TRANSSULPHURATION

As can be seen from Ella's transsulphuration pathway in Figure 5.5, she has a number of mutations, both heterozygous (grey) and homozygous (black). These mutations have the potential to reduce the conversion of homocysteine to glutathione and to produce succinyl-CoA for the citric acid cycle, necessary for porphyrin, haem and fatty acid synthesis (Leong *et al.* 2012). Recycling of glutathione may be compromised even if Ella is able to make adequate amounts. Also recall Ella had high levels of *Klebsiella* and *Pseudomonas* in her OAT profile. As *Klebsiella* specifically has been identified as a possible underlying cause of SIBO (Takakura & Pimentel 2020), it would make sense to perform a breath test to confirm SIBO or to assume it from the OAT profile, given Ella's history and symptoms of gastroparesis. It had not been possible to address dysbiosis previously due to poor detoxification as a result of underlying pyroluria.

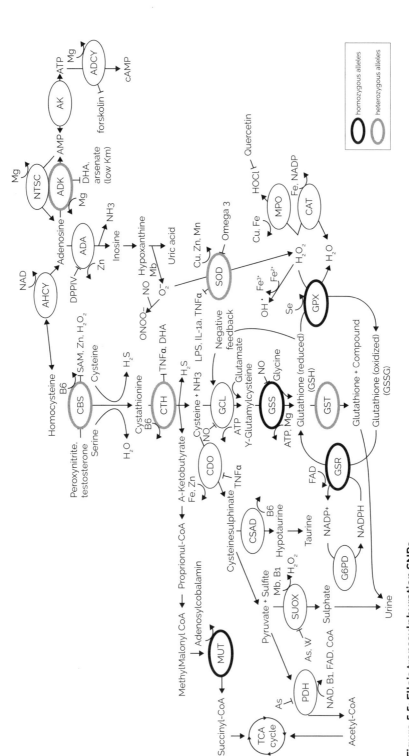

Figure 5.5: Ella's transsulphuration SNPs

Source: Methylation Planner by Dr Ben Lynch (author of Dirty Genes and creator of StrateGene)

Key: Homozygous SNPs are those with a solid black outline; heterozygous SNPs have a solid grey outline.

Metabolic markers
Urinary organic acids highlighted high levels of ammonia, citrulline, taurine and cysteine. Glutamine/glutamate were within range but very low. Whole-blood glutathione was also very low. Homocysteine was 17 (normal range 5–15). Blood analysis showed high anion gap, creatine kinase, creatine, haematocrit, LDH, MCV, platelets and liver enzymes SGOT/AST. It also showed extremely low levels of cholesterol, chloride, LDL and MCHC. This was consistent with high levels of inflammation, poor renal clearance and a distressed liver.

Symptomology
Ella had a lot of difficulty with sulphite sensitivity, generally associated with a slow SUOX. Please note this is not the same as autosomal recessive SUOX deficiency (Bindu *et al.* 2017). Her symptoms included inability to tolerate wine, which could also be due to slow ALDH enzymes (Minnick 2014), sulphite preservatives in bacon, sausage or convenience foods (could also be other additives), but her biggest reaction was to non-organic trail mix, which contains sulphites. She experienced immediate and extreme pruritus over the abdomen. However, there is no evidence of a mutation in her SUOX gene.

This is a clear case of enzyme deficiency without a mutation, which demonstrates the need for an in-depth clinical history and additional functional markers as relevant to the case. Taurine was significantly raised, suggesting sulphur metabolism was being diverted down the taurine pathway as a result of SUOX deficiency and also poor recycling of glutathione.

Sulphate needs to be produced in order to sulphate many metabolic products and systems of the body, including the CCK feedback loop that appears to bother Ella enormously. This is consistent with her endless digestive symptoms and her raised malabsorption markers on the organic acids. It may be in part responsible for her gastroparesis too. Sulphate is also needed for the phenolsulphotransferase enzymes PST-M and PST-P to detoxify amines and phenols (Moss & Waring 2003).

Interestingly, evidence points to molybdenum and thiamine being the optimal nutritional support for SUOX according to Lynch (2017) and Cohen (2015). However, Rosemary Waring's research on sulphation issues in autism spectrum disorders has clearly identified riboflavin as a more important nutrient. Waring states that thiamine is depleted rather than it being a cofactor. If this is questioned, in biochemistry textbooks the following is stated:

> Molybdenum is part of the molecular structure of the enzymes xanthine oxidase, sulphite oxidase and aldehyde oxidase. These enzymes are molybdoflavoproteins; the molybdenum is most likely involved in the linkage of flavin nucleotide (the prosthetic group, or coenzyme) to the substrate-specific protein (apoenzyme). (Burton & Foster 1988, p.164)

Ella recalled an incidence of sulphur intolerance in her diet very early on. Recall she was reacting to onions and cruciferous vegetables. She reported quite severe lower abdominal cramps about 90 minutes after eating onions. At the time this was not perceived to be a sulphur issue. However, she recalled a recent severe reaction to Nat Sulph as recommended by a homeopath. Ella recalled what she described as psychosis on taking the homeopathic remedy. This is a situation where a lot of childhood trauma was releasing from subconscious memory and she wasn't sure if her memories were real or not. The homeopathic remedy was discontinued and the surfacing memories stopped. Note this is a different reaction to the sulphites.

Ella's programme

Given Ella's endless battles with dysbiosis and these new findings of high ammonia, taurine and malabsorption with bacterial and yeast markers and her history of giving birth to a child with a diagnosed autism spectrum disorder, it could be assumed that transsulphuration is an issue. Recall there was also a mention of CCK feedback loop insufficiency from one of Ella's previous naturopathic practitioners. Ella also appeared to suffer with oestrogen imbalance in earlier years and obvious neurotransmitter balance. Basic transsulphuration support was provided at the beginning of Ella's programme, so the immediate need at this point was to recheck the transsulphuration markers on the OAT. These all came within normal ranges after six months of support.

Also, while Ella's homocysteine was slightly raised and her internalization of stress might indicate a slow BHMT enzyme and therefore a slow conversion of homocysteine to methionine via the short route, adding pyridoxine may in fact exacerbate Ella's elevated ammonia and sulphites at this time. However, this is a controversial area as pyridoxine also plays a dominant role as cofactor for the synthesis of glutamine. This has neuroprotective mechanisms in cleaving ammonia and glutamate (Häberle *et al.* 2006). It is also a cofactor for the GAD enzyme, converting glutamate to GABA (Huang *et al.* 2016).

Ammonia

- Calcium and magnesium butyrate to control ammonia; support the urea cycle and reduce gut inflammation (Canani *et al.* 2001).
- Branched-chain amino acids to support renal/muscle catabolism.
- Continue the lipids, minerals and water to help nitrogen balance (Morris & Mohiuddin 2021).

Digestion

- Epsom salts baths containing 4 cups of Epsom, 2 scoops of electrolyte minerals and 10 drops of either rose or lavender essential oil. The choice of oil was left to Ella; she was advised to use the one with the smell she was attracted to most at the time. Lavender is very calming with high levels of linalyl acetate, linalool, terpinene-4-ol, cis- and trans beta ocimene, lavandulyl acetate, beta-caryophyllene and lavandulol, giving it the therapeutic properties of being antifungal, carminative and smooth muscle relaxing (Smigielski *et al.* 2009). The oils constituents of nonadecane, nonadecene, citronellol, geraniol, heneicosane and nerol offer the therapeutic properties of rose. These offer antimicrobial antianxiety, anti-inflammatory and enhancement of GABA receptivity (Mahboubi 2015).
- Molybdenum (no more than 150mcg daily). Choose an organic form and appreciate you may need to try more than one as they are not all effective.

- Hydroxycobalamin can be used orally, as a subcutaneous injection or transdermally. This form of B12 is known to render hydrogen sulphide biologically inactive and therefore less toxic (Fujita *et al.* 2011).
- Panax (Korean red) ginseng provides HPA axis support and suppression of CBS and CSE expression, thereby reducing intrinsic production of hydrogen sulphide (Lee *et al.* 2016).
- Riboflavin and selenium were also recommended to support recycling of glutathione (Minich & Brown 2019). Incidentally, the riboflavin significantly reduced Ella's anxiety.

NB: Intestinal repair should only be initiated following healthy sulphate reestablishment.

Supplements

- Betaine HCL + pepsin reduced to 2 per meal, supporting protein digestion (Guilliams & Drake 2020).
- Digestive enzymes 1 per meal, supporting intestinal digestion of proteins, carbohydrates and fats (Ianiro *et al.* 2016).
- Potassium and sodium bicarbonate between meals x 3 supporting fluid balance and digestion and also to reduce brain fog (Popkin *et al.* 2010).
- Riboflavin-5-phosphate to support recycling of oxidized glutathione back to reduced glutathione SUOX enzyme (Minich & Brown 2019).
- Bifidobacteria x 2 to support detoxification and balancing of large intestinal microbiome and to reduce histamine (O'Callaghan & van Sinderen 2016).
- *Lactobacillus plantarum*, *L. rhamnosus* and *L. salivaricus* x 2 to support small intestine rebalancing and reduce histamine (Krzyściak *et al.* 2017; Sasikumar *et al.* 2017; Segers & Lebeer 2014).
- Broccoli seed extract powder 2 tsp to support oestrogen balance, microbiome diversity and antihistamine (Sudini *et al.* 2016).
- PC with 4:1 oil to support cell membrane integrity and gut mucin restoration (Amadei *et al.* 2018).
- Liquid molybdenum 150ug daily (Bindu *et al.* 2017).

Lifestyle

- Increase Epsom salts baths to every night for one week, then every 2–3 nights. Magnesium and sulphate are both needed to help transsulphuration.
- Continue with meditation, nature walks and gentle Dru yoga or Tai chi. Continue with rebounding daily to decrease anxiety and mobilize lymph.

PRACTITIONER NOTES

If taurine is low, this may increase sensitivity to hypochlorite which is found in swimming pools, cleaning solutions, drinking water and disinfectants. Without adequate taurine, aldehydes are also more readily increased, enhancing the need for aldehyde oxidase, a molybdenum dependent enzyme (Moss & Waring 2003).

Recap transsulphuration

To recap this section, we have considered the need for sulphur in the body to support cell membranes, hormones, neurotransmitters and both intrinsic and extrinsic toxins, and the effects of too much or too little sulphur. The genes and their respective enzymes have been discussed within the pathway that creates glutathione from homocysteine. Ella's case has demonstrated how to use nutritional support to improve the action of this pathway in order to assist the practitioner with possible approaches to support sulphation.

Neurotransmitters

Before discussing the biopterin pathway, it would seem pertinent to discuss glutamate decarboxylase (GAD). While technically not part of the biopterin pathway, a SNP on the GAD gene may have a huge impact on brain function.

Gamma-aminobutyric acid: GAD1

The GAD1 rs3828275, rs379187 and rs769391 gene encodes the enzyme glutamic acid decarboxylase to convert glutamate to gamma-aminobutyric acid (GABA). A SNP expressing in GAD1 will down-regulate the enzyme, slowing down the conversion of glutamate to GABA. Glutamate is a primary excitatory neurotransmitter. Glutamate excess also wastes glutathione and increases TNF. Glutamate is necessary for learning and both long- and short-term memory. GABA conversely is a primary inhibitory neurotransmitter. High levels of glutamate may result in high levels of energy, shortness of breath and tingling of the extremities. This may cause anxiety, low mood and an activated immune system.

Glutamate excess wastes glutathione and increases TNFα. This is likely to have a negative effect on heart health and digestion (Coghlan et al. 2012). Low levels of glutathione may manifest as fatigue and learning difficulties, excessive uncontrolled energy, and anxiousness and sleep disruption. The GAD1 enzyme seems susceptible to lead and mercury toxicity and has a requirement for pyridoxine as a nutrient cofactor. This enzyme tends to be down-regulated in autism, leading to stimulatory behaviour (Zhubi et al. 2017). It is known to lead to anxiety in adults under 40 years of age (Angst et al. 2009). Deficiencies of glutamate decarboxylase have been linked with pyridoxine-dependent epilepsy (Cotter et al. 2017), Down's syndrome, cerebral palsy (Lin et al. 2013), asthma and autism. Labouesse et al. (2015) have also found that maternal viral infections such as herpes simplex can remodel the GAD enzyme, giving rise to neurodevelopmental disorders in offspring. Low GABA levels are associated with impaired speech, anxiety, aggressive behaviour, poor socialization, poor eye contact and constipation (Coghlan et al. 2012).

Possible interventions based on GAD1 genetic expression
Nutrient cofactors to support GAD1 enzyme activity
Pyridoxine and magnesium (Lynch 2017).

Unhelpful inhibitors that reduce GAD1 enzyme activity
Mercury, aluminium, copper and lead (Lynch 2017), diuretics (furosemide, bendroflumethiazide, spironolactone), HRT, monoamine oxidase inhibitors (muclobemide, isocarboxazid), fibrates (fenofibrate) (Cohen 2015).

Practical advice

- Practitioners may need to consider restoring the balance by addressing CBS up-regulations and BHMT down-regulations to decrease alpha-ketoglutarate production.
- Check medications for interactions and refer to GP for review if necessary.
- Check for heavy metals and address as appropriate.
- Support with pyridoxine-containing foods (salmon, tuna, halibut, turkey, chicken, duck, hazelnuts and walnuts) and magnesium-rich foods (nuts, seeds, green leafy vegetables).
- Be extremely careful with pyridoxine supplementation as too much can increase sulphur thiol production leading to excessive tiredness and a feeling of overall toxicity.
- Recommend meditation (Fox *et al.* 2014; Guglietti *et al.* 2013; Hoge *et al.* 2013), walking in nature (Marselle *et al.* 2019), binaural beat music (Garcia-Argibay *et al.* 2019), taking up a creative project and/or HeartMath breathing techniques (Henriques *et al.* 2011), listening to Solfeggio sounds (Babayi & Riazi 2017). These are all practical solutions that are evidence-based to help reduce anxiety.
- Decrease food sources of glutamine (peas, parmesan cheese, milk, mushrooms, fish and foods containing monosodium glutamate). Increase foods known to support GABA production (soy, whole grains, lentils, walnuts, almonds, sunflower seeds, broccoli, potato and cocoa (Briguglio *et al.* 2018). Also consider lifestyle adaptations such as meditation (Fox *et al.* 2014; Guglietti *et al.* 2013), black seed oil (Gilhotra & Dhingra 2011) and exercise (Hill *et al.* 2010).

Biopterin cycle

The purpose of the Biopterin cycle is primarily to create tetrahydrobiopterin (BH4). This is essential for many body processes within the brain, heart, digestive and reproductive systems. Following the pathway and learning the SNPs here can really develop practitioner knowledge and confidence in dealing with the more profound and difficult cases such as autism spectrum disorders, the more severe mental health conditions and chronic fatigue.

BH4, sometimes also known as sapropterin, is essential for the biosynthesis of the neurotransmitters dopamine, serotonin, melatonin, adrenaline and noradrenaline. It also produces nitric oxide, which, as practitioners are well aware, is central to the internal milieu of the microvascular system, offering protection to humans against diabetes and heart disease (Farah *et al.* 2018). There is also evidence that connects BH4 to immune surveillance and activity via T-cell proliferation (Cronin *et al.* 2018). Clinical trials on subjects with autism undertaken by Schnetz-Boutaud *et al.* (2009) (n=403 families) genotyped 25 SNPs in nine genes on the biopterin pathway and found only nominal associations with the PST gene. However, Frye and Rossignol (2014) demonstrated low levels of BH4 in this condition and that 63% of children in the study reacted positively to supplementation with BH4 against autism rating scales. The low incidence of adverse events would suggest this might be a novel treatment for many of those with autism spectrum conditions.

BH4 is susceptible to oxidation by perioxynitrites, resulting in uncoupling of eNOS as can be seen on the pathway planner (Figure 5.6) (Lynch 2017). Oxidation of BH4 results in promoting the production of superoxide as opposed to nitric oxide. It may therefore be unwise to supplement with BH4 exogenously; naturally increasing biopterin via the salvage pathway enzyme DHFR might be preferable (recall DHFR was discussed earlier in the folate cycle).

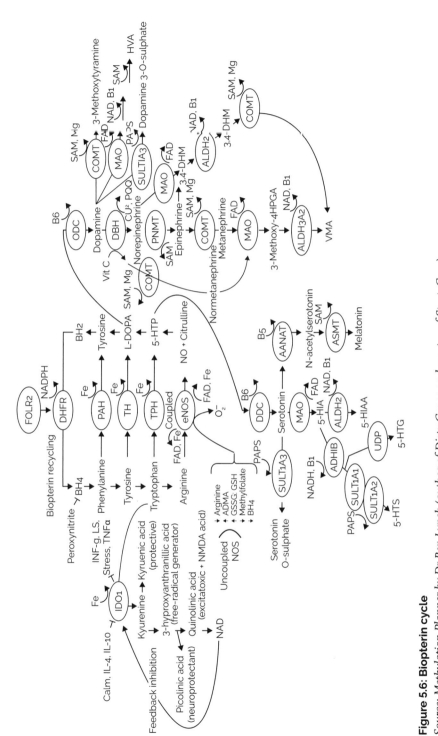

Figure 5.6: Biopterin cycle

Source: Methylation Planner by Dr Ben Lynch (author of Dirty Genes and creator of StrateGene)

SNPs to consider in this pathway:

FOLR2, DHFR, PAH, TH, TPH, eNOS, ODC, DBH, PNMT, COMT, MAO, ALDH3A2, SULT1A3, DDC, MAO, ALDH2, AANAT, ASMT, ALDH1B, SULT1A1, SULT1A2, IDO1 also GAD1.

Commencing at the top of the folate pathway, the genes FOLR2 and DHFR have already been discussed. Biopterin is oxidized, becoming BH2, at eNOS and recycled back at DHFR. Within this part of the cycle, other genes instruct their respective enzymes PAH, TH and TPH to convert their respective amino acids into neurotransmitters. These enzymes are all iron-dependent and are taken in turn below.

Nitric oxide synthase: NOS1, 2 and 3

The NOS gene encodes for the nitric oxide synthase enzyme. As previously discussed, this is a messenger molecule with diverse functions in the brain and peripheral nervous system. It has similarities with the functions of neurotransmitters. Excessive nitric oxide as a result of down-regulation of this enzyme has been implicated in neurodegenerative diseases and cerebrovascular accident or stroke. Endothelial (eNOS) or NOS3 (rs1800783, rs3918188, rs7380, 1800789, rs2070744) generates nitric oxide in the endothelial cells of the vascular epithelium. NOS then regulates leukocyte adhesion, cellular proliferation, vascular tone and platelet aggregation. This makes the function of eNOS crucial for the health of the cardiovascular system (Kietadisorn *et al.* 2011). The rs2070744 appears to be the only SNP of huge significance according to Lynch (2017). Deletion of eNOS leads to hypertension (Förstermann & Sessa 2012). eNOS needs biopterin in order to create nitric oxide, so without adequate levels of biopterin NOS will generate superoxide instead. This is responsible for the increased oxidative stress that causes endothelial dysfunction (McNeill & Channon 2012).

Possible interventions based on NOS genetic expression
Nutrient cofactors to support NOS enzyme activity for eNOS
Haem, FAD, FMN, tetrahydrobiopterin (Hill Erdei & Ledowski 2015; Lynch 2017).

Unhelpful inhibitors that reduce NOS enzyme activity
Hypoxia, low folate or BH4, increased asymmetric dimethyl arginine, green tea catechins, lipopolysaccharides, insulin resistance, standard American diet, sodium chloride, raised C-reactive protein, heavy alcohol intake (Lynch 2017).

Inducible NOS: iNOS
Inducible NOS (iNOS) or NOS2 (rs2297518, rs2248814, rs2274894) is a reactive free radical that mediates several processes including neurotransmission, antimicrobial and antitumour activity. Lipopolysaccharides and certain cytokines induce the expression of this allele. It is therefore typically induced in inflammatory disease.

Possible interventions based on iNOS genetic expression
Nutrient cofactors to support iNOS enzyme activity
Calcium, haem, flavin mononucleotide and NADPH (Förstermann & Sessa 2012).

Unhelpful inhibitors that reduce iNOS enzyme activity
Lipopolysaccharides and cytokines (Förstermann & Sessa 2012).

Neuronal NOS: nNOS

Neuronal NOS (nNOS) or NOS1 (rs7298903, rs3782206, rs 2293054) encodes for the enzyme NOS1. It is protective against acute cerebrovascular accident or stroke (Chen *et al.* 2017) due to its neuronal regulation of smooth muscle and endothelium-derived relaxing factor, regulating blood pressure.

Possible interventions based on nNOS genetic expression
Nutrient cofactors to support nNOS enzyme activity
Haem, FAD, FMN and tetrahydrobiopterin.

Unhelpful inhibitors that reduce nNOS enzyme activity
None confirmed yet.

Practical advice

- Possible testing: nitrotyrosine in serum, measure of peroxynitrite and oxidative stress.
- Check arginine and citrulline on organic acids to assess expression.
- Encourage anti-inflammatory nutritional approach where testing has confirmed high inflammatory markers such as homocysteine, c-reactive protein, erythrocyte sedimentation rate. Balance blood glucose levels, include organic fresh food where possible. Eliminate all processed foods.
- Rebalance microbiome to reduce lipopolysaccharides on the outer membrane of gram-negative bacteria (DellaGioia & Hannestad 2010).
- Encourage food high in riboflavin (milk, yogurt, cheese, chicken, beef, fish and eggs), niacin (beef, fish, poultry, beans, peas and lentils).
- Test for haem, riboflavin and niacin in serum or urine organic acids and supplement as appropriate.
- Support endothelium with polyphenol-rich foods when sulphation allows (Auger *et al.* 2016).
- Possible butyrate to neutralize ammonia.

PRACTITIONER NOTES

A dysfunctional NOS enzyme has difficulty breaking down ammonia and generating nitric oxide. There is therefore an increased risk of cardiovascular disease. The practitioner may wish to consider the use of vitamin C to neutralize superoxide and to stabilize collagen, also 5-methylfolate, assuming safety with dopamine pathway SNPs, to neutralize peroxynitrites. Statins are also known to increase peroxynitrites (Gorabi *et al.* 2019), so if the patient is suffering adverse side effects from statins, consider peroxynitrites as an underlying factor. Both BH2 and BH4 bind with eNOS equally; BH4-bound eNOS promotes nitric oxide, whereas BH2-bound eNOS promotes uncoupling and eNOS-derived superoxide instead of nitric oxide. This increases oxidative stress significantly, and administering high doses of arginine daily can stimulate this mechanism. Citrulline, red wine extract and pomegranate may also stimulate uncoupling. If BH4 is low, please support DHFR by stopping all inhibitors of DHFR and folic acid (Lynch 2017). Also discontinue all folic acid, especially for those with MTHFD1 and MTHFR SNPs. Folic acid is said to block the folate receptors making it more difficult for the body to attain good levels of 5-MTHF for methylation to occur (Lynch 2017).

Phenylalanine hydroxylase: PAH

The PAH gene encodes for the phenylalanine hydroxylase enzyme. PAH deficiency was traditionally viewed as an autosomal recessive condition, as deficiency of this enzyme may lead to phenylketonuria (Blau *et al.* 2010). This results in demyelination of the brain. However, a more modern view is that the condition may present along a continuum, with milder forms such as mild phenylketonuria and hyperphenylalaninemia. These lesser forms of the condition appear to be treatable with nutritional and lifestyle medicine (Mitchell *et al.* 2011). Phenylalanine is plentiful in meats, milk products and chocolate. PAH provides the rate-limiting step in the catabolism of phenylalanine to tyrosine. Practitioners may need to analyze chocolate addiction in depth. Is the addiction due to sugar (processed chocolate bingers) or phenylalanine need (70% or raw chocolate bingers)?

Tetrahydrobiopterin (BH4) has been found to be low in conditions such as autism, depression and heart disease. Supplementation with BH4 has been shown to reduce excessive inflammation in autism (Frye & Rossignol 2014). It has also been shown to improve endothelial function (Mäki-Petäjä *et al.* 2014). Folate administered via foods and/or supplementation may also increase BH4 (Zhang *et al.* 2014).

Possible interventions based on PAH genetic expression
Nutrient cofactors to support PAH enzyme activity
Iron and BH4 (Hill Erdei & Ledowski 2015; Lynch 2017), also pyridoxine, cobalamin and vitamin E (Cohen 2015).

Unhelpful inhibitors that reduce PAH enzyme activity
Excessive tyrosine, dopamine or tryptophan supplementation (Litwack & Litwack 2018).

Tyrosine hydroxylase: TH

The TH gene encodes the protein for the tyrosine hydroxylase enzyme. This is involved with the conversion of tyrosine to L-dopa, the precursor to dopamine. This is a rate-limiting enzyme in the synthesis of catecholamines; hence it plays a key role in the physiology of adrenergic neurons. Alterations may be seen in enzyme activity in conditions such as Parkinson's disease as the characteristic stop/start walking called tardive dyskinesia is understood to be due to tyrosine hydroxylase deficiency (Tabrez *et al.* 2012) and schizophrenia (Schuhmacher *et al.* 2012).

Possible interventions based on TH genetic expression
Nutrient cofactors that support TH enzyme activity
Iron and BH4 (Hill Erdei & Ledowski 2015; Lynch 2017), also magnesium, copper, niacin pyridoxine, vitamin C (Cohen 2015).

Unhelpful inhibitors that reduce TH enzyme activity
Increased nitric oxide, dopamine, adrenaline, noradrenaline, catechol oestrogens, panax ginseng, apomorphine levels and chronic low-grade stress (Lynch 2017).

Tryptophan-5-hydroxylase1: TPH1 and 2

TPH1 and 2 encode the enzyme tryptophan 5-hydroxylase. TPH1 is expressed in the body peripheral system and TPH2 in the brain. This neurotransmitter synthesizing enzyme converts L-tryptophan to serotonin. Serotonin is found in the gastrointestinal tract, blood platelets and the central nervous system, but also in the kidney, adrenal glands and the pineal gland (Waløen *et al.* 2017). Interestingly, serotonin is thought to be the contributor of wellbeing and happiness. However, 90% of serotonin in humans is located in the enterochromaffin cells within the gastrointestinal tract, where it regulates intestinal movements. The remaining 10% is synthesized in the serotonergic neurons of the central nervous system, regulating mood, appetite and sleep, with some cognitive function such as learning and memory. The alleles rs4570625, rs7305115 and rs4290270 have been associated with schizophrenia (Zhang *et al.* 2011).

Possible interventions based on TPH genetic expression
Nutrient cofactors that support TPH enzyme activity
Iron, BH4 and oxygen.

Unhelpful inhibitors that reduce TPH enzyme activity
High levels of tryptophan and/or dopamine, aflotoxins, lithium carbonate, acute heavy (binge) drinking and chronic low-level stress (Lynch 2017).

Practical advice

- The avoidance of aspartame in individuals with a PAH polymorphism is crucial as aspartame is known to contain phenylalanine.
- Check neurotransmitters in urine or dried urine. Lombard's neurotransmitter quiz could also be a useful tool (Lombard n.d.; Lombard *et al.* 2003). However, do be aware this has not yet been evaluated as a clinical tool so it can only be used as guidance.
- Ensure adequate methylation in order to create biopterin.

- Encourage foods high in iron (red meat and lentils), pyridoxine (salmon, halibut, tuna, turkey, chicken, duck, walnuts and hazelnuts), cobalamin (clams, red meat, chicken and turkey) and vitamin E (vegetable oils, nuts, seeds).
- Support HPA axis function.

Having explored TPH1 and 2, it would seem pertinent to now track to the left of the pathway into the kynurenine pathway.

TPH to indoleamine 2,3-dehydrogenase: IDO1

The IDO1 gene encodes the enzyme indoleamine 2,3-dioxygenase. This is another haem enzyme that converts tryptophan into kynurenine. The kynurenine pathway creates NAD+ by converting kynurenine to 3-hypoxathranillic acid, then to quinolinic acid and lastly NAD+. The balance of NAD produced is governed by the feedback loop from NAD back to IDO1. Within the pathway, certain products are protective (kynurenic acid) while others (quinolinic acid) may be detrimental. Quinolinic acid acts as a N-methyl-D-aspartate receptor (NMDA) receptor antagonist. This is a glutamate receptor and ION channel protein found in nerve cells. It is crucial for controlling synaptic plasticity and memory function (Li & Tsien 2009). Quinolinic acid's excitotoxicity effects have been linked to many psychiatric and neurodegenerative conditions (Lugo-Huitrón *et al.* 2013). Slow genes or enzymes further down the pathway at TPH, DDC or MAO may increase levels of kynurenine and quinolinic acid, as tryptophan may be unable to be converted into 5-HTP so a backlog occurs.

Possible interventions based on IDO1 genetic expression
Nutrient cofactors to support IDO1 enzyme activity
Iron, pyridoxine, NADPH (Cohen 2015).

Unhelpful inhibitors that reduce IDO1 enzyme activity

- Interleukin-4 and interleukin-10, non-steroidal anti-inflammatory medications (NSAIDs), diuretics, methotrexate (Williams 2013).

- Trimethoprim, triamterene, folates (Engin & Engin 2017).
- EGCG and grapefruit seed (Cheng *et al.* 2010).

Practical advice

- Investigate possible causes of inflammation and address. This is likely to be gastrointestinal dysbiosis and/or stress.
- Check medication interactions and depletions and address as appropriate. Refer to GP if appropriate for a medicine review.
- Eliminate any EGCG supplementation and reduce green tea to one or two cups daily.
- Eliminate grapefruit seed extract if taking and exchange for a different plant-based antimicrobial.
- Encourage anti-inflammatory diet high in iron (red meat and lentils), pyridoxine (salmon, halibut, turkey, chicken, duck, hazelnuts and walnuts) and niacin (beef, fish, poultry, beans, peas and lentils).
- Balance blood glucose levels to support mood and inflammation (Penckofer *et al.* 2012).
- Test for nutrient deficiencies (iron, pyridoxine and niacin) in blood or urine and correct if appropriate, taking into account other SNPs in the pathway and their impact.

Dopa decarboxylase: DDC

This gene encodes the enzyme dopa decarboxylase to make three conversions:

- L-2, 4 dihydroxyphenylalanine (L-dopa) to dopamine
- L-5-hydroxytryptophan to serotonin
- L-tryptophan to tryptamine.

DDC has been identified as a risk factor in many central nervous system disorders (Toma *et al.* 2012). Down-regulations of SNPs in this gene and SLC6A3 have been known to affect motor response. As such they have been studied in the area of Parkinson's disease where rs921451 and rs3837091 are said to influence the motor response to L-dopa but not change pharmacokinetic parameters for L-dopa and dopamine (Moreau *et al.* 2015).

Hypothetically speaking, the DDC gene splits at this point in effect and commences the individual pathways of serotonin and dopamine assimilation. There are far more studies on the effects of DDC on dopamine than on serotonin. For the purpose of clarity, the serotonin pathway will be addressed first.

Possible interventions based on DDC genetic expression
Nutrient cofactor to support DDC enzyme activity
Pyridoxine (Lynch 2017).

Unhelpful inhibitors that reduce DDC enzyme activity:
Dopamine, diuretics, HRT, fibrates (Lynch 2017).

Serotonin pathway

Sulphotransferase 1A3: SULT1A3

SULT genes encode for the sulphotransferase family cytosolic (1A) phenol-preferring member (3), which provide its name. Serotonin can be converted to serotonin-O-sulphate via sulphotransferase 1A (SULT1A3). The sulphotransferase enzymes assist the conjugation of sulphate to all the metabolic waste such as hormones, medications and xenobiotic compounds. 3'-phospho-5'-adenylylsulphate (PAPS) is utilized as a sulphate donor. When down-regulated, this gene has been associated with sudden cardiac death (Eagle 2012), neurodegenerative diseases and autism (Butcher *et al.* 2018).

Possible interventions based of SULT genetic expression
Nutrient cofactor to support SULT enzyme activity
3'-phosphoadenosine-5'-phosphosulphate (PAPS) (Harris & Waring 2008).

Unhelpful inhibitors that reduce SULT enzyme activity
Oestrogen, non-alcoholic fatty liver disease, cirrhosis (Yalcin *et al.* 2013), halogenated organic compounds, cigarette smoke toxicants, astralagus, curcumin, piperine (Zeng *et al.* 2017), flavonoids, polyphenols (Harris & Waring 2008), chlorogenic acid, green and black teas, heavy alcohol intake (Nishimula *et al.* 2007), winter (Eagle 2012).

Serotonin-N-acetyltransferase: AANAT

This gene (rs11077820, rs28697191, rs7360138) encodes the seroto-nin-N-acetyltransferase enzyme to create N-acetyl serotonin, the penultimate step in the production of melatonin. This enzyme is essential for the function of the circadian rhythm that influences the sleep–wake cycle as it controls the day and night rhythm of melatonin production in the pineal gland. AANAT activity increases 10–100-fold at night. Soria *et al.* (2010) and Kripke *et al.* (2011) identified AANAT down-regulation as a major contributor to the major forms of depression.

Possible interventions based on AANAT genetic expression
Nutrient cofactors to support AANAT enzyme activity
Pantothenic acid (Lynch 2017; Cohen 2015).

Animal studies have proven the importance of all B vitamins, magnesium and zinc in the production of melatonin. There is also evidence that essential fatty acids can positively influence melatonin synthesis (Peuhkuri *et al.* 2012).

Unhelpful inhibitors that reduce AANAT enzyme activity
Light (Lynch 2017; Pozdeyev *et al.* 2006), progesterone in luteal phase, bisphenol-A (Lynch 2017).

Acetylserotonin-O-methyltransferase: ASMT

This gene encodes the enzyme that transfers a methyl group on to acetylserotonin to produce melatonin. Jonsson *et al.* (2014) found an association between ASMT expression (rs5949028) and traits of autism, in particular the fact that those with ASD traits generally have low serotonin. This association was specifically related to females and not related to language impairment or repetitive behaviour.

Possible interventions based on ASMT genetic expression
Nutrient cofactor to support ASMT enzyme activity
SAM (Lynch 2017).

Unhelpful inhibitors that reduce ASMT enzyme function
Light exposure at night, depression, N-acetylserotonin (Lynch 2017), anything that hinders methylation (Cohen 2015).

Practical advice

- Check likely expression of all SNPs in this aspect of the pathway with organic acids markers or neurotransmitter testing to assess expression.
- Encourage good blood glucose regulation with diet and lifestyle in order to support oestrogen and the HPA axis (SULT1A3) (Si *et al.* 2015).
- Eliminate alcohol and smoking where necessary and address expressing ALDH genes (Byeon & Back 2016).
- Support liver detoxification with plenty of green leafy vegetables and good-quality protein (Guan & He 2015).
- Check medications, nutrients and herbs that slow down these enzymes further (Hodges & Minich 2015). Eliminate nutrients and herbs, refer to GP for medication review as appropriate.
- Ensure foods rich in the pantothenic acid (milk, yogurt, cheese, organ meats, fish, beef and sunflower seeds) and pyridoxine (turkey, chicken, duck, salmon, tuna, halibut, hazelnuts and walnuts) to support AANAT and DDC enzymes.
- Ensure good sleep hygiene by relaxing for two hours before bedtime, turning off all computers and limiting white light. Suggest guided meditation or reading to quieten the mind for sleep. Wear earplugs and eye mask or use blackout blinds for light sleepers. Early-morning walking in the sunshine, light box.

The final serotonin assimilation pathway is down through MAO, the aldehyde genes and sulphation for those following on the planner. To recap, DDC converts 5-HTP to serotonin at the beginning of the central assimilation pathway.

Monoamine oxidase: MAOA and B

Known affectionately as the warrior gene, MAO, which encodes the monoamine oxidase enzyme, has been in the literature for many years. It encodes an enzyme that breaks down the neurotransmitters noradrenaline, adrenaline and dopamine and serotonin. Sometimes this enzyme is termed as running fast or slow. They present in this way on testing:

MAO gene	Allele presentation	Fast or slow
MAOA/B	+/+	Slow
MAOA/B	+/−	Average
MAOA/B	−/−	Fast

These terms indicate the speed at which neurotransmitters are broken down. For example, if the enzyme is fast −/−, this means your client will have more of the enzyme and less available neurotransmitters. With a slow MAOA +/+, the reverse is true: low levels of the enzyme and higher levels of these neurotransmitters. Ideally, this needs to be balanced. MAOA resides in the pathway converting dopamine to vanillylmandelic acid, and serotonin to 5-HIAA, while MAOB resides in the pathway converting dopamine to homovanillic acid.

For the purposes of practitioner research, you may also see the MAO gene classified as 2R, 3R or 4R. The 2R version is the slow MAOA, which results in the lowest amount of MAOA and more circulating dopamine, adrenaline and noradrenaline. Those with this presentation are more prone to aggression and violence that can take hours to dissipate (Volavka *et al.* 2004). Other common symptoms of a slow MAO may include inability to fall asleep, highly charged startle reflex, headaches, irritability, mood swings and prolonged episodes of rage/aggression with difficulty in calming down. However, these patients can be much more focused, energetic, attentive and productive when not under pressure.

The 4R version, or fast MAO –/–, results in the highest amount of MAO and less adrenaline, noradrenaline and dopamine, so these people will be more passive. Common signs for these patients include a greater propensity towards addiction in the form of alcohol, sugar, food and carbohydrates, and towards ADHD (Malmberg *et al.* 2008). They have a tendency towards flat affect, low motivation and depression with fatigue. These patients can still get angry but they calm down very quickly. They are generally more easy-going.

The 3R version is in the middle, more likely to become aggressive than passive, just less so than 2R. Females with fast MAO may be huge chocolate and carbohydrate eaters and be quite overweight. This type of eating is also associated with low mood and waking in the night desperate to eat in order to get back to sleep. While a clear connection between carbohydrates and serotonin can be seen in this scenario, good-quality chocolate contains high levels of phenylalanine. This converts to tyrosine and L-dopa, then dopamine. Asking the client if he/she craves cheap chocolate (for the sugar) or good-quality chocolate (phenylalanine) may offer more clues for the practitioner.

Prior to the introduction of SSRIs, monoamine oxidase inhibitors (befloxatone and clorgyline) were the treatment of choice for many forms of clinical depression and anxiety disorder. MAO is an isozyme of monoamine oxidase that effectively assists in the deamination of noradrenaline, adrenaline and dopamine. Monoamine oxidase inhibitors failed to address a fast- or slow-processing COMT (more on this later) or vitamin D status, which both medications impact, so this is possibly why those drugs were never 100% successful.

Polymorphisms in the MAOA gene have been linked to alcohol and cigarette dependence in women (Philibert *et al.* 2008) and selective inhibition of this gene can promote an increase in arterial blood pressure, known as a pressor response, when foods high in tyramine are consumed. Very old studies have shown that inhibition of MAOA has also been linked to poor impulse control (Kolla *et al.* 2017).

Possible interventions based on MAO genetic expression

Nutrient cofactors to support MAO enzyme activity

Flavin adenine dinucleotide (FAD) (Gaweska & Fitzpatrick 2011).

MAO inhibitors that reduce enzyme activity (helpful
for fast MAO and unhelpful for slow)

MAO inhibitors. HRT, potassium-sparing diuretics, antidepressants, methotrexate, tricyclic antidepressants (Cohen 2015), quinolinic acid, heavy alcohol intake, smoking, caffeine, high-tyramine foods, quercetin, many herbs, acute stress, male gender.

Practical advice

- There is a need for a good intake of protein at breakfast for both the fast and slow MAO. This is in order to balance blood glucose levels and take the stress factor off the neurotransmitters so the body isn't heading into fight or flight, exacerbating the issue (Si *et al.* 2015).
- Check medication inhibitions and depletions of nutrients. Refer to GP for medicine review if appropriate.
- Eliminate alcohol and limit caffeine to one serving daily; encourage ceasing smoking by referring to smoking cessation clinic.
- Test gastrointestinal function, rebalance microbiome and heal the gut to reduce inflammation (Clapp *et al.* 2017).
- Encourage foods rich in riboflavin (milk, yogurt, cheese, chicken, beef, fish and egg) to support enzyme function.
- Test for riboflavin levels in serum or urine and replace as appropriate.

PRACTITIONER NOTES

Practitioners should ideally teach the patient to monitor their stress levels by listening to their body. Ensure you work with them to identify enjoyable activities that will assist in stress reduction. A fairly brisk walk in nature, cycling, HeartMath, Buteyko or yoga breathing or meditation can be undertaken at home for little cost. There are some potential tools to assist with this aspect in the Appendix. If the patient requires more than basic help to reduce stress, then a referral to a suitable practitioner identified from Klinghardt's 5 levels of healing or Network Spinal care may be suitable.

Alcohol dehydrogenase2 family: ALDH2

ALDH2 (rs4767939, rs7311852, rs4646778, rs16941667, rs2238152, rs2238151, rs968529) encodes the conversion of 5-HIA to 5-HIAA in the mitochondria, transforming acetaldehyde to acetic acid. As the second enzyme in the major oxidative pathway of alcohol, it functions as an antioxidant, protecting against oxidative stress, and is generally down-regulated, making the enzyme slower. This can leave the individual with higher levels of alcohol than normal and that may mean alcohol tolerance is lowered overall. The individual may feel a hangover quickly if they drink or if they suffer with yeast overgrowth. Various alleles have been identified in this gene, linking them to gastric cancer (rs16941667) (Wang *et al.* 2014), colorectal cancer, coronary artery disease and pharyngeal cancer (Yokoyama *et al.* 2015), and Parkinson's disease following pesticide exposure (Zhang *et al.* 2015). Poor metabolism of acetaldehydes needs to be taken into consideration when a patient has dysbiosis (Zeng *et al.* 2017; Leclercq *et al.* 2014).

Possible interventions based on ALDH genetic expression
Nutrient cofactor to support ALDH enzyme activity
NAD and thiamine (Lynch 2017; Cohen 2015).

Unhelpful inhibitors that reduce ALDH enzyme activity

- Methotrexate, trimethoprim, triamterene, folic acid, EGCG and grapefruit seed (Cohen 2015).
- Reactive nitrogen species, fungicides, acetylsalicylic acid, acetaminophen (Tylenol), carbon tetrachloride, excess omega 6 fatty acids (Lynch 2017).

Practical advice

- Encourage good blood glucose control and eliminate all pro-cessed foods to control aldehyde production in the gut (Painter *et al.* 2021).
- Test for evidence of dysbiosis and rebalance as appropriate to the case.
- Eliminate alcohol.
- Check for environmental exposure to paint and paint removers, cleaning solutions and degreasers, adhesives and sealants. Iden-tify the presence via lymphocyte sensitivity testing or toxic screen if suspected, address as appropriate.
- Check medications and natural products that may reduce enzyme function. Refer to GP for medication review as appropriate and replace antimicrobials with alternatives.
- Reduce green tea intake if high amounts ingested. There are some tentative suggestions that excessive intake of green tea also blocks the uptake of B12 from the gut, but these are mostly case studies (Fan 2016).
- Encourage foods rich in niacin (beef, fish, poultry, beans, peas, lentils) and thiamine (beans, peas, lentils, whole grains, pork).
- Test niacin and thiamine levels in serum or urine and supplement if appropriate.

PRACTITIONER NOTES

Serotonin is released by carcinoid tumours and metabolized by MAO in the lungs, liver and brain to 5-HIAA (Pandit *et al.* 2021). However, it doesn't seem to affect bone metabolism (van Dijk *et al.* 2012). Please check very high levels of 5-HIAA on organic acids and refer as necessary. Please also be aware that certain foods are known serotonin precursors; these include pineapple, banana, kiwi, plum, tomato, avocado, walnut and eggplant. Certain medications and supplements such as acetaminophen, nicotine and caffeine also may elevate 5-HIAA.

Alcohol dehydrogenase B1: ADH1B

This gene (rs17028834, rs6413413, rs042026, rs1353621, rs229983, rs2075633, rs1798883, rs2075633, rs1789883, rs1235416, rs1041969) encodes the alcohol dehydrogenase enzyme B1 to take 5-HIA into the SULT and UDP enzymes for sulphation. It metabolizes ethanol, retinal, hydroxysterols and lipid peroxidases, having a higher affinity for ethanol oxidation. Previously, this gene was known as ADH2. Polymorphisms in this gene are generally down-regulated or slow, and therefore associated with alcohol sensitivity, which may in part be due to the formation of acetaldehyde in the body. Also, those people with genetic susceptibility to alcohol sensitivity were seen to have a higher risk of depression (Yoshimasu *et al.* 2015).

Possible interventions based on ADH1B genetic expression
Nutrient cofactors to support ADH1B enzyme activity

- Zinc (Hill Erdei & Ledowski 2015).
- NAD and thiamine (Lynch 2017).

Unhelpful inhibitors that reduce ADH1B enzyme activity
Mercury, lead, elevated T4, being female, proton pump inhibitors, dioxin-like compounds, fasting and high alcohol intake, salicylates from food or medication (Lee *et al.* 2015).

Practical advice

- Check functional digestion and use of PPIs (may reduce B12 and iron absorption).
- Check for heavy metals in serum and/or urine and address as appropriate.
- Encourage good blood glucose control and eliminate all processed foods to control aldehyde production in the gut.
- Test for evidence of dysbiosis and rebalance as appropriate to the case.
- Eliminate alcohol.

- Check for environmental exposure to paint and paint removers, cleaning solutions and degreasers, adhesives and sealants. Lymphocyte sensitivity or toxic screen if suspected and address as appropriate.
- Check medications and natural products that may reduce enzyme function. Refer to GP for medication review as appropriate and replace antimicrobials with alternatives.
- Reduce green tea intake if high amounts are ingested. There are some tentative suggestions that excessive intake of green tea also blocks the uptake of B12 from the gut, but these are mostly case studies (Fan 2016).
- Encourage foods rich in niacin (beef, fish, poultry, beans, peas and lentils), thiamine (beans, peas, lentils, whole grains, pork) and zinc (oysters, crab, beef, dark meat, pork, chickpeas and black beans).
- Test niacin, thiamine and zinc levels in serum or urine and supplement if appropriate.

Sulphotransferase family1A1 and 1A2: SULT1A1 and 1A2

These genes encode for two more enzymes of the sulphotransferase family that catalyze the sulphation of neurotransmitters, hormones, medications and xenobiotic compounds. In this case, sulphation mostly of serotonin is occurring.

Possible interventions based on SULT1A1 and 1A2 genetic expression
Nutrient cofactor to support SULT1A1 and 1A2 enzyme activity
PAPS – the universal sulfate donor PAPS is synthesized by PAPS synthase (PAPSs), a bifunctional protein including ATP-sulfurylase and APS-kinase activities (Venkatachalam 2003).

Unhelpful inhibitors that reduce SULT1A1 and 1A2 enzyme activity
Oestrogen, non-alcoholic fatty liver disease, cirrhosis (Yalcin et al. 2013), halogenated organic compounds, cigarette smoke toxicants, astralagus,

curcumin, piperine (Zeng *et al.* 2017), flavonoids, polyphenols (Harris & Waring 2008), chlorogenic acid, green and black teas, heavy alcohol intake (Nishimuta *et al.* 2007), winter (Eagle 2012).

Practical advice

- PAPS are produced from sulphate at the end of transsulphuration so the need to ensure adequate sulphation is key.
- Eliminate alcohol.
- Ensure good blood glucose control with nutritional intervention, optimizing digestive function and reducing dysbiosis to help balance endocrine system.
- Encourage Epsom salts baths as appropriate.
- Check for environmental exposure to halogenated organic compounds (trichloromethane, dioxins and furans). Most contain bromine or chlorine, which can displace iodine, leading to unbalanced thyroid function. SULT1 family members have been identified as sulphating the simple phenols of estradiol and thyroid hormones. Other phenols sulphated by SULT1 are environmental xenobiotics and drugs (Lindsay *et al.* 2008).

UDP glucoronosyltransferase family 1: UGT1A6/UDP

The UGT/UDP enzyme is found in the cells of the liver. It is a membrane bound protein localized to the endoplasmic reticulum (Konopnicki *et al.* 2013). This gene encodes the enzyme UDP glucoronosyltransferase as part of the glucuronidation pathway. The enzyme is generally down-regulated or running slow, thereby compromising detoxification via glucuronidation. Adding D-glucarate to a toxic molecule can make it:

- more water soluble
- less toxic and reactive
- easily transported through the body
- possible to eliminate via urine (Stein *et al.* 2013).

Glucuronic acid is conjugated with a number of different substances. UGT1A1 and 1A6 are the only enzymes that conjugate glucuronidase bilirubin from its toxic (unconjugated) form, making it more soluble for excretion in bile via the digestive tract. The enzyme is of major importance for the conjugation of potentially toxic xenobiotics and endogenous compounds such as 17beta-estradiol, 17alpha-ethinylestradiol, 1-hydroxypyrene and 1-naphthol (Jancova et al. 2010). UGT1A6 is related to angina pectoris, non-small-cell lung carcinoma, diarrhoea, drug toxicity, Gilbert's syndrome, heart failure, genital female neoplasms, hepatitis, HIV, hyperbilirubinemia, neonatal jaundice, neutropenia thrombocytopenia and tuberculosis (Barbarino et al. 2014). Dopamine and serotonin are also processed by UGTs (Ouzzine et al. 2014).

Possible interventions based on UGT/UDP genetic expression

Nutrient cofactors to support UGT/UDP enzyme activity
UDP-α-D-glucarate.

Unhelpful inhibitors that reduce UGT/UDP enzyme activity
Organochlorides, bisphenol-A and food dyes, phosphatidylcholine, lipopolysaccharides, green and black tea, quercetin, rutin, naringenin, allspice, peppermint oil, cacao and silymarin (Jenkinson et al. 2013).

Practical advice

- Encourage organic eating of whole foods, especially brassicas for liver support; add beets including stalks and leaves (Hodges & Minich 2015) and lemons (Cherng et al. 2016) to assist bile flow.
- Eliminate environmental exposure to organochlorides via organic eating and avoiding farmland where regular crop-spraying occurs.
- Reduce inflammation via rebalancing gut microbiome, stress-reducing techniques and spending time in nature.
- Reduce green and black tea if intake is excessive.
- Remove food dyes and polyphenols as above if supplementing.

- Encourage good blood glucose regulation to support hormones and neurotransmitters.
- D-glucarate is sound in fruits and vegetables, especially Brussels sprouts, cabbage, broccoli, oranges and apples, so encourage these on a daily basis.
- Recommend D-glucarate as appropriate. Some organic acid testing companies test for glucaric acid but not all (Lord & Bralley 2008).

Serotonin assimilation and sulphation is now complete, so please go back up the pathway planner to L-dopa where the dopamine pathway will be discussed.

Dopamine pathway

Ornithine decarboxylase and dopa decarboxylase: ODC/DDC

The ODC gene encodes for the ornithine decarboxylase enzyme. This enzyme catalyzes the conversion of ornithine, from the urea cycle, to putrescine. DDC conversely is responsible for the conversion of L-dopa to dopamine. They both initiate the biosynthesis of amines and particularly dopamine. Learning about this metabolic pathway is crucial for those practitioners specializing in supporting patients with autism spectrum diagnoses, schizophrenia, major hormone imbalance and chronic fatigue/myalgic encephalitis. DDC regulation is tightly controlled and varies according to environmental stimuli (Pegg 2006), so practitioners will need to carefully assess symptoms and use functional testing to assess expression. A novel pathway described by Asher *et al.* (2005) is responsible for degradation of ODC during oxidative stress; NADH regulates the pathway.

Aspirin also influences the breakdown of amines within this pathway. The variant ODC influences how many polyamines are produced and how quickly they are broken down. There may be synergistic effects between aspirin and the ODC gene as they act via different mechanisms in the same pathway (Martinez *et al.* 2003). In fact, in the Martinez *et al.* study, a homozygous presentation of the A-allele of ODC was consistent with a lower risk of colorectal adenoma recurrence, associated with aspirin use.

Dopa decarboxylase: DDC

Dopamine is formed by removing a carboxyl group from a molecule of L-dopa. Dopamine plays a number of very important roles in the body. In the brain it is the neurotransmitter associated with reward. Most types of reward stimulate the production of dopamine in the brain. Individuals with low dopamine may be addicted to all manner of things that might stimulate them to feel better temporarily, and this may not at first glance be obvious as practitioners tend to associate drugs, cigarettes and alcohol with low dopamine. Other factors could be overeating (Volkow *et al.* 2011; De Weijer et al. 2011), sugar and stimulant addiction (Nutt *et al.* 2015), being 'driven'. We look for reward in so many different ways: for some this means the highest educational accomplishment; for others it's the job of our dreams, striving for perfection. For those who teach, it may be the feedback, so they may work endless hours producing the most amazing teaching sessions. Individuals may be looking for the reward because they cannot create the reward within themselves, or other aspects of life are less than satisfactory. Dopamine is the most studied neurotransmitter in relation to personality traits, which is outside the scope of this book. For those interested, DeYoung (2013) has explored this well. Also, as practitioners, don't forget movement disorders. Are we becoming a nation of low-dopamine humans due to dependence on the instant gratification received from information and communications technology? Do not miss this when considering mood disorders and dopamine.

Possible interventions based on ODC/DDC genetic expression
Nutrient cofactor to support ODC/DDC enzyme activity
ODC and DDC: pyridoxine P-5-P (Pegg 2006; Bassiri *et al.* 2015), NADH (Asher *et al.* 2005).

Unhelpful inhibitors that reduce ODC/DDC enzyme activity

- ODC: difluoromethylornithine (DMFO) anticancer agent (Alexiou *et al.* 2017; Bassiri *et al.* 2015).
- DDC: carbidopa (Montioli *et al.* 2016).

Practical advice

- Encourage eating of organic whole foods.
- Reduce inflammation via rebalancing gut microbiome, stress-reducing techniques (see Appendix) and spending time in nature.
- Encourage good blood glucose regulation to support hormones and neurotransmitters.
- Check medications for possible interactions and nutrient depletions.
- Check folate and methionine SNPs and metabolic markers (serum active B12 and folate, urine methylmalonic acid, FiGlu or uracil, homovanillic acid and vanillylmandelic acid) to ensure adequate neurotransmitters can be produced. Consider urine or dried urine neurotransmitter testing for a comprehensive evaluation.
- Encourage foods high in pyridoxine (salmon, halibut, turkey, chicken, duck, hazelnuts and walnuts) for DDC and niacin (beef, fish, poultry, beans, peas and lentils) for ODC.
- Test for nutrient deficiencies in serum or urine and address any imbalances.

Dopamine beta-hydroxylase: DBH

This gene encodes the dopamine beta-hydroxylase enzyme that converts dopamine to noradrenaline. It can be found in the brain, sympathetic nerves and the adrenal medulla. DBH within the serum originates from the sympathetic nervous system, while DBH from the cerebrospinal fluid originates from the central noradrenergic neurons. The latter form is found in soluble and membrane forms in the medulla. DBH is released into the circulation with neurotransmitters during synaptic transmission.

It inhibits tyrosine hydroxylase, which reduces dopamine production. As a result of its importance in the dopamine pathway, this gene is a novel target for pharmaceutical intervention (Punchaichira *et al.* 2020).

If DBH is under-expressing, the conversion of dopamine to noradrenaline is slow, but dopamine can also be assimilated down the right-hand side pathway to 3-methoxytryamine via COMT, to homovanillic acid via MAOB or be sulphated to dopamine 3-0-sulphate by SULT1A3. Alternatively, dopamine can be diverted down the left-hand pathway via COMT to be converted to normetanephrine, to be converted by MAO lower down, thereby bypassing the main pathway. HPA axis function may become compromised and with a slow COMT there may still be dopamine trapping. At this point, dopamine receptors DRD2 may express as a compensatory mechanism, preventing dopamine adhesion and allowing the excess dopamine to be excreted in urine. Practitioners will need to check all these parameters to gain a thorough understating of expression and risk to the patient.

Methoxytyramine and normetanephrine rise in rare cases of pheochromocytomas and paragangliomas and can be measured in serum (Gupta *et al.* 2015). Pheochromocytomas are tumours that arise in the adrenal glands, creating excess catecholamines noradrenaline and adrenaline. Paragangliomas are neuroendocrine tumours found in the head, neck, abdomen, pelvis and chest (Costa *et al.* 2015).

PRACTITIONER NOTES

If an individual has extremely high levels of salivary cortisol on daily samples, one must rule out methoxytyramine and normetanephrine as a cause and refer as necessary.

Noradrenaline provides an important role in the autonomic nervous system by controlling involuntary processes such as blood pressure regulation and regulation of body temperature. According to Hill Erdei and Ledowski (2015), at least six mutations on the DBH gene have been identified that interfere with the normal function of dopamine ß-hydroxylase, leading to a shortfall in noradrenaline, causing poor blood pressure control or postural orthostatic tachycardia syndrome (Crnošija *et al.* 2012; Wassenburg *et al.* 2021). At least six alleles have been identified as causing dopamine ß-hydroxylase deficiency when expressing.

SNPs in the DBH gene are thought to increase the incidence of psychosis in individuals with schizophrenia (Park *et al.* 2007) or unipolar major depression (Mustapić *et al.* 2007). Kwon and Lim (2013) also explored the association between DBH and ADHD and found a possible association.

As a little sidestep to show practitioners what can happen in this pathway, a small case study may help.

Ed was a young person with a diagnosis of autism spectrum disorder who presented with gender dysphoria. This is a feeling of distress or discomfort with the gender they were assigned at birth and one they identify with. These people may be referred to as transgender or non-binary. This caused more anxiety than the ASD diagnosis; hence Ed was currently on a medical programme for gender reassignment. Ed's gut was so dysfunctional, mostly due to the anxiety, that direct tube feeding into the stomach was in situ. Consultants responsible for Ed's care fully appreciated the need for nutritional and lifestyle coaching, so Ed was referred.

Many attempts to initiate testosterone exogenously as a transdermal cream resulted in suicide ideation, which Ed hadn't shared with the medical consultants due to Ed's fear that treatment might be postponed. Ed knew they felt otherwise well with a testosterone level of around 11ng/dl; nevertheless, Ed started feeling suicidal.

When Ed came for advice, they had their genetic results already. A test for organic acids and urinary neurotransmitters revealed a very slow DBH enzyme, and less problematic COMT enzymes which translate to poor ability to break down dopamine pathway products. Once the exogenous testosterone was delivered and Ed's levels built up to around 11ng/dl, this compromised further an already heavily loaded pathway. The best analogy to describe this would be a four-lane motorway full and moving at regular motorway speed limits. A crash in one lane slows traffic down to the minimum as cars move out of the blocked lane. The other lanes slow as drivers slow down to view the incident. Once the emergency services arrive, the motorway section is closed for investigation and all cars are diverted off the motorway or on to the hard shoulder until the debris from the incident has been cleared. In effect, administering the extra testosterone severely compromised Ed's dopamine pathway, creating dopamine trapping above the DBH enzyme (Ryding *et al.* 2008). Supporting the DBH enzyme with the interventions below, while finely tuning a much lower dose of testosterone to keep Ed's serum testosterone level around 11 achieved the neurotransmitter balance. Addressing serious dysbiosis of parasites, yeast and clostridia, and addressing cell membrane integrity over the long term allowed the introduction of oral foods.

Possible interventions based on DBH genetic expression
Nutrient cofactors to support DBH enzyme activity

- Vitamin C and copper (Cohen 2015; Lynch 2017).
- Pyrroloquinoline quinone (PQQ) (Lynch 2017). PQQ stimulates mitochondriogenesis (the production of mitochondria) and plays a positive role in redox signalling. It is often added to coenzyme Q10.

Unhelpful inhibitors that reduce DBH enzyme activity
Excess copper/hydrogen peroxide (Parvez *et al.* 2013), cysteine, panax ginseng (Kim *et al.* 2008), hypericum perfoliatum (Denke *et al.* 2000), disulfiram for the treatment of alcoholism and nepicostat for the treatment of cardiovascular disease and posttraumatic stress disorder (PTSD) (Manvich *et al.* 2013).

Practical advice

- Encourage organic or follow the dirty dozen/clean fifteen foods list where possible.

- Check medication interactions and nutrient depletions that may impact on enzyme function.
- Reduce alcohol intake and rebalance microbiome.
- Check copper levels (serum) or zinc-to-copper ratios.
- Encourage foods high in vitamin C (kiwi, strawberries, sweet red peppers, citrus fruits and vegetables), copper (oysters, clams, crabs, hazelnuts, almonds, peas, beans and lentils) and PQQ (parsley, papaya, green peppers (Robertson *et al.* 1989), spinach and fermented soy beans or natto (Noji *et al.* 2007)).
- Check folate and methionine SNPs and metabolic markers (serum active B12 and folate, urine methylmalonic acid, FiGlu or uracil, homovanillic acid and vanillylmandelic acid) to ensure adequate neurotransmitters can be produced. Consider urine or dried urine neurotransmitter testing for a comprehensive evaluation.

Phenylethonolamine N-methyltransferase: PNMT

PNMT (rs5638, rs876493) encodes the enzyme phenylethonolamine N-methyltransferase, in the adrenal medulla, to convert noradrenaline to adrenaline. It makes the conversion by transferring a methyl group from SAM to noradrenaline. If expressing, it is generally down-regulated, meaning a slower conversion of noradrenaline to adrenaline. This may manifest as anxiety and/or depression, changes in blood pressure, changes in heart rate, hypoglycaemia, migraine headaches and sleep issues.

PNMT shares some similarities in structure with COMT, but the evidence from its structure would suggest PNMT is a more recent adaptation to the catecholamine-synthesizing family. It is seen as evolving later than COMT but prior to GNMT (Martin *et al.* 2001). In Caucasians, PNMT SNPs are associated with the development of acute kidney injury, disease severity and in-hospital mortality (Alam *et al.* 2010), essential hypertension (Millis 2011) and neurocardiovascular disorders (Chaudhari *et al.* 2012). There are some animal studies on the effects of PNMT polymorphisms on HPA axis dysfunction associated disorder but so far no human studies. PNMT has been shown to be both hormonally and neutrally regulated by the HPA axis and the sympathoadrenal system (Wong 2003). Glucocorticoids are known to increase the half-life of the enzyme (Križanová *et al.* 2001).

Possible interventions based on PNMT genetic expression
Nutrient cofactors to support PNMT enzyme activity
SAM acts as a cofactor but also stabilizes the enzyme by increasing its half-life (Lynch 2017; Cohen 2015).

Unhelpful inhibitors that reduce PNMT enzyme activity
S-adenosyl homocysteine, excess adrenaline, Cushing syndrome and medication-induced Cushing syndrome, phenylethylamines and meth-amphetamine (Lynch 2017).

Practical advice

- Encourage organic eating or follow the dirty dozen/clean fifteen foods list where possible.
- Check medication interactions and nutrient depletions that may impact on enzyme function.
- Reduce alcohol intake and rebalance microbiome.
- Check folate and methionine SNPs and metabolic markers (serum active B12 and folate, urine methylmalonic acid, FiGlu or uracil, homovanillic acid and vanillylmandelic acid) to ensure adequate neurotransmitters can be produced. Consider urine or dried urine neurotransmitter testing for a comprehensive evaluation.
- Optimize methylation to provide methyl groups and SAM for enzyme support.

PRACTITIONER NOTES

When considering low levels of adrenaline, please note the following:

- low adrenaline and high noradrenaline
- evaluate cortisol levels
- consider HPA axis dysfunction
- consider a methylation deficiency.

Symptoms of low adrenaline:

- HPA axis dysfunction
- weight gain
- depression
- poor concentration.

Catechol-0-methyltransferase: COMT

Encoded by the COMT gene, catechol-0-methyltransferase is another one of the enzymes that degrade the catecholamines dopamine, noradrenaline and adrenaline. COMT adds a methyl group to dopamine, noradrenaline and adrenaline, after SAM has donated this. Having too little SAM and too much SAH means COMT will be compromised (Zhu & Liehr 1996). COMT is found in two forms: S-COMT, which is in soluble form, and MB-COMT, which is membrane bound. COMT also plays a role in oestrogen breakdown when paired with certain CYP enzymes. These were discussed under detoxification. Some medications and xenoestrogens are also broken down via COMT and the other enzymes in this pathway. Recall earlier it was mentioned that this pathway was exciting and really useful to understand? Well, this is why.

The two most important SNPs are the H62H (rs4633) and V158M (rs4680). There are many others, but these have not been evaluated in the evidence base. That is not to say the others should be ignored, especially if there is clear expression not assigned to these two specific alleles. The V158M AA allele, or homozygous +/+ presentation, is said to be 'slow'-running COMT and may be down-regulated by as much as 70%. This can elevate dopamine levels, so by comparison the GG allele or wild card –/– presentation is 'fast', meaning dopamine can be broken down more quickly. GG +/– is in the mid-range (Heyer *et al.* 2009). Dopamine needs to be homeostatic because levels that are either too high or too low can impede cognitive performance. COMT breaks down dopamine in the prefrontal cortex, which is the area of the brain responsible for executive functioning. V158M rs4680 has been associated with differences in intelligence, personality and disease risk, with a 3–4-fold decrease in activity (Tiihonen *et al.* 1999). Very high and very low levels of dopamine have both been associated with lower cognitive performance (Mitaki *et al.* 2013).

COMT activity in the prefrontal cortex is reduced by 30% in women. This is due to oestrogen being a down-regulator of the enzyme. This translates to a 30% increase in dopamine for women versus men (Woods *et al.* 2014; Schendzielorz *et al.* 2011; Coman *et al.* 2010). Dopamine increases under stressful conditions, so those with expressing COMT +/+ are likely to perform less well under stress while others will likely perform better due to a potentially optimal dopamine level (Dobryakova *et al.* 2015). It has been hypothesized that this may be why female performance generally declines under stress while male performance is generally better. In essence, an expressing COMT V158M AA allele +/+ may be helpful for males but detrimental for females (Woods *et al.* 2014). Is this one of the reasons why males often achieve higher ranks in promotions or attain promotion more quickly?

In addition, Schendzielorz *et al.* (2011) hypothesized that COMT may also inactivate oestrogen, offering a positive effect on oestrogen-dominant cancers. However, administering both tamoxifen and estradiol only affected COMT in the prefrontal cortex and the kidneys, where COMT is physiologically important for dopamine metabolism. Having excessive levels of S-adenosyl homocysteine and too little SAM can also inhibit the COMT enzyme.

On a more positive note, the COMT V158M AA allele +/+ has been shown to increase creativity (Zhang *et al.* 2014), improve working memory (Aguilera *et al.* 2008), better reading comprehension

(Landi *et al.* 2013), increased brain plasticity in the elderly (Heinzel *et al.* 2014), increased ability to refocus after making an error and better response to the placebo effect (Hall *et al.* 2012).

However, these individuals may be more prone to anxiety (Montag *et al.* 2012), have lower emotional resilience and more impulsivity (Soeiro-De-Souza *et al.* 2013), have a higher homocysteine (Gellekink *et al.* 2007), be more introverted (Hoth *et al.* 2006). Males are said to be at higher risk for mercury sensitivity and were more likely than girls to suffer cognitive impairment as a result of mercury toxicity (Woods *et al.* 2014).

Those with a COMT GG –/– allele were found conversely to be good at handling stress and pain (Zubieta *et al.* 2003), had more emotional resilience (Smolka 2005) and a more empathetic nature (Baeken *et al.* 2014). While they may have received less pleasure from life and have poorer executive function, this improved under stress (Mier *et al.* 2010).

SO WHICH COMT ARE YOU?
Try this test and see.
Imagine you are driving along a road.
    The police suddenly emerge in your rear-view mirror with sirens and flashing lights.
    How long does it take you to calm down?

Possible interventions based on COMT genetic expression
Nutrient cofactors to support COMT enzyme activity
SAM, magnesium (Lynch 2017).

Inhibitors that reduce COMT enzyme activity (may be helpful with fast COMT and unhelpful with slow COMT depending on symptomology)
Corticosteroids, HRT/oral contraceptives, sulphonamides (Cohen 2015).

Practical advice

- Encourage organic eating or follow the dirty dozen/clean fifteen foods list where possible.

- Check medication interactions and nutrient depletions that may impact on enzyme function.
- Reduce alcohol intake and rebalance microbiome.
- Check folate and methionine SNPs and metabolic markers (serum active B12 and folate, urine methylmalonic acid, FiGlu or uracil, homovanillic acid and vanillylmandelic acid) to ensure adequate neurotransmitters and SAM can be produced.
- If dopamine is high, optimize this pathway as a priority before addressing methionine and folate cycles.
- Consider urine or dried urine neurotransmitter testing for a comprehensive evaluation.
- Optimize methylation to provide methyl groups and SAM for enzyme support.
- Encourage foods high in magnesium (green leafy vegetables, nuts and seeds, whole grains) (Linus Pauling Institute n.d.).

PRACTITIONER NOTES

In the slow COMT individual, practitioners may also wish to consider adequate levels of pyridoxine, cobalamin and folate as these support the formation of S-adenosylmethionine, which supports COMT (Jatana *et al.* 2014), and prevent the rise of homocysteine. Consider indole-3-carbinol, broccoli seed extract or D-glucarate as relevant to the case if oestrogen is high as oestrogens also inhibit COMT (Schendzielorz *et al.* 2011). Consider preventing the oxidation of dopamine with antioxidants but not quercetin, rutin, luteolin, EGCG, catechins, epicatechins as these may inhibit COMT (Wang *et al.* 2012). It is really important to explore stress-reduction techniques with COMT expression, and if they have BHMT too, they may be completely internalizing all the stress. Stress hormones complete with oestrogens and require COMT for their breakdown.

Drugs metabolized by COMT include adrenaline, alpha-methyl drugs, apomorphine, dobutamine, dopamine, 2-hydroxyesotrogens, 4-hydroxyestrogens, isoprenaline, levetiracetam, zonisamide.

If COMT is fast, the practitioner may need to consider increasing dopamine with phenylethylamine (PEA) (Ash 2010) DL-phenylala-nine (Kapalka 2010), tyrosine (Daubner *et al.* 2011), EGCG, luteolin, quercetin, rutin (Chen *et al.* 2013), olive leaf extract (Sarbishegi *et al.* 2014) or the essential oils of oregano and thyme (Zotti *et al.* 2013) as required, depending on the case. Incidentally, carvacrol from oregano and thyme essential oils is also reputed to be useful in removing biofilms (Dos Santos Rodrigues *et al.* 2017).

Oxytocin and dopamine share roles in a limited way but oxytocin doesn't appear to burn out in the same way (Baskerville & Douglas 2010) so if raising dopamine for an individual seems impossible, do consider increasing oxytocin levels naturally. Nutritional options include vitamin D and sunshine (Patrick & Ames 2014), vitamin C, magnesium, Epsom baths and taurine (Ebner *et al.* 2004), caffeine, oestrogen, chamomile (Gholami *et al.* 2016), oleoylethanolamide (OEA), melatonin, fenugreek, jasmine essential oil, clary sage essen-tial oil diffused (Tadokoro *et al.* 2017) and increased fluid intake.

Possible first-line clinical tools

- Adaptogens: ashwaganda (*Withania*), tulsi, ginseng, *Rhodiola*, *Cordyceps*, *Astralagus*, liquorice to help reduce anxiety (Salve *et al.* 2019).
- Magnesium: glycinate (less laxative producing and transsulphura-tion supporting), taurate (heart muscle), malate (fibromyalgia), citrate (constipation). Consider transdermal (Nielsen *et al.* 2010).
- Check in on the TCA cycle intermediaries in the organic acids.

Other considerations

- Coconut vinegar to support liver (Mohamad *et al.* 2018) and microbiome (Mohamad *et al.* 2017).
- Balanced electrolytes to regulate nerve and muscle function (Shrimanker & Bhattarai 2021).
- Consider pyridoxine P-5-P to balance SAM/SAH and GAD.

- Mitochondria – there are lots in the brain and eyes, so if there is vision loss, consider mitochondria and fatty acids (visual acuity tests are available online) and indicate the need for cell membrane rescue with PC and EFAs.
- Consider astaxanthin for eyes (mitochondria), phosphatidylserine if not depressed, red blood cell fatty acid analysis and the use of a nut- and seed-based smoothie as a medium for fatty acid delivery.

Dopamine receptors 1, 2, 3 and 4: DRD2, 3 and 4

It would be remiss not to discuss DRD2 receptors here with COMT and DBH because when COMT is slow, the DRD receptors can sometimes down-regulate, releasing dopamine in the urine to compensate. A number of rs alleles have been identified in each receptor the DRD1 alleles include rs4867798, rs251937, rs686, rs5326, rs4532 and rs265981. DRD1 receptors regulate neuronal growth and development. DRD1 is a G-protein couple receptor that stimulates adenylyl cyclase and cAMP-dependent protein kinases. They are widely expressed throughout the brain. Rs4352 and rs5326 may contribute to the development of schizophrenia (Yao *et al.* 2015) by interacting with other genes. SNPs rs686 and rs265981 have been associated with maternal orienting away from the infant. This translates as poor or lack of maternal social bonding or lack of attachment (Mileva-Seitz *et al.* 2012). Oxytocin is also involved (De Dreu 2012).

G-proteins that inhibit adenylyl cyclase mediate DRD2 receptor activity. Reducing the activity of DRD2 may therefore treat schizophrenia (Göllner & Fielder 2015). A number of alleles of DRD2 have been associated with certain conditions. Examples include rs4245146 and generalized anxiety disorder that is worse with comorbid alcohol abuse (Sipilä *et al.* 2010), smoking and nicotine dependence (Laucht *et al.* 2008) and sleep disturbance, obesity and impulsivity in children (Chan *et al.* 2014).

DRD3 is also mediated by the G-proteins that regulate DRD2 and is specific to the limbic centre of the brain. The limbic system is associated with emotional, cognitive and endocrine functions. Again, a number of alleles have been identified in relation to schizophrenia (rs963488) (Domínguez *et al.* 2007), stimming behaviour in autism such as rs167771 (Staal *et al.* 2015), early-onset heroin dependence relating to rs324029 (Kuo *et al.* 2014). However, rs6280 was associated with a lower risk for Parkinson's disease but with a higher risk of aberrant decision making (Rajan *et al.* 2018).

DRD4 is responsible for neuronal signalling in the mesolimbic system of the brain, thereby helping regulate emotion and complex behaviour. This gene is again regulated by the G-proteins that inhibit adenylyl cyclase. DRD4 has been linked to a number of neurological and psychiatric conditions such as bipolar disorder, addictive behaviours, eating disorders such as anorexia nervosa and bulimia nervosa (Ptacek *et al.* 2011). The DRD enzymes are found in the cellular membranes.

Possible interventions based on DRD genetic expression
Nutrient cofactors to support DRD enzyme activity
Stephania – a Chinese herb (Wei *et al.* 2007) that is outside the remit of the nutrition therapist and would need a referral. There are no known nutrient cofactors available at this time.

Unhelpful Inhibitors that reduce DRD enzyme activity:
Metoclopramide (DiPalma 1990).

PRACTITIONER NOTES

Is it low dopamine or low serotonin?

Table 5.1: Low dopamine or serotonin?

Low dopamine	Low serotonin
Anhedonia (lack of joy)	Anxiety
Lack of motivation	Insomnia

Apathy	Depression
Procrastination	Uncontrolled appetite
Low libido	Headaches
Prolonged sleeping/excessive tiredness	Unexplained gastrointestinal pathology
Memory loss	

Taken from Young (2007), Lombard Pauling Institute (n.d.) and Armine (2014)

Aldehyde dehydrogenase 3A2: ALDH3A2

ALDH3A2 encodes the enzyme aldehyde dehydrogenase, which in turn plays a major role in the detoxification of aldehydes that are generated from alcohol metabolism and lipid peroxidation. Down-regulation of this enzyme as a result of a SNP may therefore result in an increase of aldehydes in the system. This particular gene of the aldehyde family is a fatty acid aldehyde dehydrogenase (rs72547575, rs8069576, 72547566, rs1800869, rs72547564). The enzyme functions by catalyzing the oxidation of long-chain aliphatic aldehydes into fatty acids. It acts upon both unsaturated and saturated forms of fatty acids, between six and 24 carbons in length (Kelson *et al.* 1997).

Aberrant microbial populations within the gut generate some of these aldehydes, so please consider the evidence for this as a practitioner. ALDH3A2 has been documented here due to the impact it has on the metabolism of catecholamines, but aldehyde genes found in the aldehyde pathway where yeast may be a major issue include ALDH1, ALDH2, ALDH1B1 and ALDH3A2.

Alterations in aldehyde metabolism may manifest as hydroxybutyric aciduria, hyperammonia (can be found on organic acid markers), hypoprolinemia or pyridoxine-dependent seizures, because, of course, pyridoxine is also an aldehyde. Mutations and deletions have been associated with the autosomal recessive form of Sjögren-Larsson syndrome (Nakahara *et al.* 2012).

Possible interventions based on ALDH3A2 genetic expression
Nutrient cofactors to support ALDH3A2 enzyme activity
NAD and thiamine (Lynch 2017).

Unhelpful inhibitors that reduce ALDH3A2 enzyme activity
Psoriasis (Lynch 2017), alcohol, antibiotics, antacids, PPIs, other acid-reducing medications (Cohen 2015).

Practical advice

- Advise eating an organic diet or follow the dirty dozen/clean fifteen lists of foods.
- Check medication interactions and nutrient depletions that may impact on enzyme function.
- Check digestive function and correct as appropriate.
- Reduce alcohol intake and rebalance microbiome.
- Check folate and methionine SNPs and metabolic markers (serum active B12 and folate, urine methylmalonic acid, FiGlu or uracil, homovanillic acid and vanillylmandelic acid) to ensure adequate neurotransmitters and SAM can be produced.
- If dopamine is high, optimize this pathway as a priority before addressing methionine and folate cycles.
- Consider urine or dried urine neurotransmitter testing for a comprehensive evaluation.
- Optimize methylation to provide methyl groups and SAM for enzyme support.
- Encourage foods high in thiamine (peas, beans, lentils, whole grains and pork) and niacin (beef, poultry, fish, beans, peas and lentils) (Linus Pauling Institute n.d.).
- Interestingly, fasting, toxicants from cigarette smoke, amiodarone and valproic acid (Epilim) can increase the activity of this enzyme.

PRACTITIONER NOTES

Rebalance BH4

Excess ammonia and oxidative stress both deplete BH4, so address these first. Work on nutritional intake as a starting point. Repair cell membrane and then support mitochondrial function. Leaky blood–brain barrier = leaky gut = leaky cell membranes. Consider methionine and folate cycles once transsulphuration and biopterin stability has returned.

Dopamine diet and lifestyle

- Eat regular meals that are balanced with good amounts of proteins, complex carbohydrates and healthy fats. This supports blood glucose levels so they don't swing or cause hunger in the evening.
- Eat a good amount of protein at breakfast to ensure you start your day in good balance. Breakfast for many is the most important meals of the day. Eggs, smoked salmon, mackerel or yogurt with seeds and fruit are all good choices.
- Aim for low glycaemic load carbohydrates such as rye or porridge. These are higher in fibre to support appetite control, detoxification and blood glucose levels.
- Include healthy fats such as nut and seed oils in addition to avocado, chia, flaxseeds and oily fish such as herring, trout and pilchards for their anti-inflammatory benefits.
- Eat lean proteins at lunch and dinner such as lentils and pulses, chicken, fish or lean beef.
- Exercise and laughing with friends is known to raise dopamine, so indulge in yoga classes and time outdoors with friends. Why not try forest bathing (Li *et al.* 2016)?

ELLA'S CASE: BIOPTERIN PATHWAY

As can be observed in Ella's biopterin pathway, this could potentially be the worst area for exploration. This system could be very slow-running, and if considered alone, one might suspect dopamine trapping leading to the symptoms such as suicide ideation, poor impulse control, obsessive compulsive disorder, psychosis and/or aggression. Ella displays none of these symptoms, although she can be prone to suppressing anger.

Looking at Ella's mutations in Figure 5.7, it can be clearly seen that issues with biopterin cycling may be apparent. Also slow breakdown of both dopamine and serotonin may be an issue. However, due to Ella's methylation being slow, this slow breakdown seems to be having a positive effect.

Analysis of Ella's SNPs and functional test results

Kynurenic acid is very high on the organic acid result, indicating backward flow of tryptophan into the kynurenine pathway. Thankfully, this is not being converted to quinolinic acid, so we can assume a degree of neuroprotection at this point. Arginine is low, while citrulline is very high, indicating a possible urinary tract infection or eNOS uncoupling, leading to generation of superoxide free radicals that may impede endothelial function (Kietadisorn *et al.* 2011). There were no other indictors of oxidative stress and no incidence of atheroma in Ella's family members, but it still is something to be mindful of.

There are high levels of 5-HIAA in the organic acids, possibly as a result of dysbiosis. Ella was presenting with anxiety and changeable mood, with cycling episodes of euphoria and flat affect without provocation. This may suggest neurotransmitter imbalances. Vanillylmandelic acid and homovanillic acid were also low, linked to her slow COMT, MAO and ALDH enzymes. It would be easy to take the stance that Ella is producing insufficient levels of neurotransmitters and so increasing methylation with B12 and folate should be a priority. However, Ella's homocysteine was already 17 with compromised transsulphuration, so the decision to address transsulphuration while supporting neurotransmitter levels with amino acids seemed prudent.

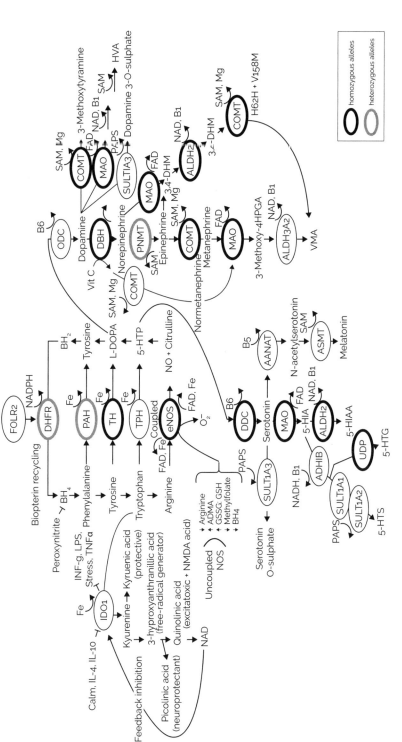

Figure 5.7: Ella's Biopterin SNPs

Source: Methylation Planner by Dr Ben Lynch (author of Dirty Genes and creator of StrateGene)

Key: Black outlined SNPs are homozygous; grey outlined SNPs are heterozygous.

In order to further assess neurotransmitter and dopamine pathway status, specific biogenic amines were performed, which showed low levels of free dopamine, noradrenaline, adrenaline, serotonin, tryptamine and tyramine. These results would suggest low levels of the precursor amino acids phenylalanine or tyrosine or a DBH enzyme deficiency, consistent with hypochlorhydria and CCK feedback loop insufficiency. This was also consistent with Ella's SNPs in the biopterin cycle (DHFR, PAH and TH). Interestingly, Ella's pyroluria would have likely left her struggling to create and recycle biopterin due to B6, zinc, manganese and magnesium deficiencies and also difficulties with haem processing. There is also the issue of long-term low stomach acid, reducing amino acid availability, and the issue of down-regulated methylation.

At this point, Ella's intermittent physical exhaustion was still a major issue along with symptoms of brain exhaustion, poor attention, flat affect, low drive and motivation, difficulty completing tasks, sleeping too much and never feeling refreshed. Ella remembered her mum always saying she could sleep on a clothesline and likened herself to the same theme. Her deceased mother was also an alcoholic with Hashimoto's thyroiditis. Ella's most pressing symptom was what she called brain death. As she was speaking to clients in her daily routine, she would literally forget her whole train of thought mid-sentence. Her father had recently passed away with dementia, so it was a huge concern when this happened to Ella. It was therefore decided to also run a comprehensive thyroid and iron panel. The iron panel consisting of iron, ferritin, caeruloplasmin, transferrin saturation, serum copper, red cell magnesium and plasma zinc. Iron and red cell magnesium were very low. Ferritin was borderline low and the rest were mid-range with the exception of a low zinc. This was despite supporting Ella's pyroluria. As zinc has strong antiviral properties, one could argue that the need for excess zinc may be indicative of a high viral load (Sandstead & Prasad 2010).

Ella's thyroid results were interesting. She presented with a mid-range normal TSH, extremely low free T4 and slightly less low free T3. Reverse T3 was also normal and she had no thyroid antibodies. At this point, Ella realized that like her mother, she also had an addictive personality. In her case she was driven by a need to succeed and she channelled this through academia. She was also a compulsive over-eater who had to curb herself every few weeks when her digestive system started to feel heavy and sluggish. She also admitted to her chocolate addiction at this point, saying that she could eat as much as £30 worth of raw chocolate in one sitting but her gut would feel very raw in the few days afterwards. Mycotoxins are formed during the manufacture and storage of chocolate, so this could be why the inflammation occurred. Ella's mould status did in fact encourage her to stop the chocolate bingeing.

While Ella doesn't appear to have mutations in the SULT1A1, 2, and 3 genes, she is not sulphating well, so may not be producing PAPS to sulphate her serotonin. This may mean she isn't able to use the serotonin she has in her system because she lacks the ability to suphate this (Lozda & Purviņš 2014), hence a further reason for her anxiety.

Ella's plan

Support dopamine and thyroid with dopamine pathway nutrients
D-L-phenylalanine DLPA: On researching for the nutrients to support this pathway it became apparent that phenylalanine is also a CCK feedback loop stimulator (Alamshah *et al.* 2017) used to tackle obesity by improving glucose tolerance and suppressing food intake. As phenylalanine is converted to tyrosine, then L-dopa or thyroxine, it would seem a key nutrient for Ella. However, there are no human studies informing of the successful conversion of phenylalanine to tyrosine, so a small dose only was given for the express use of cholecystokinin stimulation.

Improvements in digestion were seen quite quickly as transsulphuration was already being addressed and Ella was attending her chiropractic sessions twice weekly for spinal structural support and stress reduction to improve digestion. DLPA enhanced this process. No improvement was seen in brain exhaustion or other low-dopamine symptoms.

As a result the following nutrients were recommended:

- L-tyrosine in the morning and at lunchtime to support brain energy, dopamine, serotonin and thyroid (Pereira *et al.* 2010).
- DL-phenylalanine (DLPA) 2 caps daily to support CCK feedback loop (Fitzgerald *et al.* 2020).
- Methylated multivitamin and mineral to support overall general health, energy and brain function (Tardy *et al.* 2020).

- The symptoms on the neurotransmitter questionnaire (Lombard n.d.; Lombard *et al.* 2003) were revisited every two weeks and the doses adjusted accordingly.
- These were taken in addition to Ella's digestive support supplements (betaine, digestive enzymes, probiotics, bicarbonate and beet concentrate).

Within two weeks Ella reported a great improvement in brain alertness from MYMOP 5/5 to MYMOP 2/5. She also reported no further episodes of brain shutdown in mid-flow.

FINAL PRACTITIONER NOTES TO CONSOLIDATE ELLA'S NUTRIGENOMIC CASE

Once Ella's levels of amino acids had reached an appropriate level, they were reduced. On the second organic acid test six months later, all yeast and bacterial markers were within normal limits without having to resort to antimicrobial intervention, which was encouraging. She was, in her own words, 80% better. For many patients, this would be enough, but Ella wasn't in favour of needing long-term nutrient and amino acid support. She described her situation accurately as being 'held up with pills'. Exploring her nutritional intake related to genes may afford more, as discussed in Chapter 6. As mentioned previously, Ella had embarked on paleo and ketogenic/neurolipid keto diets and always felt a failure because her digestion would not support either approach for longer than one or two weeks. It was clear that the potential for a diagnosis of gastroparesis, although unconfirmed at the time, was a strong reason for this difficulty.

There appeared to be a huge emotional aspect to Ella's health challenges that required crucial input outside nutritional therapy in order to support effective digestion and assimilation. Woodhouse *et al.* (2017) discussed the correlation between gastroparesis and psychological distress. While there isn't overwhelming evidence to suggest a psychological rationale for the development of gastroparesis, Masaoka and Tack (2009) report that 62% of patients with a diagnosis of idiopathic gastroparesis associated with a history of physical or sexual abuse. The concept of gastroparesis associated with a history of abuse is not new: Soykan *et al.* (1998) also saw this profile in 70% of their females with idiopathic gastroparesis. It is interesting that this appears to be very much a feminine condition (Dickman *et al.* 2014). It was felt that there was too much evidence on the prospect of a psychological aspect to Ella's persistent and progressive digestive symptomology for this to be ignored. In Ella's timeline, there was clear indication of birth trauma with separation and attachment trauma at the ages of six and 16 years. Heenan *et al.* (2020) explored this and found it to be an independent risk factor and a determinate of poor prognosis in relation to cardiac health. This area of exploration into health is gaining momentum and as such academia is at the precipice of interrelating these concepts. This was the rationale for the use of Klinghardt's model.

Following a combined approach of NSA chiropractic care and DLPA to support the unconfirmed diagnosis of gastroparesis, Ella's digestion improved exponentially over the next 9–12 months. A very interesting finding evolved out of the NSA sessions that shed light on her health timeline. Her NSA sessions brought Ella's body into parasympathetic dominance and at the same time released feelings she hadn't been aware of. They were feelings of abandonment, hypervigilance, rejection and fear. She also reported split-second flashbacks of being pulled out into bright lights and extreme 'metal on metal' noise that she assumed to be her birth. The insight she gained from this identified how her relationship with her own mother, which was very turbulent, may have been affected. It also highlighted for Ella how she had fear-of-abandonment behaviour patterns that plagued her social life. She was able to work through this with her NSA practitioner, thereby positively influencing her compliance and progress with the nutrigenomics programme. McLaughlin *et al.* (2017) have explored the possibility of PTSD from early childhood trauma. The memories unconsciously surface in adulthood as a result of repeated triggers. It would seem from Ella's history of birth trauma and subsequent thoughts and feelings about herself had a significant impact on her biochemistry as Butnariu and Sarac (2019) purport.

At her final appointment, Ella reported that she felt better in her overall health than at any point in her life. She became completely symptom-free.

A methylated multivitamin and mineral specifically targeted to pyroluria was continued as a baseline ongoing support with the intent to reduce and discontinue the amino acids. Her iron levels were corrected over two months and Ella no longer needed the betaine after her chiropractic sessions. Digestive enzymes and pro-biotics were continued for a further three months alongside bone broths daily for gut healing. Ella felt her socialization had improved markedly on the broccoli seed and it has benefits for the microbi-ome (Kaczmarek *et al.* 2019), so she wanted to keep that as a super-food for daily use. There was no need to recommend antimicrobials as supporting digestion and reducing stress allowed the body to reduce inflammation. The bacteria and yeast came back into bal-ance as a result. Ella's nutritional intake improved dramatically. It was then much easier to gain her compliance with a more balanced approach of 70–80% plant with protein intake at 1–1.2g per kg body weight daily. Specific genes in the next section were considered in making this choice.

This case has followed the structure of the pathways in a famil-iar pattern to allow the case to flow for practitioner understanding. There is no finite way to address these cycles due to biochemical individuality. In Ella's case, it was important to address transsul-phuration, neurotransmitter and hormone imbalances so that it was possible to achieve the mindset change, motivation and energy to complete the programme. Achieving this meant there was no need for aggressive gut-rebalancing programmes or aggressive heavy-metal detoxification. Methylation and pyroluria were addressed in the final stages.

Recap of neurotransmitters and biopterin

This section covered how biopterin synthesizes neurotransmitters and nitric oxide. Also discussed was the susceptibility to oxidation by peroxynitrites, which can uncouple NOS, leading to excessive oxidative stress. The genes of the pathway were all discussed in order to provide clarity. Two case studies were provided to assist the practitioner in polar aspects of the issues that can present in this pathway. The chapter was concluded with the programme constructed for Ella and her respective progress.

References

Adams JB, Audhya T, Geis E *et al.* (2018) Comprehensive nutritional and dietary intervention for autism spectrum disorder – a randomized, controlled 12-month trial. *Nutrients 10*, 3, 369. doi:10.3390/nu10030369

Adams MA, Shearer G Jr. (2020) Cysteine dioxygenase enzyme activity and gene expression in the dimorphic pathogenic fungus *Histoplasma capsulatum* is in both the mold and yeast morphotypes and exhibits substantial strain variation. *Journal of Fungi 6*, 1, 24. doi:10.3390/jof6010024

Aguilera M, Barrantes-Vidal N, Arias B *et al.* (2008) Putative role of the COMT gene polymorphism (Val158Met) on verbal working memory functioning in a healthy population. *American Journal of Medical Genetics Part B Neuropsychiatric Genetics 147B*, 6, 898–902. doi:10.1002/ajmg.b.30705

Akinyemi AJ, Okonkwo PK, Faboya OA *et al.* (2017) Curcumin improves episodic memory in cadmium induced memory impairment through inhibition of acetylcholinesterase and adenosine deaminase activities in a rat model. *Metabolic Brain Disease 32*, 1, 87–95. doi:10.1007/s11011-016-9887-x

Aksungar FB, Eren A, Ure S *et al.* (2005) Effects of intermittent fasting on serum lipid levels, coagulation status and plasma homocysteine levels. *Annals of Nutrition and Metabolism 49*, 2, 77–82. doi:10.1159/000084739

Alam A, O'Connor DT, Perianayagam MC *et al.* (2010) Phenylethanolamine n-methyl-transferase gene polymorphisms and adverse outcomes in acute kidney injury. *Nephron Clinical Practice 114*, 34, c253–c259. doi:10.1159/000276577

Alamshah A, Spreckley E, Norton M *et al.* (2017) L-phenylalanine modulates gut hormone release and glucose tolerance, and suppresses food intake through the calcium-sensing receptor in rodents. *International Journal of Obesity 41*, 11, 1693–1701. doi:10.1038/ijo.2017.164

Al-Baradie RS, Chaudhary MW (2014) Diagnosis and management of cerebral folate deficiency. A form of folinic acid-responsive seizures. *Neurosciences 19*, 4, 312–316.

Alexiou GA, Lianos GD, Ragos V *et al.* (2017) Difluoromethylornithine in cancer: New advances. *Future Oncology 13*, 9, 809–819. doi:10.2217/fon-2016-0266

Allocati N, Masulli M, Di Ilio C *et al.* (2018) Glutathione transferases: Substrates, inihibitors and pro-drugs in cancer and neurodegenerative diseases. *Oncogenesis 7*, 8. doi:10.1038/s41389-017-0025-3

Alur VC, Raju V, Vastrad B *et al.* (2019) Mining featured biomarkers linked with epithelial ovarian cancer based on bioinformatics. *Diagnostics 9*, 2, 39. doi:10.3390/diagnostics9020039

Amadei F, Fröhlich B, Stremmel W *et al.* (2018) Nonclassical interactions of phosphatidylcholine with mucin protect intestinal surfaces: A microinterferometry study. *Langmuir: The ACS Journal of Surfaces and Colloids 34*, 46, 14046–14057. doi:10.1021/acs.langmuir.8b03035

Angst J, Gamma A, Baldwin DS *et al.* (2009) The generalized anxiety spectrum: Prevalence, onset, course and outcome. *European Archives of Psychiatry and Clinical Neuroscience 259*, 1, 37-45. doi:10.1007/s00406-008-0832-9

Aoyama K, Nakaki T (2013) Impaired glutathione synthesis in neurodegeneration. *International Journal of Molecular Sciences 14*, 10, 21021–21044. doi:10.3390/ijms141021021

Ardalan B, Subbarayan PR, Ramos Y *et al.* (2010) A phase I study of 5-fluorouracil/leucovorin and arsenic trioxide for patients with refractory/relapsed colorectal carcinoma. *Clinical Cancer Research 16*, 11, 3019–3027. doi:10.1158/1078-0432.CCR-09-2590

Armine J (2014) The Brainwall. Poster presentation delivered by Dr Armine regularly and available from www.methylationsupport.com/wp-content/uploads/2015/07/brain-wall-lect-7-6-15.pdf

Ash M (2010) PEA – a natural antidepressant. www.clinicaleducation.org/resources/reviews/pea-a-natural-antidepressant

Ash M (2011) Oral glutathione equivelant to IV therapy. www.clinicaleducation.org/resources/reviews/oral-glutathione-equivalent-to-iv-therapy/#_ftn19

Asher G, Bercovich Z, Tsvetkov T *et al.* (2005) 20S proteasomal degradation of ornithine decarboxylase is regulated by NQO1. *Molecular Cell 17*, 5, 645–655 doi:10.1016/j.molcel.2005.01.020

Ashoori M, Saedisomeolia A (2014) Riboflavin (vitamin B_2) and oxidative stress: A review. *British Journal of Nutrition 111*, 11, 1985–1991. doi:10.1017/S0007114514000178

Askari BS, Krajinovic M (2010) Dihydrofolate reductase gene variations in susceptibility to disease and treatment outcomes. *Current Genomics 11*, 8, 578–583. doi:10.2174/138920210793360925

Assies J, Pouwer F, Lok A *et al.* (2010) Plasma and erythrocyte fatty acid patterns in patients with recurrent depression: A matched case-control study. *PLOS ONE 5*, 5, e10635. doi:10.1371/journal.pone.0010635

Auger C, Said A, Nguyen PN *et al.* (2016) Potential of food and natural products to promote endothelial and vascular health. *Journal of Cardiovascular Pharmacology 68*, 1, 11–18. doi:10.1097/FJC.0000000000000382

Babayi T, Riazi GH (2017) The effects of 528 Hz sound wave to reduce cell death in human astrocyte primary cell culture treated with ethanol. *Journal of Addiction Research and Therapy 8*, 335. doi:10.4172/2155-6105.1000335

Baeken C, Claes S, De Raedt R (2014) The influence of COMT Val[158]Met genotype on the character dimension cooperativeness in healthy females. *Brain and Behavior 4*, 4, 515–520. doi:0.1002/brb3.233

Bai J, Meng Z (2011) Effect of sulfur dioxide on expression of proto-oncogenes and tumor suppressor genes from rats. *Environmental Toxicology 25*, 3, 272–283. doi:10.1002/tox.20495

Bailey LB, Stover PJ, McNulty H *et al.* (2015) Biomarkers of nutrition for development–Folate review. *Journal of Nutrition 145*, 7, 1636S–1680S. doi:10.3945/jn.114.206599

Bailey RL, Mills JL, Yetley EA *et al.* (2010) Unmetabolized serum folic acid and its relation to folic acid intake from diet and supplements in a nationally representative sample of adults aged > or =60 y in the United States. *American Journal of Clinical Nutrition 92*, 2, 383–389.

Ballatori N, Krance SM, Notenboom S *et al.* (2009) Glutathione dysregulation and the etiology and progression of human diseases. *Biological Chemistry 390*, 3, 191–214. doi:10.1515/BC.2009.033

Baltgalvis, KA, Greising SM, Warren GL *et al.* (2010) Estrogen regulates estrogen receptors and antioxidant gene expression in mouse skeletal muscle. *PLOS ONE 5*, 4, e10164. doi:10.1371/journal.pone.0010164

Banci L, Bertini I, Boca M *et al.* (2008) SOD1 and amyotrophic lateral sclerosis: mutations and oligomerization. *PLOS ONE 3*, 2, e1677. doi:10.1371/journal.pone.0001677

Banik GD, De A, Som S *et al.* (2016) Hydrogen sulphide in exhaled breath: A potential biomarker for small intestinal bacterial overgrowth in IBS. *Journal of Breath Research 10*, 2, 026010. doi:10.1088/1752-7155/10/2/026010

Barbarino JM, Haidar CE, Klein TE *et al.* (2014) PharmGKB summary: Very important pharmacogene information for UGT1A1. *Pharmacogenetics and Genomics 24*, 3, 177–183.

Barić I, Erdol S, Saglam H *et al.* (2017) Glycine N-methyltransferase deficiency: A member of dysmethylating liver disorders? *JIMD Reports 31*, 101–106. doi:10.1007/8904_2016_543

Barile M, Giancaspero TA, Leone P *et al.* (2016) Riboflavin transport and metabolism in humans. *Journal of Inherited Metabolic Disorders 39*, 4, 545–557. doi:10.1007/s10545-016-9950-0

Baskerville TA, Douglas AJ (2010) Dopamine and oxytocin interactions underlying behaviors: Potential contributions to behavioral disorders. *CNS Neuroscience and Therapeutics 16*, 3, e92–e123. doi:10.1111/j.1755-5949.2010.00154.x

Bassiri H, Benavides A, Haber M *et al.* (2015) Translational development of difluoromethylornithine (DFMO) for the treatment of neuroblastoma. *Translational Pediatrics 4*, 3, 226–238. doi:10.3978/j.issn.2224-4336.2015.04.06

Bazan NG, Scott BL (1990) Dietary omega-3 fatty acids and accumulation of docosahexanoic in rod photoreceptor cells of the retina and at synapses. *Upsala Journal of Medical Sciences Supplement 48*, 97–107

Bazzocco S, Dopeso H, Carton-Garcia F *et al.* (2015) Highly expressed genes in rapidly proliferating tumor cells as new targets for colorectal cancer treatment. *Clinical Cancer Research 21*, 16, 3695–3704. doi:10.1158/1078-0432.CCR-14-2457

Bedford A, Gong J (2018) Implications of butyrate and its derivatives for gut health and animal production. *Animal Nutrition 4*, 2, 151–159. doi:10.1016/j.aninu.2017.08.010

Bellé LP, De Bona KS, Abdalla FH *et al.* (2009) Comparative evaluation of adenosine deaminase activity in cerebral cortex and hippocampus of young and adult rats: Effect of garlic extract (*Allium sativum* L.) on their susceptibility to heavy metal exposure. *Basic and Clinical Pharmacology and Toxicology 104*, 5, 408–413. doi:10.1111/j.1742-7843.2009.00390.x

Belužić L, Grbeša I, Belužić R *et al.* (2018) Knock-down of AHCY and depletion of adenosine induces DNA damage and cell cycle arrest. *Scientific Reports 8*, 14012. doi:10.1038/s41598-018-32356-8

Berry T, Abohamza E, Moustafa AA (2020) Treatment-resistant schizophrenia: Focus on the transsulfuration pathway. *Reviews in the Neurosciences 31*, 2, 219–232. doi:10.1515/revneuro-2019-0057

Bindu PS, Nagappa M, Bharath RD *et al.* (2017) Isolated Sulfite Oxidase Deficiency. Sep 21. In: MP Adam, HH Ardinger, RA Pagon *et al.* (eds) *GeneReviews®* [Internet]. Seattle, WA: University of Washington, Seattle; 1993–2021. Available from: www.ncbi.nlm.nih.gov/books/NBK453433

Biswas SK, McClure D, Jimenez LA *et al.* (2005) Curcumin induces glutathione biosynthesis and inhibits NF-κB activation and interleukin-8 release in alveolar epithelial cells: Mechanism of free radical scavenging activity. *Antioxidant and Redox Signaling 7*, 1–2, 32–41. doi:10.1089/ars.2005.7.32

Blau N, van Spronsen FJ, Levy HL (2010) Phenylketonuria. *Lancet 376*, 9750, 1417–1427. doi:10.1016/S0140-6736(10)60961-0

Blits M, Jansen G, Assaraf YG *et al.* (2013) Methotrexate normalizes up-regulated folate pathway genes in rheumatoid arthritis. *Arthritism and Rheumatism 65*, 11, 2791–2802. doi:10.1002/art.38094

Board RE, Knight L, Greystoke A *et al.* (2007) DNA methylation in circulating tumour dna as a biomarker for cancer. *Biomark Insights 2*, 307–319.

Bocedi A, Noce A, Marrone G *et al.* (2019) Glutathione transferase P1-1 an enzyme useful in biomedicine and as biomarker in clinical practice and in environmental pollution. *Nutrients 11*, 1741. doi:10.3390/nu11081741

Bolton JL, Dunlap T (2017) Formation and biological targets of quinones: Cytotoxic versus cytoprotective effects. *Chemical Research in Toxicology 30*, 1, 13–37. doi:10.1021/acs.chemrestox.6b00256

Breit S, Kupferberg A, Rogler G *et al.* (2018) Vagus nerve as modulator of the brain-gut axis in psychiatric and inflammatory disorders. *Frontiers in Psychiatry 9*, 44. doi:10.3389/fpsyt.2018.00044

Briguglio M, Dell'Osso B, Panzica G *et al.* (2018) Dietary neurotransmitters: A narrative review on current knowledge. *Nutrients 10*, 5, 591. doi:10.3390/nu10050591

Burdelski C, Strauss C, Tsourlakis MC *et al.* (2015) Overexpression of thymidylate synthase (TYMS) is associated with aggressive tumor features and early PSA recurrence in prostate cancer. *Oncotarget 6*, 10, 8377–8387. doi:10.18632/oncotarget.3107

Burhanettin K, Nihal A, Ersin F *et al.* (2012) Elements levels and glucose- 6-phosphate dehydrogenase activity in blood of patients with schizophrenia. *Journal of Psychiatry and Neurological Sciences 25*, 198–205. doi:10.5350/DAJPN2012250301

Burton BT, Foster WR (1988) *Human Nutrition.* New York, NY: McGraw-Hill.

Butcher NJ *et al.* (2018) Sulfotransferase 1A3/4 copy number variation is associated with neurodegenerative disease. *The Pharmacogenomics Journal 18*, 2, 209.

Butnariu M, Sarac J (2019) Biochemistry of hormones that influences feelings. *Annals of Pharmacovigilance & Drug Safety*, review article. www.remedypublications.com/open-access/biochemistry-of-hormones-that-influences-feelings-4862.pdf

Byeon Y, Back K (2016) Low melatonin production by suppression of either serotonin N-acetyltransferase or N-acetylserotonin methyltransferase in rice causes seedling growth retardation with yield penalty, abiotic stress susceptibility, and enhanced coleoptile growth under anoxic conditions. *Journal of Pineal Research 60*, 3, 348–359. doi:10.1111/jpi.12317

Canani RB, Costanzo MD, Leone L *et al.* (2011) Potential beneficial effects of butyrate in intestinal and extraintestinal diseases. *World Journal of Gastroenterology 17*, 12, 1519–1528. doi:10.3748/wjg.v17.i12.1519

Carballo JJ, Akamnonu CP, Oquendo MA (2008) Neurobiology of suicidal behavior: An integration of biological and clinical findings. *Archives of Suicide Research 12*, 2, 93–110. doi:10.1080/13811110701857004

Cario H, Smith DE, Blom H *et al.* (2011) Dihydrofolate reductase deficiency due to a homozygous DHFR mutation causes megaloblastic anemia and cerebral folate deficiency leading to severe neurologic disease. *American Journal of Human Genetics 88*, 2, 226–231.

Castro-Rojas CA, Esparza-Mota AR, Hernandez-Cabrera F *et al.* (2017) Thymidylate synthase gene variants as predictors of clinical response and toxicity to fluoropyrimidine-based chemotherapy for colorectal cancer. *Drug Metabolism and Personalized Therapy 32*, 4, 209–218. doi:10.1515/dmpt-2017-0028

Chan T, Bates J, Lansford J *et al.* (2014) Impulsivity and genetic variants in *DRD2* and *ANKK1* moderate longitudinal associations between sleep problems and overweight from ages 5 to 11. *International Journal of Obesity 38*, 404–410. doi:10.1038/ijo.2013.123

Chandra P, Wolfenden LL, Ziegler TR *et al.* (2007) Treatment of vitamin D deficiency with UV light in patients with malabsorption syndromes: A case series. *Photodermatology, Photoimmunology and Photomedicine 23*, 5, 179–185. doi:10.1111/j.1600-0781.2007.00302.x

Chanseaume E, Malpuech-Brugère C, Patrac V *et al.* (2006) Diets high in sugar, fat, and energy induce muscle type-specific adaptations in mitochondrial functions in rats. *Journal of Nutrition 136*, 8, 2194–2200. doi:10.1093/jn/136.8.2194

Chao YL, Anders CK (2018) TYMS Gene polymorphisms in breast cancer patients receiving 5-fluorouracil-based chemotherapy. *Clinical Breast Cancer 18*, 3, e301–e304. doi:10.1016/j.clbc.2017.08.006

Chattopadhyay MK, Chen W, Tabor H (2013) *Escherichia coli* glutathionylspermidine synthetase/amidase: phylogeny and effect on regulation of gene expression. *FEMS Microbiology Letters 338*, 2, 132–140. doi:10.1111/1574-6968.12035

Chaudhari SA, Sacerdote A, Bahtiyar G (2012) 1-α hydroxylation defect in postural ortho-static tachycardia syndrome: Remission with calcitriol supplementation. *BMJ Case Reports*. doi:10.1136/bcr.02.2012.5730

Chen B, Rao X, House MG *et al.* (2011) GPx3 promoter hypermethylation is a frequent event in human cancer and is associated with tumorigenesis and chemotherapy response. *Cancer Letters 309*, 1, 37–45. doi:10.1016/j.canlet.2011.05.013

Chen I, Hsieh T, Thomas T *et al.* (2001) Identi-fication of estrogen-induced genes down-regulated by AhR agonists in MCF-7 breast cancer cells using suppression subtractive hybridization. *Gene 262*, 1–2, 207–214. doi:10.1016/s0378-1119(00)00530-8

Chen ZJ, Dai YQ, Kong SS *et al.* (2013) Luteolin is a rare substrate of human catechol-O-methyltransferase favoring a para-methylation. *Molecular Nutrition and Food Research 57*, 5, 877–885. doi:10.1002/mnfr.201200584

Chen ZQ, Mou RT, Feng DX *et al.* (2017) The role of nitric oxide in stroke. *Medical Gas Research 7*, 3, 194–203. doi:10.4103/2045-9912.215750

Cheng CW, Shieh PC, Lin YC *et al.* (2010) Indoleamine 2,3-dioxygenase, an immunomodulatory protein, is suppressed by (-)-epigallocatechin-3-gallate via blocking of gamma-interferon-induced JAK-PKC-delta-STAT1 signaling in human oral cancer cells. *Journal of Agricultural and Food Chemistry 58*, 2, 887–894.

Cherng SC, Chen YH, Lee MS *et al.* (2006) Acceleration of hepatobiliary excretion by lemon juice on 99mTc-tetrofosmin cardiac SPECT. *Nuclear Medicine Communica-tions 27*, 11, 859–864. doi:10.1097/01. mnm.0000243377.57001.33

Chow HHS, Garland LL, Hsu CH *et al.* (2010) Resveratrol modulates drug- and carcin-ogen-metabolizing enzymes in a healthy volunteer study. *Cancer Prevention Research 3*, 9, 1168–1175,

Circu ML, Aw TY (2012) Glutathione and modulation of cell apoptosis. *Biochimica et Biophysica Acta 1823*, 10, 1767–1777. doi:10.1016/j.bbamcr.2012.06.019

Claerhout H, Witters P, Régal L *et al.* (2018) Isolated sulfite oxidase deficiency. *Journal of Inherited Metabolic Disease 41*, 1, 101–108. doi:10.1007/s10545-017-0089-4

Clapp M, Aurora N, Herrera L *et al.* (2017) Gut microbiota's effect on mental health: The gut-brain axis. *Clin Pract 7*, 4, 987. doi:10.4081/cp.2017.987

Coghlan S, Horder J, Inkster B *et al.* (2012) GABA system dysfunction in autism and related disorders: From synapse to symptoms. *Neuroscience and Biobehavioral Reviews 36*, 9, 2044–2055.

Cohen S (2015) America's pharmacist. www.SuzyCohen.com

Cole BF, Baron JA, Sandler RS *et al.* (2007) Folic acid for the prevention of colorectal adenomas: A randomized clinical trial. *JAMA 297*, 2351–2359.

Coles LD, Tuite PJ, Öz G *et al.* (2017) Repeated-dose oral N-acetylcysteine in Parkinson's disease: Pharmacokinetics and effect on brain glutathione and oxidative stress. *Journal of Clinical Pharmacology 58*, 2, 158–167. doi:10.1002/jcph.1008

Coman IL, Gnirke MH, Middleton FA *et al.* (2010) The effects of gender and catechol O-methyltransferase (COMT) Val108/158Met polymorphism on emotion regulation in velo-cardio-facial syndrome (22q11.2 deletion syndrome): An fMRI study. *NeuroImage 53*, 3, 1043–1050.

Conklin DJ, Bhatnagar A (2011) Are glutathione S-transferase null genotypes 'null and void' of risk for ischemic vascular disease? *Circulation: Cardiovascular Genetics 4*, 4, 339–341.

Cook I, Wang T, Leyh TS (2017) Tetrahydrobiop-terin regulates monoamine neurotransmit-ter sulfonation. *PNAS 114*, 27, E5317–E5324. doi:10.1073/pnas.1704500114

Costa MH, Ortiga-Carvalho TM, Violante AD *et al.* (2015) Pheochromocytomas and paragangliomas: Clinical and genetic approaches. *Frontiers in Endocrinology 6*, 126. doi:10.3389/fendo.2015.00126

Cotter D, Kelso A, Neligan A (2017) Genetic biomarkers of posttraumatic epilepsy: A systematic review. *Seizure 46*, 53–58. doi:10.1016/j.seizure.2017.02.002

Crnošija L, Adamec I, Mišmaš A *et al.* (2012) Postural orthostatic tachycardia syndrome. *European Neurology 77*, 5–6, 253–257. doi:10.1159/000469707

Cronin SJF, Seehus C, Weidinger A *et al.* (2018) The metabolite BH4 controls T cell proliferation in autoimmunity and cancer. *Nature 563*, 564–568.

Dabai NS, Pramyothin P, Holick MF (2012) The effect of ultraviolet radiation from a novel portable fluorescent lamp on serum 25-hydroxyvitamin D3 levels in healthy adults with Fitzpatrick skin types II and III. *Photodermatology, Photoimmunology and Photomedicine 28*, 6, 307–311. doi:10.1111/phpp.12000

Daubner SC, Le T, Wang S (2011) Tyrosine hydroxylase and regulation of dopamine synthesis. *Archives of Biochemistry and Biophysics 508*, 1, 1–12. doi:10.1016/j.abb.2010.12.017

De Dreu CKW (2012) Oxytocin modulates the link between adult attachment and cooperation through reduced betrayal aversion. *Psychoneuroendocrinology 37*, 7, 871–880.

de Groot NS, Burgas MT (2015) Is membrane homeostasis the missing link between inflammation and neurodegenerative diseases? *Cellular and Molecular Life Sciences 72*, 24, 4795–4805. doi:10.1007/s00018-015-2038-4

De Mattia E, Toffoli G (2009) C677T and A1298C MTHFR polymorphisms, a challenge for antifolate and fluoropyrimidine-based therapy personalisation. *European Journal of Cancer 45*, 8, 1333–1351. doi:10.1016/j.ejca.2008.12.004

De Weijer BA, Van de Giessen E, Van Amelsvoort TA (2011) Lower striatal dopamine D2/3 receptor availability in obese compared with non-obese subjects. *EJNMMI Research 1*, 37. doi:10.1186/2191-219X-1-37

Dean L (2016) Methylenetetrahydrofolate reductase deficiency. *Medical Genetics Summaries*. NCBI. www.ncbi.nlm.nih.gov/books/NBK66131

DellaGioia N, Hannestad J (2010) A critical review of human endotoxin administration as an experimental paradigm of depression. *Neuroscience and Biobehavioral Reviews 34*, 1, 130–143. doi:10.1016/j.neubiorev.2009.07.014

Denke A, Schempp H, Weiser D *et al.* (2000) Biochemical activities of extracts from Hypericum perforatum L. 5th communication: dopamine-beta-hydroxylase-product quantification by HPLC and inhibition by hypericins and flavonoids. *Arzneimittelforschung 50*, 5, 415–419. doi:10.1055/s-0031-1300225

DeYoung CG (2013) The neuromodulator of exploration: A unifying theory of the role of dopamine in personality. *Frontiers in Human Neuroscience.* doi:10.3389/fnhum.2013.00762

Dickman R, Wainstein J, Glezerman M *et al.* (2014) Gender aspects suggestive of gastroparesis in patients with diabetes mellitus: A cross-sectional survey. *BMC Gastroenterology 14*, 34. doi:10.1186/1471-230X-14-34

DiPalma JR (1990) Metoclopramide: A dopamine receptor antagonist. *American Family Physician 41*, 3, 919–924.

Dobryakova E, Genova HM, DeLuca J *et al.* (2015) The dopamine imbalance hypothesis of fatigue in multiple sclerosis and other neurological disorders. *Frontiers in Neurology 6*, 52. doi:10.3389/fneur.2015.00052

Dolan LC, Matulka RA, Burdock GA (2010) Naturally occurring food toxins. *Toxins 2*, 9, 2289–2332. doi:10.3390/toxins2092289

Domínguez E, Loza MI, Padín F *et al.* (2007) Extensive linkage disequilibrium mapping at HTR2A and DRD3 for schizophrenia susceptibility genes in the Galician population. *Schizophrenia Research 90*, 1–3, 123–129. doi:10.1016/j.schres.2006.09.022

Dominy JE, Hwang J, Guo S *et al.* (2008) Synthesis of amino acid cofactor in cysteine dioxygenase is regulated by substrate and represents a novel post-translational regulation of activity. *The Journal of Biological Chemistry 283*, 18, 12188–12201.

Dos Santos Rodrigues JB, De Carvalho RJ, De Souza NT *et al.* (2017) Effects of oregano essential oil and carvacrol on biofilms of *Staphylococcus aureus* from food-contact surfaces. *Food Control*, 1237–1246. doi:10.1016/j.foodcont.2016.10.043

Drexel University (2016) At any skill level, making art reduces stress hormones: Cortisol lowers significantly after just 45 minutes of art creation. *Science Daily.* www.sciencedaily.com/releases/2016/06/160615134946.htm

Ducker GS, Ghergurovich JM, Mainolfi N *et al.* (2017) Human SHMT inhibitors reveal defective glycine import as a targetable metabolic vulnerability of diffuse large B-cell lymphoma. *PNAS 114*, 43, 11404–11409. doi:10.1073/pnas.1706617114

Dunna NR, Vure S, Sailaja K *et al.* (2013) Deletion of GSTM1 and T1 genes as a risk factor for development of acute leukemia. *Asian Pacific Journal of Cancer Prevention 14*, 4, 2221–2224.

Durak I, Biri H, Devrim E *et al.* (2004) Aqueous extract of Urtica dioica makes significant inhibition on adenosine deaminase activity in prostate tissue from patients with prostate cancer. *Cancer Biology and Therapy 3*, 9, 855–857. doi:10.4161/cbt.3.9.1038

Eagle K (2012) Hypothesis: Holiday sudden cardiac death: food and alcohol inhibition of SULT1A enzymes as a precipitant. *Journal of Applied Toxicology 32*, 10, 751–755. doi:10.1002/jat.2764

Ebner K, Bosch OJ, Krömer SA *et al.* (2004) Release of oxytocin in the rat central amygdala modulates stress-coping behavior and the release of excitatory amino acids. *Neuropsychopharmacology 30*, 223–230. doi:10.1038/sj.npp.1300607

Engin AB, Engin A (2017) The interactions between kynurenine, folate, methionine and pteridine pathways in obesity. *Obesity and Lipotoxicity*, 511–527. doi:10.1007/978-3-319-48382-5_22

Erasmus U (1993) *Fats that Heal, Fats that Kill.* Summertown, TN: Alive Books.

Esin E, Necat Y, Ozgur A (2013) Functionally defective high-density lipoprotein and paraoxonase: A couple for endothelial dysfunction in atherosclerosis. *Cholesterol 2013*, 792090. doi:10.1155/2013/792090

Fan FS (2016) Iron deficiency anemia due to excessive green tea drinking. *Clinical Case Reports 4*, 111053–1056. doi:10.1002/ccr3.707

Farah C, Michel LYM, Balligand JL (2018) Nitric oxide signalling in cardiovascular health and disease. *Nature Reviews: Cardiology 15*, 5, 292–316.

Fei Z, Gao Y, Qiu M *et al.* (2016) Down-regulation of dihydrofolate reductase inhibits the growth of endothelial EA.hy926 cell through induction of G1 cell cycle arrest via up-regulating p53 and p21(waf1/cip1) expression. *Journal of Clinical Biochemistry and Nutrition 58*, 2, 105–113. doi:10.3164/jcbn.15-64

Felker P, Bunch R, Leung AM (2016) Concentrations of thiocyanate and goitrin in human plasma, their precursor concentrations in brassica vegetables, and associated potential risk for hypothyroidism. *Nutrition Reviews 74*, 4, 248–258. doi:10.1093/nutrit/nuv110

Figueiredo JC, Grau MV, Haile RW *et al.* (2009) Folic acid and risk of prostate cancer: Results from a randomized clinical trial. *Journal of the National Cancer Institute 101*, 6, 432–435. doi:10.1093/jnci/djp019

Fischer LM, da Costa KA, Kwock L *et al.* (2010) Dietary choline requirements of women; effects of estrogen and genetic variation. *American Journal of Clinical Nutrition 92*, 5, 1113–1119.

Fitzgerald PCE, Manoliu B, Herbillon B *et al.* (2020) Effects of L-phenylalanine on energy intake and glycaemia – Impacts on appetite perceptions, gastrointestinal hormones and gastric emptying in healthy males. *Nutrients 12*, 6, 1788. doi:10.3390/nu12061788

Förstermann U, Sessa WC (2012) Nitric oxide synthases: Regulation and function. *European Heart Journal 33*, 7, 829–837. doi:10.1093/eurheartj/ehr304

Fowler B (2001) The folate cycle and disease in humans. *Kidney Int Suppl, 78*, S221–229. doi: 10.1046/j.1523-1755.2001.59780221.x

Fox KC, Nijeboer S, Dixon ML *et al.* (2014) Is meditation associated with altered brain structure? A systematic review and meta-analysis of morphometric neuroimaging in meditation practitioners. *Neuroscience and Biobehavioral Reviews 43*, 48–73. doi:10.1016/j.neubiorev.2014.03.016

Fransquet PD, Lacaze P, Saffery R *et al.* (2018) Blood DNA methylation as a potential biomarker of dementia: A systematic review. *Alzheimer's and Dementia 14*, 1, 81–103. doi:10.1016/j.jalz.2017.10.002

Fraternale A, Brundu S, Magnani M (2017) Glutathione and glutathione derivatives in immunotherapy. *Biological Chemistry 398*, 2, 261–275. doi:10.1515/hsz-2016-0202

Frye RE, Rossignol DA (2014) Treatments for biomedical abnormalities associated with autism spectrum disorder. *Frontiers in Pediatrics 2*, 66. doi:10.3389/fped.2014.00066

Fujita Y, Fujino Y, Onodera M *et al.* (2011) A fatal case of acute hydrogen sulfide poisoning caused by hydrogen sulfide: Hydroxoco-balamin therapy for acute hydrogen sulfide poisoning. *Journal of Analytical Toxicology 35*, 2, 119–123.

Furujo M, Kinoshita M, Nago M *et al.* (2012) Methionine adenosyltransferase I/III deficiency: Neurological manifestations and relevance of S-adenosylmethionine. *Molecular Genetics and Metabolism 107*, 3, 253–256. doi:10.1016/j.ymgme.2012.08.002

Gaita L, Manzi B, Sacco R *et al.* (2010) Decreased serum arylesterase activity in autism spectrum disorders. *Psychiatry Research 180*, 2–3, 105–113. doi:10.1016/j.psychres.2010.04.010

Gao S, Li H, Xiao H *et al.* (2012) Association of MTHFR 677T variant allele with risk of intracerebral haemorrhage: A meta-analysis. *Journal of the Neurological Sciences 323*, 1–2, 40–45. doi:10.1016/j.jns.2012.07.038

Gao X, van der Veen JN, Vance JE *et al.* (2015) Lack of phosphatidylethanolamine N-methyltransferase alters hepatic phospholipid composition and induces endoplasmic reticulum stress. *Biochimica et Biophysica Acta 1852,* 12, 2689–2699. doi:10.1016/j.bbadis.2015.09.006

Garcia-Argibay M, Santed MA *et al.* (2019) Efficacy of binaural auditory beats in cognition, anxiety, and pain perception: a meta-analysis. *Psychological Research 83*, 357–372 doi:10.1007/s00426-018-1066-8

García-Giménez JL, Romá-Mateo C, Pérez-Machado G *et al.* (2017) Role of glutathione in the regulation of epigenetic mechanisms in disease. *Free Radical Biology and Medicine 112*, 36–48. doi:10.1016/j.freeradbiomed.2017.07.008

García-Minguillán CJ, Fernandez-Ballart JD, Ceruelo S *et al.* (2014) Riboflavin status modifies the effects of methylenetetrahydrofolate reductase (MTHFR) and methionine synthase reductase (MTRR) polymorphisms on homocysteine. *Genes and Nutrition 9*, 6, 435. doi:10.1007/s12263-014-0435-1

Gaweska H, Fitzpatrick PF (2011) Structures and mechanism of the monoamine oxidase family. *Biomolecular Concepts 2*, 5, 365–377. doi:10.1515/BMC.2011.030

Gellekink H, Muntjewerff JW, Vermeulen SHHM *et al.* (2007) Catechol-O-methyltransferase genotype is associated with plasma total homocysteine levels and may increase venous thrombosis risk. *Thrombosis and Haemostasis 98*, 6, 1226–1231.

Gerritsen RJS, Band GPH (2018) Breath of life: The respiratory vagal stimulation model of contemplative activity. *Frontiers in Human Neuroscience 12*, 397. doi:10.3389/fnhum.2018.00397

Ghazali RA, Waring RH (1999) The effects of flavonoids on human phenolsulphotransferases: Potential in drug metabolism and chemoprevention. *Life Sciences 65*, 16, 1625–1632.

Gholami F, Neisani Samani L, Kashanian M *et al.* (2016). Onset of labor in post-term pregnancy by chamomile. *Iranian Red Crescent Medical Journal 18*, 11, e19871. doi:10.5812/ircmj.19871

Gilhotra N, Dhingra D (2011) Thymoquinone produced antianxiety-like effects in mice through modulation of GABA and NO levels. *Pharmacological Reports 63*, 3, 660–669. doi:10.1016/s1734-1140(11)70577-1

Göllner T, Fieder M (2015) Selection in the dopamine receptor 2 gene: A candidate SNP study. *PeerJ 3*, e1149. doi:10.7717/peerj.1149

Gorabi AM, Kiaie N, Hajighasemi S *et al.* (2019) Statin-induced nitric oxide signaling: mechanisms and therapeutic implications. *Journal of Clinical Medicine 8*, 12, 2051. doi:10.3390/jcm8122051

Griffiths R (2018) *Mitochondria in Health and Disease: Personalized Nutrition and Lifestyle Medicine for Healthcare Practitioners.* London and Philadelphia, PA: Singing Dragon.

Guan YS, He Q (2015) Plants consumption and liver health. *Evidence-Based Complementary and Alternative Medicine 2015*, 824185. doi:10.1155/2015/824185

Guglietti CL, Daskalakis ZJ, Radhu N *et al.* (2013) Meditation-related increases in GABAB modulated cortical inhibition. *Brain Stimulation 6*, 3, 397–402. doi:10.1016/j.brs.2012.08.005

Guilford FT, Hope J (2014) Deficient glutathione in the pathophysiology of mycotoxin-related illness. *Toxins 6*, 2, 608–623. doi:10.3390/toxins6020608

Guilliams TG, Drake LE (2020) Meal-time supplementation with betaine HCl for functional hypochlorhydria: What is the evidence? *Integrated Medicine 1*, 1, 32–36.

Günal S, Hardman R, Kopriva S *et al.* (2019) Sulfation pathways from red to green. *Journal of Biological Chemistry 294*, 33, 12293–12312. doi:10.1074/jbc. REV119.007422

Guo QN, Wang HD, Tie LZ *et al.* (2017) Parental genetic variants, MTHFR 677C>T and MTRR 66A>G, associated differently with fetal congenital heart defect. *BioMed Research International 2017*, 3043476. doi:10.1155/2017/3043476

Gupta P, Khurana ML, Khadgawat R (2015) Plasma free metanephrine, normeta-nephrine, and 3-methoxytyramine for the diagnosis of pheochromocytoma/paragan-glioma. *Indian Journal of Endocrinology and Metabolism 19*, 5, 633–638.

Haag M (2003) Essential fatty acids and the brain. *Canadian Journal of Psychiatry 48*, 3. doi:10.1177%2F070674370304800308

Häberle J *et al.* (2006) Inborn error of amino acid synthesis: Human glutamine synthetase deficiency. *Journal of Inherited Metabolic Disorders 29*, 352–358.

Hall KT, Lembo AJ, Kirsch I *et al.* (2012) Catechol-O-methyltransferase val158met polymorphism predicts placebo effect in irritable bowel syndrome. *PLoS One 7*, 10, doi: 10.1371/journal.pone.0048135

Harel M, Aharoni A, Gaidukov L *et al.* (2004) Structure and evolution of the serum paraoxonase family of detoxifying and anti-atherosclerotic enzymes. *Nature Structural and Molecular Biology 11*, 5, 412–419. doi:10.1038/nsmb767

Harris RM, Waring RH (2008) Sulfotransferase inhibition: potential impact of diet and environmental chemicals on steroid metabolism and drug detoxification. *Current Drug Metabolism 9*, 4, 269–275. doi:10.2174/138920008784220637

Hatcher HC, Singh RN, Torti FM *et al.* (2009) Synthetic and natural iron chelators: Therapeutic potential and clinical use. *Future Medicinal Chemistry 1*, 9, 1643–1670. doi:10.4155/fmc.09.121

He Z, Zhang R, Jiang F *et al.* (2018) Role of genetic and environmental factors in DNA methylation of lipid metabolism. *Genes and Diseases 5*, 1, 9–15. doi:10.1016/j. gendis.2017.11.005

Heber D, Li Z, Garcia-Lloret M *et al.* (2014) Sulforaphane-rich broccoli sprout extract attenuates nasal allergic response to diesel exhaust particles. *Food and Function 5*, 1, 35–41. doi:10.1039/c3fo60277j

Heenan A, Greenman PS, Tassé V *et al.* (2020) Traumatic stress, attachment style, and health outcomes in cardiac rehabilitation patients. *Frontiers in Psychology 11*, 75. doi:10.3389/fpsyg.2020.00075

Heinzel S, Riemer TG, Schulte S *et al.* (2014) Catechol-O-methyltransferase (COMT) genotype affects age-related changes in plasticity in working memory: A pilot study. *BioMed Research International 2014*, 313351. doi:10.1155/2014/414351

Hellmich MR, Coletta C, Chao C *et al.* (2015) The therapeutic potential of cystathionine β-synthase/hydrogen sulfide inhibition in cancer. *Antioxidants and Redox Signaling 22*, 5, 424–448. doi:10.1089/ars.2014.5933

Henriques G, Keffer S, Abrahamson C *et al.* (2011) Exploring the effectiveness of a computer-based heart rate variability biofeedback program in reducing anxiety in college students. *Applied Psychophysiology and Biofeedback 36*, 101–112. doi:10.1007/ s10484-011-9151-4

Hershfield M (2017) Adenosine deaminase deficiency. *GeneReviews*. www.ncbi.nlm.nih. gov/books/NBK1483

Heyer NJ, Echeverria D, Martin MD *et al.* (2009) Catechol O-methyltransferase (COMT) VAL158MET functional polymorphism, dental mercury exposure, and self-reported symptoms and mood. *Journal of Toxicology and Environmental Health Part A 72*, 9, 599–609.

Hickey SE, Curry CJ, Toriello HV (2013) ACMG practice guideline: Lack of evidence for MTHFR polymorphism testing. *Genetics in Medicine 15*, 2, 153–156. doi:10.1038/ gim.2012.165

Hildebrandt TM, Grieshaber MK (2008) Three enzymatic activities catalyze the oxidation of sulfide to thiosulfate in mammalian and invertebrate mitochon-dria. *FEBS Journal 275*, 13, 3352–3361. doi:10.1111/j.1742-4658.2008.06482.x

Hill Erdei S (2014) What floxies should be aware of and some important updates. https://mthfrsupport.com/2014/03/what-floxies-should-be-aware-of

Hill Erdei S, Ledowski C (2015) *SNPBit Compendium 1*. Chicago, IL: Lifezone Wellness.

Hill L, Droste S, Nutt D *et al.* (2010) Voluntary exercise alters GABAA receptor subunit and glutamic acid decarboxylase-67 gene expression in the rat forebrain. *Journal of Psychopharmacology 24*, 5, 745–756. doi:10.1177/0269881108096983

Hirata F, Axelrod J (1978) Enzymatic methylation of phosphatidylethanolamine increases erythrocyte membrane fluidity. *Nature 275*, 219–220.

Hirsch A (2015) *Nutrition and Sensation*. Boco Raton, FL: CRC Press.

Hobson EE, Thomas S, Crofton PM *et al.* (2005) Isolated sulphite oxidase deficiency mimics the features of hypoxic ischaemic encephalopathy. *European Journal of Pediatrics 164*, 11, 655–659. doi:10.1007/s00431-005-1729-5

Hodges RE, Minich DM (2015) Modulation of metabolic detoxification pathways using foods and food-derived components: A scientific review with clinical application. *Journal of Nutrition and Metabolism 2015*, 760689. doi:10.1155/2015/760689

Hoge EA, Bui E, Marques L *et al.* (2013) Randomized controlled trial of mindfulness meditation for generalized anxiety disorder: effects on anxiety and stress reactivity. *Journal of Clinical Psychiatry 74*, 8, 786–792. doi:10.4088/JCP.12m08083

Horita M, Bueno CT, Horimoto AR *et al.* (2016) *MTRR* rs326119 polymorphism is associated with plasma concentrations of homocysteine and cobalamin, but not with congenital heart disease or coronary atherosclerosis in Brazilian patients. *International Journal of Cardiology, Heart and Vasculature 14*, 1–5. doi:10.1016/j.ijcha.2016.11.004

Hoth KF, Paul RH, Williams LM *et al.* (2006) Associations between the COMT Val/Met polymorphism, early life stress, and personality among healthy adults. *Neuropsychiatric Disease and Treatment 2*, 2, 219–225. doi:10.2147/nedt.2006.2.2.219

Hreljac I, Filipic M (2009) Organophosphorus pesticides enhance the genotoxicity of benzo(a)pyrene by modulating its metabolism. *Mutation Research 671*, 1–2, 84–92. doi:10.1016/j.mrfmmm.2009.09.011

Hu T, Zhang C, Tang Q *et al.* (2013) Variant G6PD levels promote tumor cell proliferation or apoptosis via the STAT3/5 pathway in the human melanoma xenograft mouse model. *BMC Cancer 13*, 251. doi:10.1186/1471-2407-13-251

Hua Y, Zhao H, Kong Y *et al.* (2011) Association between the MTHFR gene and Alzheimer's disease: A meta-analysis. *International Journal of Neuroscience 121*, 8, 462–471. doi:10.3109/00207454.2011.578778

Huang L, Teng T, Zhao J *et al.* (2017) The relationship between serum zinc levels, cardiac markers and the risk of acute myocardial infarction by zinc quartiles. *Heart, Lung and Circulation 27*, 1, 66–72. doi:10.1016/j.hlc.2017.01.022

Huang Y, Su L, Wu J (2016) Pyridoxine supplementation improves the activity of recombinant glutamate decarboxylase and the enzymatic production of gama-aminobutyric acid. *PLOS ONE 11*, 7, e0157466. doi:10.1371/journal.pone.0157466

Humphreys BD, Forman JP, Zandi-Nejad K *et al.* (2005) Acetaminophen-induced anion gap metabolic acidosis and 5-oxoprolinuria (pyroglutamic aciduria) acquired in hospital. *American Journal of Kidney Diseases 46*, 1, 143–146.

Ianiro G, Pecere S, Giorgio V *et al.* (2016) Digestive enzyme supplementation in gastrointestinal diseases. *Current Drug Metabolism 17*, 2, 187–193. doi:10.2174/1389200217021602160114150137

Imbard A, Benoist JF, Blom HJ (2013) Neural tube defects, folic acid and methylation. *International Journal of Environmental Research and Public Health 10*, 9, 4352–4389. doi:10.3390/ijerph10094352

Ismail AA, Ismail NA (2016) Magnesium: A mineral essential for health yet generally underestimated or even ignored. *Journal of Nutrition and Food Sciences 6*, 4. doi:10.4172/2155-9600.1000523

Iwase S, Bérubé NG, Zhou Z *et al.* (2017) Epigenetic etiology of intellectual disability. *Journal of Neuroscience 37*, 45, 10773–10782. doi:10.1523/JNEUROSCI.1840-17.2017

Izmirli M (2013) A literature review of MTHFR (C677T and A1298C polymorphisms) and cancer risk. *Molecular Biology Reports 40*, 1, 625–637. doi:10.1007/s11033-012-2101-2

James HM, Gillis D, Hissaria P *et al.* (2008) Common polymorphisms in the folate pathway predict efficacy of combination regimens containing methotrexate and sulfasalazine in early rheumatoid arthritis. *Journal of Rheumatology 35*, 4, 562–571.

Jancova P, Anzenbacher P, Anzenbacherova E (2010) Phase II drug metabolizing enzymes. *Biomedical Papers of the Medical Faculty of the University of Palacky, Olomouc, Czech Republic 154*, 2, 103–116. doi:10.5507/bp.2010.017

Jatana N, Apoorva N, Malik S *et al.* (2014) Inhibitors of catechol-O-methyl transferase in the treatment of neurological disorders. *Central Nervous System Agents in Medicinal Chemistry 13*, 3. doi:10.2174/1871524913666140109113341.

Jenkinson C, Petroczi A, Naughton DP (2013) Effects of dietary components on testosterone metabolism via UDP-glucuronosyl-transferase. *Frontiers in Endocrinology 4*, 80. doi:10.3389/fendo.2013.00080

Jethva R (2019) Sulfite oxidase deficiency and molybdenum cofactor deficiency. *Medscape.* https://emedicine.medscape.com/article/949303-overview

Ji W, Zhang Y (2017) The association of *MPO* gene promoter polymorphisms with Alzheimer's disease risk in Chinese Han population. *Oncotarget 8*, 64, 107870–107876. doi:10.18632/oncotarget.22330

Jiang H, Li B, Wang F *et al.* (2019) Expression of ERCC1 and TYMS in colorectal cancer patients and the predictive value of chemotherapy efficacy. *Oncology Letters 18*, 2, 1157–1162. doi:10.3892/ol.2019.10395

Joneidi Z, Mortazavi Y, Memari F *et al.* (2019) The impact of genetic variation on metabolism of heavy metals: Genetic predisposition? *Biomedicine and Pharmacotherarpy 113*, 108642. doi:10.1016/j.biopha.2019.108642

Jonsson L, Anckarsäter H, Zettergren A *et al.* (2014) Association between ASMT and autistic-like traits in children from a Swedish nationwide cohort. *Psychiatric Genetics 24*, 1, 21–27. doi:10.1097/YPG.0000000000000010

Joo J-HE, Andronikos RH, Saffery R (2011) Chapter 17 – Metabolic Regulation of DNA Methylation in Mammals. In T Tollefsbol (ed.) *Handbook of Epigenetics.* San Diego, CA: Academic Press. doi:10.1016/B978-0-12-375709-8.00017-4

Juul K, Tybjærg-Hansen A, Marklund S *et al.* (2004) Genetically reduced antioxidative protection and increased ischemic heart disease risk: The Copenhagen City Heart Study. *Circulation 109*, 1. doi:10.1161/01.CIR.0000105720.28086.6C

Kaczmarek JL, Liu X, Charron CS *et al.* (2019) Broccoli consumption affects the human gastrointestinal microbiota. *Journal of Nutritional Biochemistry 63*, 27–34.

Kane E (2017) Life on a membrane. Paper presented during the Membrane Medicine Seminar on 18 November.

Kang DJ, Betrapally NS, Ghosh SA *et al.* (2016) Gut microbiota drive the development of neuroinflammatory response in cirrhosis in mice. *Hepatology 64*, 4, 1232–1248. doi:10.1002/hep.28696

Kannaiyan R, Mahadevan D (2018) A comprehensive review of protein kinase inhibitors for cancer therapy. *Expert Review of Anticancer Therapy 18*, 12, 1249–1270. doi:10.1080/14737140.2018.1527688

Kao TT, Tu HC, Chang WN *et al.* (2010) Grape seed extract inhibits the growth and pathogenicity of *Staphylococcus aureus* by interfering with dihydrofolate reductase activity and folate-mediated one-carbon metabolism. *International Journal of Food Microbiology 141*, 1–2, 17–27. doi:10.1016/j.ijfoodmicro.2010.04.025

Kapalka GM (2006) Chapter 6 – Depression. In: *Practical Resources for the Mental Health Professional: Nutritional and Herbal Therapies for Children and Adolescents.* New York, NY: Academic Press. doi:10.1016/B978-0-12-374927-7.00006-6

Kelemen LE (2006) The role of folate receptor α in cancer development, progression and treatment: Cause, consequence or innocent bystander? *International Journal of Cancer* 119, 2, 243–250.

Kelson TL, Secor McVoy JR, Rizzo WB (1997) Human liver fatty aldehyde dehydrogenase: Microsomal localization, purification, and biochemical characterization. *Biochim Biophys Acta - Gen Subj 1335*, 1, 99–110. Available from: www.sciencedirect.com/science/article/pii/S0304416596001262

Kerr TA, Matsumoto Y, Matsumoto H *et al.* (2014) Cysteine sulfinic acid decarboxylase regulation: A role for farnesoid X receptor and small heterodimer partner in murine hepatic taurine metabolism. *Hepatology Research 44*, 10, E218–E228. doi:10.1111/hepr.12230

Kettle AJ, Turner R, Gangell CL et al. (2014) Oxidation contributes to low glutathione in the airways of children with cystic fibrosis. *European Respiratory Journal 44*, 1, 1222–129. doi:10.1183/09031936.00170213

Kietadisorn R, Juni RP, Moens AL (2011) Tackling endothelial dysfunction by modulating NOS uncoupling: new insights into its pathogenesis and therapeutic possibilities. *American Journal of Physiology – Endocrinology and Metabolism 302*, 5, 481–495. doi:10.1152/ajpendo.00540.2011

Kim S, Park DH, Shim J (2008) Thymidylate synthase and dihydropyrimidine dehydrogenase levels are associated with response to 5-fluorouracil in *Caenorhabditis elegans*. *Molecules and Cells 26*, 4, 344–349.

Kim YR, Hong SH (2019) Associations of MTRR and TSER polymorphisms related to folate metabolism with susceptibility to metabolic syndrome. *Genes and Genomics 41*, 8, 983–991. doi:10.1007/s13258-019-00840-8

Klerk M, Verhoef P, Clarke R *et al.* (2002) MTHFR 677C→T polymorphism and risk of coronary heart disease: A meta-analysis. *JAMA 288*, 16, 2023–2031. doi:10.1001/jama.288.16.2023

Klutstein M, Nejman D, Greenfield R *et al.* (2016) DNA methylation in cancer and aging; *Cancer Research 76*, 12, 3446–3450. doi:10.1158/0008-5472.CAN-15-3278

Ko JC, Tsai MS, Chiu YF *et al.* (2011) Up-regulation of extracellular signal-regulated kinase 1/2-dependent thymidylate synthase and thymidine phosphorylase contributes to cisplatin resistance in human non-small-cell lung cancer cells. *Journal of Pharmacology and Experimental Therapeutics 338*, 1, 184–194. doi:10.1124/jpet.111.179663

Kohlmeier, M (2013) *Nutrigenetics: Applying the Science of Personal Nutrition*. New York, NY: Elsevier.

Kolla NJ, Meyer J, Sanches M *et al.* (2017) Monoamine Oxidase-A Genetic Variants and Childhood Abuse Predict Impulsiveness in Borderline Personality Disorder. *Clinical Psychopharmacology and Neuroscience: The Official Scientific Journal of the Korean College of Neuropsychopharmacology 15*, 4, 343–351. doi:10.9758/cpn.2017.15.4.343

Konopnicki CM, Dickmann LJ, Tracy JM *et al.* (2013) Evaluation of UGT protein interactions in human hepatocytes: effect of siRNA down regulation of UGT1A9 and UGT2B7 on propofol glucuronidation in human hepatocytes. *Archives of Biochemistry and Biophysics 535*, 2, 143–149. doi:10.1016/j.abb.2013.03.012

Kooti W, Daraei N (2017) A review of the antioxidant activity of celery (*Apium graveolens* L). *Journal of Evidence-Based Complementary and Alternative Medicine 22*, 4, 1029–1034. doi:10.1177/2156587217717415

Kotnik BF, Jazbec J, Grabar PB *et al.* (2017) Association between *SLC19A1* gene polymorphism and high dose methotrexate toxicity in childhood acute lymphoblastic leukaemia and non-Hodgkin malignant lymphoma: Introducing a haplotype based approach. *Radiology and Oncology 51*, 4, 455–462. doi:10.1515/raon-2017-0040

Kou Y, Betancur C, Xu H (2012) Network- and attribute-based classifiers can prioritize genes and pathways for autism spectrum disorders and intellectual disability. *American Journal of Medical Genetics 160C*, 2, 130–142. doi:10.1002/ajmg.c.31330

Kriebitzsch C, Verlinden L, Eelen G *et al.* (2011) 1,25-dihydroxyvitamin D3 influences cellular homocysteine levels in murine preosteoblastic MC3T3-E1 cells by direct regulation of cystathionine β-synthase. *Journal of Bone and Mineral Research 26*, 12, 2991–3000. doi:10.1002/jbmr.493

Kripke DF, Nievergelt CM, Tranah GJ et al. (2011) Polymorphisms in melatonin synthesis pathways: possible influences on depression. *Journal of Circadian Rhythms 9*, 8. doi:10.1186/1740-3391-9-8

Križanová O, Mičutková L, Jeloková J et al. (2001) Existence of cardiac PNMT mRNA in adult rats: Elevation by stress in a glucocorticoid dependent manner. *American Journal of Physiology: Heart and Circulatory Physiology 281*, 3, H1372–1379. doi:10.1152/ajpheart.2001.281.3.H1372

Kruger WD, Gupta S (2015) The effect of dietary modulation of sulfur amino acids on cystathionine β synthase-deficient mice. *Annals of the New York Academy of Sciences 1363*, 1, 80–90. doi:10.1111/nyas.12967

Krzyściak W, Kościelniak D, Papież M et al. (2017) Effect of a *Lactobacillus salivarius* probiotic on a double-species *Streptococcus mutans* and *Candida albicans* caries biofilm. *Nutrients 9*, 11, 1242. doi:10.3390/nu9111242

Kuo SC, Yeh YW, Chen CY et al. (2014) DRD3 variation associates with early-onset heroin dependence, but not specific personality traits. *Progress in Neuro-Psychopharmacology and Biological Psychiatry 51*, 1–8. doi: 10.1016/j.pnpbp.2013.12.018

Kurogi K, Sakakibara Y, Suiko M et al. (2017) Sulfation of vitamin D_3-related compounds – identification and characterization of the responsible human cytosolic sulfotransferases. *FEBS Letters 591*, 16, 2417–2425. doi:10.1002/1873-3468.12767

Kwon HJ, Lim MH (2013) Association between dopamine Beta-hydroxylase gene polymorphisms and attention-deficit hyperactivity disorder in Korean children. *Genetic Testing and Molecular Biomarkers 17*, 7, 529–534. doi:10.1089/gtmb.2013.0072

Labouesse MA, Dong E, Grayson DR et al. (2015) Maternal immune activation induces GAD1 and GAD2 promoter remodeling in the offspring prefrontal cortex. *Epigenetics 10*, 12, 1143–1155. doi:10.1080/15592294.2015.1114202

Lai CQ, Parnell LD, Troen AM et al. (2010) MAT1A variants are associated with hypertension, stroke, and markers of DNA damage and are modulated by plasma vitamin B-6 and folate. *American Journal of Clinical Nutrition 91*, 5, 1377–1386. doi:10.3945/ajcn.2009.28923

Landi N, Frost SJ, Einer W et al. (2013) The COMT Val/Met polymorphism is associated with reading-related skills and consistent patterns of functional neural activation. *Developmental Science 16*, 1, 13–23. doi:10.1111/j.1467-7687.2012.01180.x

Landolt H-P (2018) Sleep homeostasis: A role for adenosine in humans? *Biochemical Pharmacology 75*, 11, 2070–2079. doi:10.1016/j.bcp.2008.02.024

Laucht M, Becker K, Frank J et al. (2008) Genetic variation in dopamine pathways differentially associated with smoking progression in adolescence. *Journal of the American Academy of Child and Adolescent Psychiatry 47*, 6, 673–681. doi:10.1097/CHI.0b013e31816bff77

Lauritano EC, Gabrielli M, Scarpellini E et al. (2008) Small intestinal bacterial overgrowth recurrence after antibiotic therapy. *American Journal of Gastroenterology 103*, 8, 2031–2035.

Lebon S, Minai L, Chretien D et al. (2007) A novel mutation of the NDUFS7 gene leads to activation of a cryptic exon and impaired assembly of mitochondrial complex I in a patient with Leigh syndrome. *Molecular Genetics and Metabolism 92*, 1–2, 104–108. doi:10.1016/j.ymgme.2007.05.010

Leclercq S, Matamoros S, Cani PD et al. (2014) Intestinal permeability, gut-bacterial dysbiosis, and behavioral markers of alcohol-dependence severity. *PNAS 111*, 42, E4485–4493. doi:10.1073/pnas.1415174111

Lee EJ, An D, Nguyen CT et al. (2014) Betalain and betaine composition of greenhouse- or field-produced beetroot (*Beta vulgaris* L.) and inhibition of HepG2 cell proliferation. *Journal of Agricultural and Food Chemistry 62*, 6, 1324–1331. doi:10.1021/jf404648u

Lee JI, Kang J, Stipanuk MH (2006) Differential regulation of glutamate-cysteine ligase subunit expression and increased holoenzyme formation in response to cysteine deprivation. *Biochemical Journal 393*, 1, 181–190. doi:10.1042/BJ20051111

Lee S, Park JM, Jeong M et al. (2016) Korean red ginseng ameliorated experimental pancreatitis through the inhibition of hydrogen sulfide in mice. *Pancreatology 16*, 3, 326–336.

Lee SL, Lee YP, Wu ML *et al.* (2015) Inhibition of human alcohol and aldehyde dehydrogenases by aspirin and salicylate: Assessment of the effects on first-pass metabolism of ethanol. *Biochemical Pharmacology 95*, 1, 71–79. doi:10.1016/j.bcp.2015.03.003

Leong XF, Salimon J, Mustafa MR *et al.* (2012) Effect of repeatedly heated palm olein on blood pressure-regulating enzymes activity and lipid peroxidation in rats. *Malaysian Journal of Medical Sciences 19*, 1, 20–29.

Levy G (1986) Sulfate conjugation in drug metabolism: Role of inorganic sulfate. *Federation Proceedings 45*, 2235–2240.

Li F, Tsien JZ (2009) Memory and the NMDA receptors. *New England Journal of Medicine 361*, 3, 302–303. doi:10.1056/NEJMcibr0902052

Li Q, Kobayashi M, Kumeda S *et al.* (2016) Effects of forest bathing on cardiovascular and metabolic parameters in middle-aged males. *Evidence-Based Complementary and Alternative Medicine*, 2587381. doi:10.1155/2016/2587381

Li X, Shen M, Cai H *et al.* (2016) Association between manganese superoxide dismutase (MnSOD) polymorphism and prostate cancer susceptibility: A meta-analysis. *International Journal of Biological Markers 31*, 4, 422–430. doi:10.5301/jbm.5000188

Lin S, Li T, Zhu D *et al.* (2013) The association between GAD1 gene polymorphisms and cerebral palsy in Chinese infants. *Cytology and Genetics 47*, 5, 22–27.

Lindsay J, Wang LL, Li Y *et al.* (2008) Structure, function and polymorphism of human cytosolic sulfotransferases. *Current Drug Metabolism 9*, 2, 99–105. doi:10.2174/138920008783571819

Linus Pauling Institute (n.d.) Micronutrient Information Center. https://lpi.oregonstate.edu/mic

Lipton, B. (2015) *Biology of Belief: Unleashing the Power of Consciousness, Matter and Miracles*. London: Hay House Publishing.

Litwack G, Litwack G (2018) Chapter 13 – Metabolism of Amino Acids. *Human Biochemistry*. New York, NY: Academic Press. doi:10.1016/B978-0-12-383864-3.00013-2

Locasale JW (2013) Serine, glycine and one-carbon units: Cancer metabolism in full circle. *National Reviews, Cancer 13*, 8, 572–583. doi:10.1038/nrc3557

Loguercio C, D'Argenio G, Delle Cave M *et al.* (2003) Glutathione supplementation improves oxidative damage in experimental colitis. *Digestive and Liver Disease 35*, 9, 635–641.

Lombard J (n.d.) A functional approach to mental health: Summary signs and symptoms associated with neurotransmitter imbalances. Accessed on 27/10/2021 at www.clinicaleducation.org/downloads/Summary%20Symptom%20%20Neurotransmitter%20Doc%20JL.pdf

Lombard J, Renna C, Brott A (2003) *The Super Mind-body Cure: Rebalance Your Body and Calm Your Mind*. New York, NY: John Wiley & Sons Inc.

Lord RS, Bralley JA (2008) Clinical applications of urinary organic acids. Part I: Detoxification markers. *Alternative Medicine Review 13*, 3, 205–215.

Lozda R, Purviņš I (2014) Quantification of serotonin O-sulphate by LC-MS method in plasma of healthy volunteers. *Frontiers in Pharmacology*. doi:10.3389/fphar.2014.00062

Lu SC (2020) Dysregulation of glutathione synthesis in liver disease. *Liver Research 4*, 2, 64–73. doi:10.1016/j.livres.2020.05.003

Luckey M (2012) *Membrane Structural Biology*. Cambridge and New York: Cambridge University Press.

Lugo-Huitrón R, Ugalde Muñiz P, Pineda B *et al.* (2013) Quinolinic acid: An endogenous neurotoxin with multiple targets. *Oxidative Medicine and Cellular Longevity*, 104024. doi:10.1155/2013/104024

Luzzatto L, Seneca E (2014) G6PD deficiency: A classic example of pharmacogenetics with on-going clinical implications. *British Journal of Haematology 164*, 4, 469–480. doi:10.1111/bjh.12665

Lynch B (2017) SHEICON 2017 Conference Proceedings And Pathway Planner v5. Seattle.

Maclean KN, Janosík M, Kraus E *et al.* (2002) Cystathionine beta-synthase is coordinately regulated with proliferation through a redox-sensitive mechanism in cultured human cells and Saccharomyces cerevisiae. *Journal of Cell Physiology 192*, 1, 81–92.

Magnusson M, Wang TJ, Clish C *et al.* (2015). Dimethylglycine deficiency and the development of diabetes. *Diabetes 64*, 8, 3010–3016.

Mahboubi M (2015) Rosa damascena as holy ancient herb with novel applications. *Journal of Traditional and Complementary Medicine 6*, 1, 10–16. doi:10.1016/j.jtcme.2015.09.005

Mahrooz A, Rashidi MR, Nouri M (2011) Naringenin is an inhibitor of human serum paraoxonase (PON1): An in vitro study. *Journal of Clinical Laboratory Analysis 25*, 395–401. doi:10.1002/jcla.20490

Mäki-Petäjä KM, Day L, Cheriyan J *et al.* (2016) Tetrahydrobiopterin supplementation improves endothelial function but does not alter aortic stiffness in patients with rheumatoid arthritis. *Journal of the American Heart Association 5*, 2, e002762. doi:10.1161/JAHA.115.002762

Malle E, Furtmüller PG, Sattler W *et al.* (2007) Myeloperoxidase: A target for new drug development? *British Journal of Pharmacology 152*, 6, 838–854.

Malmberg K, Wargelius HL, Lichtenstein P *et al.* (2008) ADHD and disruptive behavior scores: Associations with MAO-A and 5-HTT genes and with platelet MAO-B activity in adolescents. *BMC Psychiatry 8*, 28. doi:10.1186/1471-244X-8-28

Mansoori N, Tripathi M, Luthra K *et al.* (2012) MTHFR (677 and 1298) and IL-6-174 G/C genes in pathogenesis of Alzheimer's and vascular dementia and their epistatic interaction. *Neurobiology of Aging 33*, 5, 1003.e1–1003.e8. doi:10.1016/j.neurobiolaging.2011.09.018

Manvich DF, DePoy LM, Weinshenker D (2013) Dopamine β-hydroxylase inhibitors enhance the discriminative stimulus effects of cocaine in rats. *Journal of Pharmacology and Experimental Therapeutics 347*, 3, 564–573. doi:10.1124/jpet.113.207746

Markovich D, Aronson PS (2007) Specificity and regulation of renal sulphate transporters. *Annual Review of Physiology 69*, 361–375.

Marselle MR, Warber SL, Irvine KN (2019) Growing resilience through interaction with nature: Can group walks in nature buffer the effects of stressful life events on mental health? *International Journal of Environmental Research and Public Health 16*, 6, 986. doi:10.3390/ijerph16060986

Martens CR, Denman BA, Mazzo MR *et al.* (2018) Chronic nicotinamide riboside supplementation is well-tolerated and elevates NAD+ in healthy middle-aged and older adults. *Nature Communications 9*, 1286. doi:10.1038/s41467-018-03421-7

Martin JL, Begun J, McLeish MJ *et al.* (2001) Getting the adrenaline going: Crystal structure of the adrenaline-synthesizing enzyme PNMT. *Structure 9*, 10, 977–985.

Martinez ME, O'Brien TG, Fultz KE *et al.* (2003) Pronounced reduction in adenoma recurrence associated with aspirin use and a polymorphism in the ornithine decarboxylase gene. *PNAS 100*, 3, 7859–7864.

Masaoka T, Tack J (2009) Gastroparesis: current concepts and management. *Gut and Liver 3*, 3, 166–173. doi:10.5009/gnl.2009.3.3.166

McLaughlin KA, Koenen KC, Bromet EJ *et al.* (2017) Childhood adversities and post-traumatic stress disorder: evidence for stress sensitisation in the World Mental Health Surveys. *British Journal of Psychiatry 211*, 5, 280–288. doi:10.1192/bjp.bp.116.197640

McNeill E, Channon KM (2012) The role of tetrahydrobiopterin in inflammation and cardiovascular disease. *Thrombosis and Haemostasis 108*, 5, 832–839. doi:10.1160/TH12-06-0424

Mier D, Kirsch P, Meyer-Lindenberg A (2010) Neural substrates of pleiotropic action of genetic variation in COMT: A meta-analysis. *Molecular Psychiatry 15*, 9, 918–927. doi:10.1038/mp.2009.36

Mileva-Seitz V, Fleming AS, Meaney MJ *et al.* (2012) Dopamine receptors D1 and D2 are related to observed maternal behavior. *Genes, Brain and Behavior 11*, 6, 684–694. doi:10.1111/j.1601-183X.2012.00804.x

Millis RM (2011) Epigenetics and hypertension. *Current Hypertension Reports 17*, 4, 451. doi:10.3390/ijms17040451

Minich DM, Brown BI (2019) A review of dietary phytonutrients for glutathione support. *Nutrients 11*, 2073. doi:10.3390/nu11092073

Minnick F (2014) In search of a cure for the dreaded hangover. Can science help defeat the physical aftereffects of drinking too much alcohol – if not the regrets? *Scientific American*. Accessed on 27/10/2021 at www.scientificamerican.com/article/in-search-of-a-cure-for-the-dreaded-hangover

Mitaki S, Isomura M, Maniwa K *et al.* (2013) Impact of five SNPs in dopamine-related genes on executive function. *Acta Neurologica Scandinavica 127*, 1, 70–76. doi:10.1111/j.1600-0404.2012.01673.x

Mitchell JJ, Trakadis YJ, Scriver CR (2011) Phenylalanine hydroxylase deficiency. *Genetics in Medicine 13*, 8, 697–707. doi:10.1097/GIM.0b013e3182141b48

Mitchell S, Waring R (2016) Sulphate absorption across biological membranes. *Xenobiotica 46*, 2, 184–191. doi:10.3109/00498254.2015.1054921

Mitsuhashi H, Yamashita S, Ikeuchi H *et al.* (2005) Oxidative stress-dependent conversion of hydrogen sulfide to sulfite by activated neutrophils. *Shock 2*, 6, 529–534.

Mittelstraß K, Waldenberger M (2018) DNA methylation in human lipid metabolism and related diseases. *Current Opinion in Lipidology 29*, 2, 116–124. doi:10.1097/MOL.0000000000000491

Mohamad NE, Yeap SK, Beh B-K *et al.* (2018) Coconut water vinegar ameliorates recovery of acetaminophen induced liver damage in mice. *BMC Complementary Medicine and Therapies 18*, 1, 195. doi:10.1186/s12906-018-2199-4

Mohamad NE, Yeap SK, Ky H *et al.* (2017) Dietary coconut water vinegar for improvement of obesity-associated inflammation in high-fat-diet-treated mice. *Food and Nutrition Research 61*, 1, 1368322. doi:10.1080/16546628.2017.1368322

Montag C, Jurkiewicz M, Reuter M (2012) The role of the catechol-O-methyltransferase (COMT) gene in personality and related psychopathological disorders. *CNS and Neurological Disorders Drug Targets 11*, 3, 236–250.

Montioli R, Voltattorni CB, Bertoldi M (2016) Parkinson's disease: Recent updates in the identification of human dopa decarboxylase inhibitors. *Current Drug Metabolism 17*, 5, 513–518. doi:10.2174/138920021705160324170558

Moreau C, Meguig S, Corvol JC *et al.* (2015) Polymorphism of the dopamine transporter type 1 gene modifies the treatment response in Parkinson's disease. *Brain: A Journal of Neurology 138*, 5, 1271–1283. doi:10.1093/brain/awv063

Morris AL, Mohiuddin SS (2021) Biochemistry, Nutrients. *StatPearls.* www.ncbi.nlm.nih.gov/books/NBK554545

Morris MS, Jacques PF, Rosenberg IH *et al.* (2007) Folate and vitamin B-12 status in relation to anemia, macrocytosis, and cognitive impairment in older Americans in the age of folic acid fortification. *American Journal of Clinical Nutrition 85*, 1, 193–200. doi:10.1093/ajcn/85.1.193

Moss M, Waring RH (2003) The plasma cysteine/sulphate ratio: A possible clinical biomarker. *Journal of Nutritional and Environmental Medicine 13*, 4, 215–229. doi:10.1080/13590840310001642003

Motzek A, Knežević J, Switzeny OJ *et al.* (2016) Abnormal hypermethylation at imprinting control regions in patients with S-adenosylhomocysteine hydrolase (AHCY) deficiency. *PLOS ONE 11*, 3, e0151261. doi:10.1371/journal.pone.0151261

Mrozikiewicz PM, Bogacz A, Omielańczyk *et al.* (2015) The importance of rs1021737 and rs482843 polymorphisms of cystathionine gammalyase in the etiology of preeclampsia in the Caucasian population. *Ginekologia Polska 86*, 2, 119–125.

Mustapić M, Pivac N, Kozarić-Kovačić D *et al.* (2007) Dopamine beta-hydroxylase (DBH) activity and –1021c/t polymorphism of DBH gene in combat-related post-traumatic stress disorder. *American Journal of Medical Genetics Part B 144B*, 8, 1087–1089. doi:10.1002/ajmg.b.30526

Na HS, Chung YH, Hwang JW *et al.* (2012) Effects of magnesium sulphate on postoperative coagulation, measured by rotational thromboelastometry (ROTEM(®)). *Anaesthesia 67*, 8, 862–869. doi:10.1111/j.1365-2044.2012.07149.x

Nair R, Maseeh A (2012) Vitamin D: The 'sunshine' vitamin. *Journal of Pharmacolgoy and Pharmacotherapeutics 3*, 2, 118–126. doi:10.4103/0976-500X.95506

Nakahara K, Ohkuni A, Kitamura T *et al.* (2012) The Sjögren-Larsson syndrome gene encodes a hexadecenal dehydrogenase of the sphingosine 1-phosphate degradation pathway. *Molecular Cell 46*, 4, 461–471. doi:10.1016/j.molcel.2012.04.033

Navab M, Reddy ST, Van Lenten BJ et al. (2011) HDL and cardiovascular disease: Atherogenic and atheroprotective mechanisms. Nature Reviews, Cardiology 8, 222. doi:10.1038/nrcardio.2010.222

Navarro-Perán E, Cabezas-Herrera J, García-Cánovas F et al. (2005) The antifolate activity of tea catechins. Cancer Research 65, 6, 2059–2064

Naviaux RK (2013) Metabolic features of the cell danger response. Mitochondrion 16, 7–17.

Neumann M, Leimkühler S (2008) Heavy metal ions inhibit molybdoenzyme activity by binding to the dithiolene moiety of molybdopterin in Escherichia coli. FEBS Journal 2275, 22, 5678–5689.

Nielsen FH, Johnson LK, Zeng H (2010) Magnesium supplementation improves indicators of low magnesium status and inflammatory stress in adults older than 51 years with poor quality sleep. Magnesium Research 23, 4, 158–168. doi:10.1684/mrh.2010.0220

Nigh G (2019) SIBO as an adaptation: A proposed role for hydrogen sulphide, Gastrointestinal. https://ndnr.com/gastrointestinal/sibo-as-an-adaptation-a-proposed-role-for-hydrogen-sulfide

Nishimuta H, Ohtani H, Tsujimoto M et al. (2007) Inhibitory effects of various beverages on human recombinant sulfotransferase isoforms sult1a1 and sult1a3. Biopharmaceutics and Drug Disposition 28, 9, 491–500.

Noji N, Nakamura T, Kitahata N et al. (2007) Simple and sensitive method for pyrroloquinoline quinone (PQQ) analysis in various foods using liquid chromatography/electrospray-ionization tandem mass spectrometry. Journal of Agricultural and Food Chemistry 55, 18, 7258–7263. doi:10.1021/jf070483r

Nonaka H, Nakanishi Y, Kuno S et al. (2019) Design strategy for serine hydroxymethyltransferase probes based on retro-aldol-type reaction. Nature Communications 10, 876. doi:10.1038/s41467-019-08833-7

NutritionData (2018) Foods highest in choline. https://nutritiondata.self.com/foods-016144000000000000000-w.html?maxCount=36

Nutt DJ, Lingford-Hughes A, Erritzoe D et al. (2015) The dopamine theory of addiction: 40 years of highs and lows. Nature Reviews Neuroscience 16, 305. doi:10.1038/nrn3939

O'Callaghan A, van Sinderen D (2016) Bifidobacteria and their role as members of the human gut microbiota. Frontiers in Microbiology 7, 925. doi:10.3389/fmicb.2016.00925

Obeid R (2013) The metabolic burden of methyl donor deficiency with focus on the betaine homocysteine methyltransferase pathway. Nutrients 5, 9, 3481–3495. doi:10.3390/nu5093481

Ogwang S, Nguyen HT, Sherman M et al. (2011) Bacterial conversion of folinic acid is required for antifolate resistance. Journal of Biological Chemistry 286, 7, 15377–15390. doi:10.1074%2Fjbc.M111.231076

Ouzzine M, Gulberti S, Ramalanjaona N et al. (2014) The UDP-glucuronosyltransferases of the blood–brain barrier: Their role in drug metabolism and detoxication. Frontiers in Cellular Neuroscience 8, 349. doi:10.3389/fncel.2014.00349

Painter K, Cordell BJ, Sticco KL (2021) Auto-brewery syndrome. StatPearls. www.ncbi.nlm.nih.gov/books/NBK513346

Palmer AM, Kamynina E, Field MS et al. (2017) Folate rescues vitamin B 12 depletion-induced inhibition of nuclear thymidylate biosynthesis and genome instability. PNAS 114, 20, E4095–E4102. doi:10.1073/pnas.1619582114

Pandit S, Annamaraju P, Bhusal K (2021) Carcinoid syndrome. StatPearls. www.ncbi.nlm.nih.gov/books/NBK448096

Paré G, Chasman DI, Parker AN et al. (2009) Novel associations of CPS1, MUT, NOX4, and DPEP1 with plasma homocysteine in a healthy population: A| genome-wide evaluation of 13, 974 participants in the women's genome health study. Circulation: Cardiovascular Genetics 2, 2, 142–150. doi:10.1161/CIRCGENETICS.108.829804

Park JK, Kim JW, Lee HJ et al. (2007) Dopamine beta-hydroxylase gene polymorphisms and psychotic symptoms in schizophrenia. American Journal of Medical Genetics Part B Neuropsychiatric Genetics 144B, 7, 944–945. doi:10.1002/ajmg.b.30516

Parvez SH, Naoi M, Nagatsu T (2013) Methods in Neurotransmitter and Neuropeptide Research. Amsterdam: Elsevier.

Patrick RP, Ames BN (2014) Vitamin D hormone regulates serotonin synthesis. Part 1: relevance for autism. The FASEB Journal 28, 6, 2398–2413. doi:10.1096/fj.13-246546

Pegg AE (2006) Regulation of ornithine decar-boxylase. *Journal of Biological Chemistry 281*, 21, P14529–14532. doi:10.1074/jbc. R500031200

Pençe S, Erkutlu I, Kurtul N *et al.* (2009) Effects of progesterone on total brain tissue adenosine deaminase activity in experimental epilepsy. *International Journal of Neuroscience 119*, 2, 204–213. doi:10.1080/00207450802055374

Penckofer S, Quinn L, Byrn M *et al.* (2012) Does glycemic variability impact mood and quality of life? *Diabetes Technology and Therapeutics 14*, 4, 303–310. doi:10.1089/dia.2011.0191

Pereira JC Jr, Pradella-Hallinan M, Lins Pessoa H (2010) Imbalance between thyroid hormones and the dopaminergic system might be central to the pathophysiology of restless legs syndrome: A hypothesis. *Clinics (Sao Paulo) 65*, 5, 548–554. doi:10.1590/S1807-59322010000500013

Pérez-Miguelsanz J, Vallecillo N, Garrido F *et al.* (2017) Betaine homocysteine S-methyltransferase emerges as a new player of the nuclear methionine cycle. *Biochimica et Biophysica Acta: Molecular Cell Research 1864*, 7, 1165–1182. doi:10.1016/j.bbamcr.2017.03.004

Perry C, Yu S, Chen J *et al.* (2007) Effect of vitamin B6 availability on serine hydrox-ymethyltransferase in MCF-7 cells. *Archives of Biochemistry and Biophysics 462*, 1, 21–27. doi:10.1074/jbc.R500031200

Peuhkuri K, Sihvola N, Korpela R (2012) Dietary factors and fluctuating levels of melatonin. *Food and Nutrition Research 56*. doi:10.3402/fnr.v56i0.17252

Pfeifer GP (2018) Defining driver dna methyl-ation changes in human cancer. *International Journal of Molecular Sciences 19*, 4, 1166. doi:10.3390/ijms19041166

Philibert RA, Gunter TD, Beach SRH *et al.* (2008) MAOA methylation is associated with nicotine and alcohol dependence in women. *American Journal of Medical Genetics Part B: Neuropsychiatric Genetics 147B*, 5, 565–570. doi:10.1002/ajmg.b.30778

Pigatto PD, Ronchi A, Guzzi G (2016) Iron overload, G6PD deficiency, and lead levels on blood smears. *International Journal of Hematology 103*, 6, 724. doi:10.1007/s12185-016-1990-6

Pogribna M, Melnyk S, Pogribny I *et al.* (2011) Homocysteine metabolism in children with Down syndrome: In vitro modulation. *American Journal of Human Genetics 69*, 1, 88–95.

Polonikov AV, Vialykh EK, Churnosov MI *et al.* (2012) The C718T polymorphism in the 3′-untranslated region of glutathione peroxidase-4 gene is a predictor of cerebral stroke in patients with essential hyperten-sion. *Hypertension Research 35*, 5, 507–512. doi:10.1038/hr.2011.213

Pomin VH (2017) Sulfated glycans and related digestive enzymes in the Zika virus infectivity: Potential Mechanisms of virus-host interaction and perspectives in drug discovery. *Interdisciplinary Perspectives on Infectious Diseases 2017*, 4894598. doi:10.1155/2017/4894598.

Pool-Zobel B, Veeriah S, Böhmer FD (2005) Modulation of xenobiotic metabolising enzymes by anticarcinogens – focus on glutathione S-transferases and their role as targets of dietary chemoprevention in colorectal carcinogenesis. *Mutation Research 591*, 1–2, 74–92.

Popkin BM, D'Anci KE, Rosenberg IH (2010) Water, hydration, and health. *Nutrition Reviews 68*, 8, 439–458. doi:10.1111/j.1753-4887.2010.00304.x

Powers HJ, Hill MH, Mushtaq S *et al.* (2011) Correcting a marginal riboflavin defi-ciency improves hematologic status in young women in the United Kingdom (RIBOFEM). *American Journal of Clinical Nutrition 93*, 6, 1274–1284. doi:10.3945/ajcn.110.008409

Pozdeyev N, Taylor C, Haque R *et al.* (2006) Photic regulation of arylalkylamine N-acet-yltransferase binding to 14-3-3 proteins in retinal photoreceptor cells. *Journal of Neuroscience 26*, 36, 9153–9161. doi:10.1523/jneurosci.1384-06.2006

Ptacek R, Kuzelova H, Stefano GB (2011) Dopamine D4 receptor gene DRD4 and its association with psychiatric disorders. *Medical Science Monitor 17*, 9, RA215–220.

Punchaichira TJ, Mukhopadhyay A, Kukshal P *et al.* (2020) Association of regulatory variants of dopamine β-hydroxylase with cognition and tardive dyskinesia in schizophrenia subjects. *Journal of Psychopharmacology 34*, 3, 358–369. doi:10.1177/0269881119895539

Rae CD, Williams SR (2017) Glutathione in the human brain: Review of its roles and measurement by magnetic resonance spectroscopy. *Analytical Biochemistry 529*, 127–143. doi:10.1016/j.ab.2016.12.022

Rai V (2016) Association of methylenetetrahydrofolate reductase (MTHFR) gene C677T polymorphism with autism: Evidence of genetic susceptibility. *Metabolic Brain Disease 31*, 4, 727–735. doi:10.1007/s11011-016-9815-0

Rajagopalan, KV (1988) Molybdenum: An essential trace element in human nutrition. *Annual Review of Nutrition 8*, 1, 401–427.

Rajan R, Krishnan S, Sarma G *et al.* (2018) Dopamine receptor D3 rs6280 is associated with aberrant decision-making in Parkinson's disease. *Movement Disorders Clinical Practice 5*, 413–416. doi:10.1002/mdc3.12631

Ramaekers VT, Hausler M, Opladen T *et al.* (2002) Psychomotor retardation, spastic paraplegia, cerebellar ataxia and dyskinesia associated with low 5-methyltetrahydrofolate in cerebrospinal fluid: A novel neurometabolic condition responding to folinic acid substitution. *Neuropediatrics 33*, 6, 301–308.

Ramos PS, Oates JC, Kamen DL *et al.* (2013) Variable association of reactive intermediate genes with systemic lupus erythematosus in populations with different African ancestry. *Journal of Rheumatology 40*, 6, 842–849. doi:10.3899/jrheum.120989.C1

Rao NA, Ambili M, Jala VR *et al.* (2003) Structure-function relationship in serine hydroxymethyltransferase. *Biochimica et Biophysica Acta: Proteins and Proteomics 1647*, 1–2, 24–29. doi:10.1016/S1570-9639(03)00043-8

Rapoport TA (2007) Protein translocation across the eukaryotic endoplasmic reticulum and bacterial plasma membranes. *Nature 450*, 7170, 663–669. doi:10.1038/nature06384

Rees MD, Kennett EC, Whitelock JM *et al.* (2008) Oxidative damage to extracellular matrix and its role in human pathologies. *Free Radical Biology and Medicine 44*, 12, 1973–2001.

Resseguie J, Song MD, Niculescu KA *et al.* (2007) Phosphatidylethanolamine N-methyltransferase (PEMT) gene expression is induced by estrogen in human and mouse primary hepatocytes. *FASEB Journal 21*, 2622–2632.

Ristoff E, Mayatepek E, Larsson A (2001) Long-term clinical outcome in patients with glutathione synthetase deficiency. *Journal of Pediatrics 139*, 1, 79–84.

Robertson JG, Kumar A, Mancewicz JA *et al.* (1989) Spectral studies of bovine dopamine beta-hydroxylase. Absence of covalently bound pyrroloquinoline quinone. *Journal of Biological Chemistry 264, 33*, 19916–19921.

Rong XI, Albert CJ, Hong C *et al.* (2013) LXRs regulate ER stress and inflammation through dynamic modulation of membrane phospholipid composition. *Cell Metabolism 18*, 5, 685–697.

Rubinstein A (2016) Adenosine deaminase deficiency: Pathogenesis, clinical manifestations, and diagnosis. *UpToDate*. www.uptodate.com/contents/adenosine-deaminase-deficiency-pathogenesis-clinical-manifestations-and-diagnosis

Rudolph MJ, Johnson JL, Rajagopalan KV *et al.* (2003) The 1.2 Å structure of the human sulfite oxidase cytochrome b5 domain. *Acta Crystallographica Section D Structural Biology D59*, 1183–1191. doi:10.1107/S0907444903009934

Rushworth GF, Megson IL (2014) Existing and potential therapeutic uses for N-acetylcysteine: The need for conversion to intracellular glutathione for antioxidant benefits. *Pharmacology and Therapeutics 141*, 2, 150–159. doi:10.1016/j.pharmthera.2013.09.006

Ryding E, Lindström M, Träskman-Bendz L (2008) The role of dopamine and serotonin in suicidal behaviour and aggression. *Progress in Brain Research 172*, 307–315. doi:10.1016/S0079-6123(08)00915-1

Saha T, Chatterjee M, Verma D *et al.* (2018) Genetic variants of the folate metabolic system and mild hyperhomocysteinemia may affect ADHD associated behavioral problems. *Progress in Neuro-Psychopharmacology and Biological Psychiatry 84*, A, 1–10. doi:10.1016/J.PNPBP.2018.01.016

Sakata SF, Okumura S, Matsuda K *et al.* (2005) Effect of fasting on methionine adenosyltransferase expression and the methionine cycle in the mouse liver. *Journal of Nutritional Science and Vitaminology 51*, 2, 118–123. doi:10.3177/jnsv.51.118

Salve J, Pate S, Debnath K *et al.* (2019) Adaptogenic and anxiolytic effects of Ashwagandha root extract in healthy adults: A double-blind, randomized, placebo-controlled clinical study. *Cureus 11*, 12, e6466. doi:10.7759/cureus.6466

Samsel A, Seneff S (2013) Glyphosate, pathways to modern diseases II: Celiac sprue and gluten intolerance. *Interdisciplinary Toxicology 6*, 4, 159–184.

Sánchez-Santed F, Colomina MT, Herrero H *et al.* (2016) Organophosphate pesticide exposure and neurodegeneration. *Cortex 74*, 417–426. doi:10.1016/j.cortex.2015.10.003

Sandstead HH, Prasad AS (2010) Zinc intake and resistance to H1N1 influenza. *American Journal of Public Health 100*, 6, 970–971. doi:10.2105/AJPH.2009.187773

Sarbishegi M, Mehraein F, Soleimani M (2014) Antioxidant role of oleuropein on midbrain and dopaminergic neurons of substantia nigra in aged rats. *Iranian Biomedical Journal 18*, 1, 16–22. doi:10.6091/ibj.1274.2013

Sasikumar K, Kozhummal Vaikkath D, Devendra L (2017) An exopolysaccharide (EPS) from a Lactobacillus plantarum BR2 with potential benefits for making functional foods. Bioresource Technology 241, 1152–1156. doi:10.1016/j.biortech.2017.05.075

Savukaitytė A, Ugenskienė R, Jankauskaitė R *et al.* (2015) Investigation of prognostic value of polymorphisms within estrogen metabolizing genes in Lithuanian breast cancer patients. *BMC Medical Genetics 16*, 2. doi:10.1186/s12881-015-0147-4

Schachter D, Abbott RE, Cogan U *et al.* (1983) Lipid fluidity of the individual helileaflets in human erythrocyte membranes. *Annals of the New York Academy of Sciences 414*, 19–28.

Schendzielorz N, Rysa A, Reenila I *et al.* (2011) Complex estrogenic regulation of catechol-O-methyltransferase (COMT) in rats. *Journal of Physiology and Pharmacology 62*, 4, 483–490.

Schnetz-Boutaud NC, Anderson BM, Brown KD *et al.* (2009) Examination of tetrahydrobiopterin pathway genes in autism. *Genes, Brain*, 753–757. doi:10.1111/j.1601-183X.2009.00521.x

Schober AF, Mathis AD, Ingle C *et al.* (2019) A two-enzyme adaptive unit within bacterial folate metabolism. *Cell Reports 27*, 11, 3359–3370. doi:10.1016/j.celrep.2019.05.030

Schuhmacher A, Becker T, Rujescu D *et al.* (2012) Investigation of tryptophan hydroxylase 2 (TPH2) in schizophrenia and in the response to antipsychotics. *Journal of Psychiatric Research 46*, 8, 1073–1080. doi:10.1016/j.jpsychires.2012.04.021

Segers ME, Lebeer S (2014) Towards a better understanding of *Lactobacillus rhamnosus* GG – host interactions. *Microbial Cell Factories 13*, Suppl 1, S7. doi:10.1186/1475-2859-13-S1-S7

Sekine Y, Osei-Hwedieh D, Matsuda K *et al.* (2011) High fat diet reduces the expression of glutathione peroxidase 3 in mouse prostate. *The Prostate 71*, 14, 1499–1509.

Seneff S (2014) Cholesterol, sulfate, and heart disease. Wise Traditions Workshop, London, 9 February 2014. https://people. csail.mit.edu/seneff/London2014/Seneff-HeartDisease2014.pdf

Seneff S, Davidson RM, Liu J (2012) Is cholesterol sulfate deficiency a common factor in preeclampsia, autism, and pernicious anemia? *Entropy 14*, 2265–2290.

Seneff S, Lauritzen A, Davidson R *et al.* (2012) Is endothelial nitric oxide synthase a moonlighting protein whose day job is cholesterol sulfate synthesis? Implications for cholesterol transport, diabetes and cardiovascular disease. *Entropy 14*, 12, 2492–2530.

Shahvali KM, Kazemi Nezhad SR, Rajaei E *et al.* (2015) Association of the MTHFR C677T polymorphism (rs1801133) with risk of rheumatoid arthritis in the Khuzestan Province of Iran. *Gene and Cell Tissue 2*, 4, e28421. doi:10.17795/gct-28421

Sharma M, Li Y, Stoll ML *et al.* (2020) The epigenetic connection between the gut microbiome in obesity and diabetes. *Frontiers in Genetics 10*, 1329. doi:10.3389/fgene.2019.01329

Shrimanker I, Bhattarai S (2021) Electrolytes. *StatPearls*. www.ncbi.nlm.nih.gov/books/NBK541123

Si MW, Yang MK, Fu XD (2015) Effect of hypothalamic-pituitary-adrenal axis alterations on glucose and lipid metabolism in diabetic rats. *Genetics and Molecular Research 14*, 3, 9562–9570. doi:10.4238/2015.August.14.19

Sipilä T, Kananen L, Greco D *et al.* (2010) An association analysis of circadian genes in anxiety disorders. *Biological Psychiatry 67*, 12, 1163–1170.

Slomiany BL, Murty VLN, Piotrowski J *et al.* (1992) Glycosulfatase activity of *H. pylori* toward human gastric mucin: Effect of sucralfate. *American Journal of Gastroenterology 87*, 9, 1132–1137.

Smigielski K, Raj A, Krosowiak K *et al.* (2009) Chemical composition of the essential oil of *Lavandula angustifolia* cultivated in Poland. *Journal of Essential Oil Bearing Plants 12*, 3, 338–347 doi:10.1080/09720 60X.2009.10643729

Smolka MN (2005) Catechol-O-methyltransferase val158met genotype affects processing of emotional stimuli in the amygdala and prefrontal cortex. *Journal of Neuroscience 25*, 4, 836–842. doi:10.1523/jneurosci.1792-04.2005

Soeiro-De-Souza MG, Stanford MS, Bio DS *et al.* (2013) Association of the COMT met158allele with trait impulsivity in healthy young adults. *Molecular Medicine Reports 7*, 4, 1067–1072. doi:10.3892/mmr.2013.1336

Soria V, Martínez-Amorós È, Escaramís G *et al.* (2010) Resequencing and association analysis of arylalkylamine N-acetyltransferase (AANAT) gene and its contribution to major depression susceptibility. *Journal of Pineal Research 49*, 1, 35–44. doi:10.1111/j.1600-079X.2010.00763.x

Soykan, B. Sivri, I. Sarosiek, B *et al.* (1998) Demography, clinical characteristics, psychological and abuse profiles, treatment, and long-term follow-up of patients with gastroparesis. *Digestive Diseases and Sciences 43*, 11, 2398–2404.

Staal WG, Langen M, Van Dijk S *et al.* (2015) DRD3 gene and striatum in autism spectrum disorder. *British Journal of Psychiatry 206*, 5, 431–432. doi:10.1192/bjp.bp.114.148973

Stein TP, Schluter MD, Steer RA *et al.* (2013) Autism and phthalate metabolite glucuronidation. *Journal of Autism and Developmental Disorders 43*, 11, 2677–2685. doi:10.1007/s10803-013-1822-y

Strakova J, Gupta S, Kruger WD *et al.* (2011) Inhibition of betaine-homocysteine S-methyltransferase in rats causes hyperhomocysteinemia and reduces liver cystathionine β-synthase activity and methylation capacity. *Nutrition Research 31*, 7, 563–571. doi:10.1016/j.nutres.2011.06.004

Stremmel W, Merle U, Zahn A *et al.* (2005) Retarded release phosphatidylcholine benefits patients with chronic active ulcerative colitis. *Gut 54*, 7, 966–971.

Stremmel W, Staffer S, Gan-Schreier H *et al.* (2016) Phosphatidylcholine passes through lateral tight junctions for paracellular transport to the apical side of the polarized intestinal tumor cell-line CaCo2. *Biochimica et Biophysica Acta – Molecular and Cell Biology of Lipids 1861*, 9, Part A, 1161–1169. doi:10.1016/j.bbalip.2016.06.019

Strickland FM, Hewagama A, Wu A *et al.* (2013) Diet influences expression of autoimmune-associated genes and disease severity by epigenetic mechanisms in a transgenic mouse model of lupus. *Arthritis and Rheumatism 65*, 7, 1872–1881.

Sudini K, Diette GB, Breysse PN *et al.* (2016) A randomized controlled trial of the effect of broccoli sprouts on antioxidant gene expression and airway inflammation in asthmatics. *Journal of Allergy and Clinical Immunology in Practice 4*, 5, 932–940. doi:10.1016/j.jaip.2016.03.012

Sun A, Ni Y, Li X *et al.* (2014) Urinary methylmalonic acid as an indicator of early vitamin B12 deficiency and its role in polyneuropathy in type 2 diabetes. *Journal of Diabetes Research 2014*, 921616. doi:10.1155/2014/921616

Sureda A, Bibiloni MDM, Julibert A *et al.* (2018) Adherence to the Mediterranean diet and inflammatory markers. *Nutrients 10*, 1, 62. doi:10.3390/nu10010062

Tabrez S, Jabir NR, Shakil S *et al.* (2012) A synopsis on the role of tyrosine hydroxylase in Parkinson's disease. *CNS and Neurological Disorders Drug Targets 11*, 4, 395–409. doi:10.2174/187152712800792785

Tadokoro Y, Horiuchi S, Takahata K *et al.* (2017) Changes in salivary oxytocin after inhalation of clary sage essential oil scent in term-pregnant women: a feasibility pilot study. *BMC Research Notes 10*, 1, 717. doi:10.1186/s13104-017-3053-3

Takakura W, Pimentel M (2020) Small intestinal bacterial overgrowth and irritable bowel syndrome – an update. *Frontiers in Psychiatry 11*, 664. doi:10.3389/fpsyt.2020.00664

Tan W-H, Eichler FS, Hoda S *et al.* (2005) Isolated sulfite oxidase deficiency: A case report with a novel mutation and review of the literature. *Pediatrics 116*, 3, 757–766. doi:10.1542/peds.2004-1897

Tanaka S, Abe M, Kohno G *et al.* (2020) A single episode of hypoglycemia as a possible early warning sign of adrenal insufficiency. *Therapeutics and Clinical Risk Management 16*, 147–153. doi:10.2147/tcrm.s238435

Tardy AL, Pouteau E, Marquez D *et al.* (2020) Vitamins and minerals for energy, fatigue and cognition: A narrative review of the biochemical and clinical evidence. *Nutrients 12*, 1, 228. doi:10.3390/nu12010228

Tiihonen J, Hallikainen T, Lachman H *et al.* (1999) Association between the functional variant of the catechol-O-methyltransferase (COMT) gene and type 1 alcoholism. *Molecular Psychiatry 4*, 3, 286–289. doi:10.1038/sj.mp.4000509

Tobisawa Y, Imai Y, Fukuda M *et al.* (2010) Sulfation of colonic mucins by N-acetylglucosamine 6-O-sulfotransferase-2 and its protective function in experimental colitis in mice. *Journal of Biological Chemistry 285*, 9, 6750–6760. doi:10.1074/jbc.M109.067082

Toma C, Hervas A, Balmana N *et al.* (2012) Neurotransmitter systems and neurotrophic factors in autism: Association study of 37 genes suggests involvement of DDC. *World Journal of Biological Psychiatry 14*, 7, 516–527. doi:10.3109/15622975.2011.602719

Tomita LY (2016) Folate and cancer: Is there any association? *Journal of Inborn Errors of Metabolism and Screening 4*. doi:10.1177%2F2326409816661357

Traverso N, Ricciarelli R, Nitti M *et al.* (2013) Role of glutathione in cancer progression and chemoresistance. *Oxidative Medicine and Cellular Longevity 2013*, 972913. doi:10.1155/2013/972913

Troen AM, Mitchell B, Sorensen B *et al.* (2006) Unmetabolized folic acid in plasma is associated with reduced natural killer cell cytotoxicity among postmenopausal women. *Journal of Nutrition 136*, 1, 189–194. doi:10.1093/jn/136.1.189

Vally H, Misso NL (2012) Adverse reactions to the sulphite additives. *Gastroenterology and Hepatology from Bed to Bench 5*, 1, 16–23.

Van der Veen JN, Kennelly JP, Wan S *et al.* (2017) The critical role of phosphatidylcholine and phosphatidylethanolamine metabolism in health and disease. *Biochimica et Biophysica Acta – Biomembranes 1859*, 9, Part B, 1558–1572. doi:0.1016/j.bbamem.2017.04.006

van Dijk SC, de Herder WW, Kwekkeboom DJ *et al.* (2012) 5-HIAA excretion is not associated with bone metabolism in carcinoid syndrome patients. *Bone 50*, 6, 1260–1265. doi:10.1016/j.bone.2012.02.637

Vance DE (2013) Physiological roles of phosphatidylethanolamine N-methyltransferase. *Biochimica et Biophysica Acta – Molecular and Cell Biology of Lipids 1831*, 3, 626–632. doi:10.1016/j.bbalip.2012.07.017

Vance DE (2014) Phospholipid methylation in mammals: From biochemistry to physiological function. *Biochimica et Biophysica Acta (BBA) – Biomembranes 1838*, 6, 1477–1487, doi:10.1016/j.bbamem.2013.10.018

Venkatachalam KV (2003) Human 3'-phosphoadenosine 5'-phosphosulfate (PAPS) synthase: biochemistry, molecular biology and genetic deficiency. *IUBMB Life 55*, 1–11.

Vergés J, Montell E, Herrero M *et al.* (2005) Clinical and histopathological improvement of psoriasis with oral chondroitin sulfate: A serendipitous finding. *Dermatology Online Journal 11*, 1, 31. doi:10.5070/D32zh8x3vf

Volavka J, Bilder R, Nolan K (2004) Catecholamines and aggression: The role of COMT and MAO polymorphisms. *Annals of the New York Academy of Sciences 1036*, 393–398. doi:10.1196/annals.1330.023

Volkow ND, Wang G-J, Baler RD (2011) Reward, dopamine and the control of food intake: implications for obesity. *Trends in Cognitive Sciences 15*, 1, 37–46. doi:10.1016/j.tics.2010.11.001

Von Seidlein L, Auburn S, Espino F *et al.* (2013) Review of key knowledge gaps in glucose-6-phosphate dehydrogenase deficiency detection with regard to the safe clinical deployment of 8-aminoquinoline treatment regimens: A workshop report. *Malaria Journal 12*, 112. doi:10.1186/1475-2875-12-112

Waløen K, Kleppe R, Martinez A et al. (2017) Tyrosine and tryptophan hydroxylases as therapeutic targets in human disease. *Expert Opinion on Therapeutic Targets 21*, 2, 167–180. doi:10.1080/14728222.2017.1272581

Waly M, Olteanu H, Banerjee R et al. (2004) Activation of methionine synthase by insulin-like growth factor 1 and dopamine: A target for neurodevelopmental toxins and thimerosal. *Molecular Psychiatry 9*, 358–370. doi:10.1038/sj.mp.4001476

Wan L, Li Y, Zhang Z et al. (2018) Methylene-tetrahydrofolate reductase and psychiatric diseases. *Translational Psychiatry 8*, 1, 242. doi:10.1038/s41398-018-0276-6

Wang D, Curtis A, Papp A et al. (2012) Polymorphism in glutamate cysteine ligase catalytic subunit (GCLC) is associated with sulfamethoxazole-induced hypersensitivity in HIV/AIDS patients. *BMC Medical Genomics 5*, 32. doi:10.1186/1755-8794-5-32

Wang HL, Zhou PY, Liu P et al. (2014) ALDH2 and ADH1 genetic polymorphisms may contribute to the risk of gastric cancer: A meta-analysis. *PLOS ONE 9*, 3, e88779. doi:10.1371/journal.pone.0088779

Wang J, Huff AM, Spence JD et al. (2004) Single nucleotide polymorphism in CTH associated with variation in plasma homocysteine concentration. *Clinical Genetics 65*, 6, 483–486.

Wang J, Zhou W, Chen H et al. (2019) Ammonium nitrogen tolerant *Chlorella* strain screening and its damaging effects on photosynthesis. *Frontiers in Microbiology 9*, 3250. doi:10.3389/fmicb.2018.03250

Wang P, Heber D, Henning SM (2012) Quercetin increased bioavailability and decreased methylation of green tea polyphenols in vitro and in vivo. *Food and Function 3*, 6, 635–642.

Wang P, Li S, Wang M et al. (2017) Association of MTRR A66G polymorphism with cancer susceptibility: Evidence from 85 studies. *Journal of Cancer 8*, 2, 266–277. doi:10.7150/jca.17379

Wang Q, Yan ZQ, Wang HB et al. (2011) Analysis for myeloperoxidase genetic polymorphism in gastric cancer. *Zhonghua Wei Chang Wai Ke Za Zhi 14*, 7, 542–544.

Waring R (n.d.) Sulfate and Sulfation. www.epsomsaltcouncil.org/wp-content/uploads/2015/10/sulfation_benefits.pdf

Waring R, Klovrza LV (2000) Sulfur metabolism in autism. *Journal of Nutritional and Environmental Medicine 10*, 1, 25–32. doi:10.1080/13590840050000861

Waring RH (2010) Report on absorption of magnesium sulfate (Epsom salts) across the skin. www.epsomsaltcouncil.org/wp-content/uploads/2015/10/report_on_absorption_of_magnesium_sulfate.pdf

Wassenberg T, Deinum J, van Ittersum FJ et al. (2021) Clinical presentation and long-term follow-up of dopamine beta hydroxylase deficiency. *Journal of Inherited Metabolic Disease 44*, 3, 554–565. doi:10.1002/jimd.12321

Wei F, Jianhua S, Xiaimin L (2007) Dopamine D1 receptor agonist and D2 Receptor antagonist effects of the natural product (–)– stepholidine: Molecular modeling and dynamics simulations. *Biophysical Journal 93*, 1431–1441.

Weng YL, An R, Shin J et al. (2013) DNA modifications and neurological disorders. *Neurotherapeutics 10*, 4, 556–567. doi:10.1007/s13311-013-0223-4

Wieringa FT, Dijkhuizen MA, Fiorentino M et al. (2015) Determination of zinc status in humans: which indicator should we use? *Nutrients 7*, 5, 3252–3263. doi: 10.3390/nu7053252

Williams RO (2013) Exploitation of the IDO pathway in the therapy of rheumatoid arthritis. *International Journal of Tryptophan Research 6*, Suppl 1, 67–73. doi:10.4137%2FIJTR.S11737

Wilson Tang WH, Wang Z, Levison BS et al. (2013) Intestinal microbial metabolism of phosphatidylcholine and cardiovascular risk. *New England Journal of Medicine 368*, 17, 1575. doi:10.1056/NEJMoa1109400

Wong DL (2003) Why is the adrenal adrenergic? *Endocrine Pathology 14*, 1, 25–36.

Wong PT, Choi SK (2015) Mechanisms and implications of dual-acting methotrexate in folate-targeted nanotherapeutic delivery. *International Journal of Molecular Sciences 16*, 1, 1772–1790. doi:10.3390/ijms16011772

Woodhouse S, Hebbard G, Knowles SR (2017) Psychological controversies in gastroparesis: A systematic review. *World Journal of Gastroenterology 23*, 7, 1298–1309. doi:10.3748/wjg.v23.i7.1298

Woods JS, Heyer NJ, Russo JE *et al.* (2014) Genetic polymorphisms of catechol-O-methyltransferase modify the neurobehavioral effects of mercury in children. *Journal of Toxicology and Environmental Health Part A 77*, 6, 293–312.

Woodson K, Tangrea JA, Lehman TA *et al.* (2003) Manganese superoxide dismutase (MnSOD) polymorphism, α-tocopherol supplementation and prostate cancer risk in the Alpha-Tocopherol, Beta-Carotene Cancer Prevention Study (Finland). *Cancer Causes and Control 14*, 6, 513–518.

Wu G, Fang YZ, Yang S *et al.* (2004) Glutathione metabolism and its implications for health. *The Journal of Nutrition 134*, 3, 489–492, doi:10.1093/jn/134.3.489

Wu JY, Tang XW, Schloss JV *et al.* (1998) Regulation of taurine biosynthesis and its physiological significance in the brain. *Advances in Experimental Medicine and Biology 442*, 339–345. doi:10.1007/978-1-4899-0117-0_42

Xie Y, Zhou B, Lin MY *et al.* (2015) Endolysosomal deficits augment mitochondria pathology in spinal motor neurons of asymptomatic fALS mice. *Neuron 87*, 2, 355–370. doi:10.1016/j.neuron.2015.06.026

Yalcin EB, More V, Neira KL *et al.* (2013) Down-regulation of sulfotransferase expression and activity in diseased human livers. *Drug Metabolism and Disposition: The Biological Fate of Chemicals 41*, 9, 1642–1650. doi:10.1124/dmd.113.050930

Yang JP, Wang WB, Yang XX *et al.* (2013) The MPO-463G>A polymorphism and lung cancer risk: A meta-analysis based on 22 case-control studies. *PLOS ONE 8*, 6, e65778. doi:10.1371%2Fjournal.pone.0065778

Yang S, Li X, Yang F *et al.* (2019) Gut microbiota-dependent marker TMAO in Promoting cardiovascular disease: Inflammation mechanism, clinical prognostic, and potential as a therapeutic target. *Frontiers in Pharmacology 10*, 1360. doi:10.3389/fphar.2019.01360

Yao J, Pan YQ, Ding M *et al.* (2015) Association between DRD2 (rs1799732 and rs1801028) and ANKK1 (rs1800497) polymorphisms and schizophrenia: A meta-analysis. *American Journal of Medical Genetics Part B 168B*, 1, 1–13.

Yehuda Sl, Rabinovits S, Mostofsky DI (2005) Essential fatty acids and the brain: From infancy to aging. *Neurobiology of Aging 26*, Suppl 1, 98–102. doi:10.1016/j.neurobiolaging.2005.09.013

Yokoyama A, Yokoyama T, Matsui T *et al.* (2015) Alcohol dehydrogenase-1B (rs1229984) and aldehyde dehydrogenase-2 (rs671) genotypes are strong determinants of the serum triglyceride and cholesterol levels of Japanese alcoholic men. *PLOS ONE 8*, 6, e65778. doi:10.1371/journal.pone.0065778

Yoshida E, Toyama T, Shinkai Y *et al.* (2011) Detoxification of methylmercury by hydrogen sulfide-producing enzyme in mammalian cells. *Chemical Research in Toxicology 24*, 10, 1633–1635. doi:10.1021/tx200394g

Yoshimasu K, Mure K, Hashimoto M *et al.* (2015) Genetic alcohol sensitivity regulated by ALDH2 and ADH1B polymorphisms is strongly associated with depression and anxiety in Japanese employees. *Drug and Alcohol Dependence 147*, 130–136. doi:10.1016/j.drugalcdep.2014.11.034

Young SN (2007) How to increase serotonin in the human brain without drugs. *Journal of Psychiatry and Neuroscience 32*, 6, 394–399.

Yudkoff M (2012) Chapter 42 – Disorders of Amino Acid Metabolism. In ST Brady, GJ Siegel, RW Albers, DL Price (eds) *Basic Neurochemistry*, 8th edition. New York, NY: Academic Press. doi:10.1016/B978-0-12-374947-5.00042-0

Zalba S, Ten Hagen TL (2016). Cell membrane modulation as adjuvant in cancer therapy. *Cancer Treatment Reviews 52*, 48–57. doi:10.1016/j.ctrv.2016.10.008

Zeng MY, Inohara N, Nuñez G (2017) Mechanisms of inflammation-driven bacterial dysbiosis in the gut. *Mucosal Immunology 10*, 1, 18–26. doi:10.1038/mi.2016.75

Zeng X, Cai D, Zeng Q *et al.* (2017) Selective reduction in the expression of UGTs and SULTs, a novel mechanism by which piperine enhances the bioavailability of curcumin in rat. *Biopharmaceutics and Drug Disposition 38*, 3–19. doi:10.1002/bdd.2049.

Zhang C, Li Z, Shao Y et al. (2011) Association study of tryptophan hydroxylase-2 gene in schizophrenia and its clinical features in Chinese Han population. *Journal of Molecular Neuroscience 43*, 406–411. doi:10.1007/s12031-010-9458-2

Zhang S, Zhang M, Zhang J (2014) Association of COMT and COMT-DRD2 interaction with creative potential. *Frontiers in Human Neuroscience*. doi:10.3389/fnhum.2014.00216

Zhang X, Ye YL, Wang YN et al. (2015) Aldehyde dehydrogenase 2 genetic variations may increase susceptibility to Parkinson's disease in Han Chinese population. *Neurobiology of Aging 36*, 9, 2660.e9–13. doi:10.1016/j.neurobiolaging.2015.06.001

Zhang Y, Mei J, Li J et al. (2021) DNA methylation in atherosclerosis: A new perspective. *Evidence-Based Complementary and Alternative Medicine 2021*, 6623657. doi:10.1155/2021/6623657

Zhao H, Xu X, Na J et al. (2008) Protective effects of salicylic acid and vitamin C on sulfur dioxide-induced lipid peroxidation in mice. *Inhalation Toxicology 20*, 9, 865–871. doi:10.1080/08958370701861512

Zhong J, Agha G, Baccarelli AA (2016) The role of DNA methylation in cardiovascular risk and disease: Methodological aspects, study design, and data analysis for epidemiological studies. *Circulation Research 118*, 1, 119–131. doi:10.1161/CIRCRESAHA.115.305206

Zhu BT, Liehr JG (1996) Inhibition of catechol O-methyltransferase-catalyzed O-methylation of 2- and 4-hydroxyestradiol by quercetin. Possible role in estradiol-induced tumorigenesis. *Journal of Biological Chemistry 271*, 3, 1357–1363. doi:10.1074/jbc.271.3.1357

Zhubi A, Chen Y, Guidotti A et al. (2017) Epigenetic regulation of RELN and GAD1 in the frontal cortex (FC) of autism spectrum disorder (ASD) subjects. *International Journal of Developmental Neuroscience 62*, 63–72. doi:10.1016/j.ijdevneu.2017.02.003

Zotti M, Colaianna M, Morgese MG et al. (2013) Carvacrol: From ancient flavoring to neuromodulatory agent. *Molecules 18*, 6, 6161–6172. doi:10.3390/molecules18066161

Zubieta JK, Heitzeg MM, Smith YR et al. (2003) COMT val158genotype affects μ-opioid neurotransmitter responses to a pain stressor. *Science 299*, 5610, 1240–1243.

6

Genes Associated with Nutrient Metabolism

A number of genes have been associated with overall health and fitness and a number of genetic testing companies have seen the potential for improving fitness, weight management and basic food metabolism. From these particular genes, associations are made on body shape, muscle function, stress and burnout, cortisol and sleep. In this chapter, the relevant genes will be discussed:

FTO, MC4R, PPARG, APOA2, TNFα, ADBR2, ACTN3, COMT V158M, GSTT1, GSTM1, ADBR2, TCF7L2, MTHFR C677T.

Fat mass and obesity-associated protein: FTO

It has to be said that a lot of the early research on the FTO gene has been undertaken on mouse and rat models that have highlighted high levels of FTO expression in the hypothalamus. This is now showing consistency with human studies (Fawcett & Borosso 2010). Hypothalamic FTO expression appears to be down-regulated under fasting conditions and up-regulated during feeding. However, the exact mechanism remains elusive, according to Speakman (2015).

The FTO gene has gained a lot of attention in the media and in the NHS domain as the gene purported to make humans fat. Carriers of the variant rs9939609 AA allele are said to be less satiated but do not expend the energy gained from overeating. Western medicine markets this gene exceptionally well, suggesting those with the AA rs1421085 variant may be more vulnerable to becoming obese as they age. The gene has been studied to find associations with changes in body mass index (BMI) and personality traits such as impulsivity. Original studies on FTO date back to 1958.

Chuang *et al.* (2014) performed a longitudinal study on the effects of this gene on obesity, analyzing those with one, two or no FTO variants for age, BMI, brain activity, diet and personality traits.

Findings included the following:

- 20% of participants had two copies of the FTO gene variants
- 48% carried one copy.

Carriers were more likely to have:

- higher BMI with age
- reduced brain activity in the area involved in impulse control with age.

All participants reported eating less fat and more carbohydrates over time; however, those with the FTO variant still ate more fat.

Possible dietary interventions for FTO mutations

- Higher protein, lower carbohydrate (de Luis *et al.* 2015).
- Mediterranean diet for the rs9939609 risk allele (Wood *et al.* 2016; Yang *et al.* 2012).
- High fat, low carbohydrate for variants rs1558902 and rs9939609 (Zheng *et al.* 2015).

It is worth noting that many studies have shown inconclusive evidence for one consistent nutritional approach. This is due to small-scale studies, short duration of intervention, measurement of different outcomes and the focus on single variant genes on outcomes (Tan *et al.* 2019).

Melanocortin 4 receptor: MC4R

The MC4R gene encodes the melanocortin 4 receptor enzyme. Defects in this gene have been associated with autosomal dominant obesity. It has been identified as playing a role in appetite, metabolic regulation and satiation, involving the hormone leptin. This hormone allows us to feel full for longer. However, if this gene is expressing, this may lead to increased snacking or indeed overeating and therefore obesity and hyperinsulinemia. Again, this gene is expressed in the hypothalamus. Those with BMI above 30 tend to be more likely to have issues with this gene.

Leptin is produced in adipose tissue and is an indicator of nutritional status. Leptin levels fall in response to fasting, triggering the expression of agouti-related peptide (AgRP) to increase food intake. Concurrently, leptin inhibits POMC neurons, reducing melanocyte-stimulating hormone. Second-order neurons intercept this reaction, encouraging expression of the MC4R gene and thereby increasing food intake. Homozygous presentations of MC4R genes have been ubiquitously associated with inherited obesity in various ethnic groups (Stutzman *et al.* 2008; Farooqi *et al.* 2003; Farooqi *et al.* 2000).

Individuals with MC4R deficiency have a tendency towards obesity from early childhood, meditated by early hyperinsulinemia. Adults with MC4R deficiency have been shown to experience impaired sympathetic nervous system activation, resulting in low blood pressure and lower measure of sympathovagal tone (Greenfield *et al.* 2009).

Bariatric surgery may be the only viable option for many with MC4R deficiency, as they tend to be very poorly responsive to diet and exercise. However, Hatoum *et al.* (2012) purport that bariatric surgery is only effective in those with heterozygous presentation. MC4R antagonists are currently being trialled (Collet *et al.* 2017).

Inducers and inhibitors are unavailable due to lack of evidence.

Peroxisome proliferator-activated receptors: PPARG

This gene encodes for a member of the peroxisome proliferator-activated receptor. It is expressed in adipose tissue. PPARG is a very important gene in famine as it has helped humans survive due to its role in shunting fat from the blood into cells and using glucose for energy. In today's world of overabundance of dietary sugar and refined carbohydrates, however, this gene can be a significant downfall. Individuals who have this gene are encouraged to eliminate all foods that contain a combination of fats and refined carbohydrate. The doughnut is a prime example. PPARG has been associated with a number of aberrant metabolic processes, namely insulin resistance (Hu *et al.* 2006), obesity and colorectal cancer (Motawi *et al.* 2017) and dyslipidemia (Nohara *et al.* 2007); this is also a gene that has been associated with biliary tract cancer. These are cancers of the gallbladder, extrahepatic ducts and the ampulla of Vater. While these cancers are relatively rare, they do carry a high risk of fatality (Chang *et al.* 2008). As obesity in women has been strongly associated with cholestasis and other biliary insufficiencies, it would be pertinent to consider supporting the biliary system when considering the PPARG gene in relation to weight loss and body composition. The importance of the use of foods and nutrients that may support bile flow, such as apple (malic acid and pectin), lemon juice (limonene) and beetroot, cannot be overstated. Assessment of biliary status should be of primary concern before embarking on programmes to significantly or quickly reduce weight in susceptible individuals.

PPARG is abundant in adipose tissue, playing a significant role in adipogenesis cell differentiation and inflammatory response (Feige *et al.* 2006). These qualities allow PPARG to exert antineoplastic effects (Wang *et al.* 2006; Panigrahy *et al.* 2002), with obesity being reported as a potential inducer of gene expression (Diradourian *et al.* 2005).

Cofactors that support PPARG enzyme activity
Weight loss, blood glucose management and biliary flow (Gardner *et al.* 2018).

Practical advice
Follow a low-carbohydrate diet while supporting biliary flow with apples, lemon and beets (Contreras *et al.* 2013). Include healthy fats (AlSaleh *et al.* 2011).

Apolipoprotein A2: APOA2

APOA2 encodes for the enzyme apolipoprotein A2. Fatty acid and glucose metabolism is this gene's claim to fame. APOA2 is a signalling molecule that supports healthy HDL cholesterol in its journey back to the liver. If this gene is down-regulated, then HDL transport back to the liver may be compromised, giving rise to inflammation when fats are eaten in excess or unhealthy fats are consumed (Lai *et al.* 2018).

Possible interventions based on APOA2 genetic expression
Promoters to support APOA2 enzyme activity
Healthy fats from nuts, seeds, oily fish and olives, along with their raw oils taken uncooked (Zamani *et al.* 2017).

Unhelpful inhibitors that reduce APOA2 enzyme activity
Trans fats such as hydrogenated oils used to make margarine, also found in meat and dairy; and high oleic vegetable oils from the diet are very important (Basiri *et al.* 2015).

Practical advice

- Follow a high-fat, low-carbohydrate diet or neurolipid keto diet (Kane 2017).
- Low saturated fats are associated with weight loss, whereas diets in high saturated fats with ADBR2 are associated with adiposity and high BMI (Corella *et al.* 2009).

Tumour necrosis factor alpha: TNFα

The TNFα gene encodes for the tumour necrosis factor alpha enzyme. This is a multifunctional pro-inflammatory enzyme associated with inflammation. This cytokine is mainly secreted by macrophages. It can bind to and function through its receptors and is involved in the regulation of a wide spectrum of biological processes. Medications such as monoclonal antibodies target TNFα in order to reduce or even dispel inflammation. This has made treatment for severe rheumatoid arthritis possible (Monaco *et al.* 2014). TNFα expression can create inflamed arteries that subsequently predisposes to atheroma and poor circulatory health. However, knockout mice studies have suggested some neuroprotective elements (Figiel 2008). This gene has also been included in the section on inflammation in Chapter 7 for completion.

Possible interventions based on TNF genetic expression
Promoters to support TNF enzyme activity
Exercise (Smart *et al.* 2011).

Unhelpful inducers that increase TNF enzyme activity
Sugar and stress increase CD33, a membrane receptor containing lectin. CD33 expression triggers the release of TNFα (Gonzalez *et al.* 2012).

Practical advice
Follow a low-carbohydrate or autoimmune paleo diet (Konijeti *et al.* 2017).

Adreno beta 2: ADBR2

This gene codes for the beta 2 adrenergic receptor, which binds adrenaline. Two alleles are important, Arg16Gly and Gin27Glu, as both of these have been identified as being influential in VO2max trainability, or the amount of oxygen a person can take up during intense exercise, and carbohydrate sensitivity. Due to the effects this gene may have on adrenaline, effects on the heart and lungs can be quite profound.

Increased heart rate and blood pressure, transportation of nutrients and oxygen around the body and increased bronchus/bronchiole sizing to effect the oxygen increase are noted, alongside the ability to break down fat for fuel, which makes this an interesting gene for the fitness industry. If this gene is down-regulated, hunger appears to be the key symptom. When this is up-regulated, the individual can exercise more efficiently for longer. Smoking and high sugar intake can cause this gene to express negatively.

Possible interventions based on ADBR2 genetic expression
Promoters to support ADBR2 enzyme activity
Low-carbohydrate diet, blood glucose regulation supplements (Gardner *et al.* 2018).

Unhelpful inhibitors that reduce ADBR2 enzyme activity
Cigarette smoke, excess sugar intake and excess stress (Nielsen *et al.* 2018).

Practical advice

- Follow a low-carbohydrate diet; remove all extrinsic sugars (Gardner *et al.* 2018).
- Advise and refer to smoking cessation clinic (Nielsen *et al.* 2018).
- Ensure a PUFA-rich diet (Mitra *et al.* 2019).

α-actinin-3: ACTN3

This gene encodes for α-actinin-3, an actin-binding protein that has a pivotal role in muscle metabolism (Ben-Zaken *et al.* 2015). Genetic testing companies appear to be saying that expression of this gene allows advice on whether slow endurance or fast explosive exercise is best for the individual as it appears to determine the rate of muscle twitching. However, Ben-Zaken *et al.* would argue that this is not the case and that physique, tactics and mindset are more likely to influence the type of exercise. The ACTN3-deficient person is the one who functions better as an endurance athlete rather than for speed (Yang *et al.* 2003).

ACTN3 deficiency has been associated with muscle wasting and loss of muscle strength in the elderly (Delmonico *et al.* 2008). The R allele appears to be protective for sarcopenia (Cho *et al.* 2017). However, from a dietary perspective a high fat diet does not appear to contribute to alterations in BMI or obesity (Houweling *et al.* 2017).

Inducers and inhibitors have been omitted for ACTN3 due to lack of evidence.

Transcription factor 7-like-2: TCF7L2

This gene encodes a high mobility box-containing transcription factor gene implicated in blood glucose homeostasis. It has been suggested that TCF7L2 regulates proglucagon (Shao *et al.* 2013). The allele rs7903146 has been identified as the most significant in its association with non-insulin-dependent diabetes mellitus (NIDDM) (Vaquero *et al.* 2012). Zhou *et al.* (2014) reviewed 29 genes in their study and found TCF7L2 to be a key regulator of pro-insulin and its subsequent conversion of mature insulin. The two pro-hormones responsible for this conversion were also regulated by TCF7L2.

TCF7L2 has been implicated in other conditions that in part are associated with blood glucose dysregulation. Schizophrenia was identified in the Chinese Han population rs12573128 (Liu *et al.* 2017). Three alleles were found to be associated with gestational diabetes – rs7903146, rs12255372 and rs7901695 (Chang *et al.* 2017).

Possible interventions based on TCF7L2 genetic expression
Promoters to support TCF7L2 enzyme activity
Zinc (Boroujeni *et al.* 2018).

Unhelpful inhibitors that reduce TCF7L2 enzyme activity
Refined carbohydrates. (Vaquero *et al.* 2012).

Practical advice
Enjoy a low-carbohydrate, Mediterranean-style diet that is lower in fat
(Mattei *et al.* 2012) as a higher-fat diet with this gene expression leads to
increased adipose tissue storage as a result.

Solute carrier 2 family 4: SLC2A4/GLUT4

Practitioners may see this gene under either of these two names. The
gene encodes an integral membrane protein that functions as a glucose
transporter, regulated by insulin. In the presence of insulin, the protein
moves to the cell surface to transport glucose into the cell. Mutations
have been associated with NIDDM. Expression of GLUT4 has also been
identified in bone and cancer tissues, where insulin-like growth factor
regulates it. (Schwartzenberg-Bar-Yoseph *et al.* 2004). Expression has
been under extensive investigation and found to be very tightly regulated at mRNA and protein levels (Armoni *et al.* 2007) with a strong
interplay between GLUT4, PPARgamma and FOXO1. Tissue-specific
GLUT4 expression is amplified in altered metabolic states. Experiments
using mouse models have indicated that modifying the expression of
GLUT4 affects glucose and lipid metabolism in a profound way, affecting whole-body insulin action and utilization. In the Armoni studies,
GLUT4 protein levels were 30% lower in those with hyperlipidaemia
and/or non-insulin dependent diabetes compared to controls.

Practical advice
Responds well to a high-fat, low-carbohydrate diet that will maximize
insulin resistance (Atkinson *et al.* 2013).

Fatty acid desaturase 2: FADS2

FADS2 encodes for the enzyme fatty acid desaturase 2. The enzyme
regulates the unsaturation of fatty acids by introducing double bonds
between defined carbons of the fatty acyl chain. It is therefore related
to dyslipidemia and therefore levels of triglycerides. The rs174570 allele

research suggests normal levels of triglycerides with a TT (–/–) presentation and increased levels with CT (+/–) and CC (+/+) presentations.

Tian *et al.* (2016) found an association between decreased expression of FADS2 and incidence of polycystic ovarian syndrome (PCOS), using data from their previous GWAS studies of 1918 PCOS cases with 1989 age-matched controls. PCOS subjects carrying the CC genotype had higher testosterone and similar lipid/glucose levels than those carrying CT or TT genotypes. This may also infer a higher risk of cardiovascular incident and the need for lipid management practices. As PCOS is also associated with non-insulin dependent diabetes and obesity, this gene may be worth considering within the framework of weight management.

Practical advice
Encourage a diet high in omega 3 fatty acids in the form of alpha linolenic acid and EPA/DHA from oils fish (Sanders 2016).

COMT V158M, MTHFR C677T, GSTT1, GSTM1

These genes have all been discussed in full in the section on methylation in Chapter 5. Suffice to say here that all these genes are implicated as part of detoxification of intrinsic and extrinsic metabolic substances from steroid hormones to xenobiotics, to medications. A sluggish liver may not effectively metabolize these substances. Cortisol and oestrogen not being metabolized by the body contribute to weight gain and cellulite deposition. Addressing dysfunction via methylation as appropriate may support weight loss in some clients.

ELLA'S GENETIC DETERMINANTS

Ella had the CC allele or homozygous presentation for PPARgamma, which suggests she is compromised in her ability to absorb fats into her cells. Excessive fat or sugar intake may predispose Ella to arterial inflammation, obesity and a higher risk of non-insulin dependent diabetes. Recall her father has dementia, so there was some concern about Ella's possible risk. However, her nutritional intake was clean and balanced more towards 80% plant or Mediterranean-style eating, as this is what her digestive system found the easiest approach and ultimately how she maintained a steady weight. TNFα and GLUT2 genes were homozygous, indicating a potential for increased sensitivity to refined carbohydrates, greater levels of fatigue and slower recovery. Endurance exercise was recommended, which Ella would not have been able to undertake given her exercise ability. However, her exercise routines increased and her aim was to succeed in undertaking the 'Couch to 5K' initiatives. (www. nhs.uk/live-well/exercise/couch-to-5k-week-by-week).

APOA2 was heterozygous for Ella, and as this is a signalling molecule that assists healthy HDL cholesterol back to the liver. Ella's HDL was slightly low, so the suggestion to only eat healthy unprocessed fats from nuts, seeds and fish, while avoiding transfats and vegetable oils, would be good advice.

Due to homozygous presentation of GSTM1 and GSTT1 genes and COMT (all discussed in the section on methylation in Chapter 5), a high-sulphur diet was recommended. This would be a direct contradiction of her transsulphuration difficulties as laid out above. However, this was possible at a later date. The importance of a thorough case history is paramount here, as is the limitation of choosing a small number of genes from any given pathway. This is because when the focus is too narrow the resulting programme may be ineffective due to inability to see the impact on all relevant pathways.

References

AlSaleh A, O'Dell SD, Frost GS et al. (2011) Interaction of PPARG Pro12Ala with dietary fat influences plasma lipids in subjects at cardiometabolic risk. *Journal of Lipid Research 52*, 12, 2298–2303. doi:10.1194/jlr. P019281

Armoni M, Harel C, Karnieli E (2007) Transcriptional regulation of the GLUT4 gene: From PPAR-gamma and FOXO1 to FFA and inflammation. *Trends in Endocrinology and Metabolism 18*, 100–107.

Atkinson BJ, Griesel BA, King CD et al. (2013) Moderate GLUT4 overexpression improves insulin sensitivity and fasting triglyceridemia in high-fat diet-fed transgenic mice. *Diabetes 62*, 7, 2249–2258. doi:10.2337/db12-1146

Basiri MG, Sotoudeh G, Alvandi E et al. (2015) APOA2 −256T>C polymorphism interacts with saturated fatty acids intake to affect anthropometric and hormonal variables in type 2 diabetic patients. *Genes and Nutrition 10*, 3, 464. doi:10.1007/s12263-015-0464-4

Ben-Zaken S, Eliakim A, Nemet D et al. (2015) ACTN3 polymorphism: Comparison between elite swimmers and runners. *Sports Medicine – Open 1*, 1, 13. doi:10.1186/s40798-015-0023-y

Boroujeni MB, Fazilati M, Salavati H et al. (2018) Investigation of blood selenium and zinc in type 2 diabetes with TCF7L2 (rs7903146 C/T) genotypes. *Journal of Biology and Today's World 7*, 8–15.

Chang S, Wang Z, Wu L et al. (2017) Association between TCF7L2 polymorphisms and gestational diabetes mellitus: A meta-analysis. *Journal of Diabetes Investigation 8*, 4, 560–570. doi:10.1111/jdi.12612

Chang SC, Rashid A, Gao Y et al. (2008) Polymorphism of genes related to insulin sensitivity and the risk of biliary tract cancer and biliary stone: A population-based case-control study in Shanghai, China. *Carcinogenesis 29*, 5, 944–948, doi:10.1093/carcin/bgn025

Cho J, Lee I, Kang H (2017) ACTN3 gene and susceptibility to sarcopenia and osteoporotic status in older Korean adults. *Biomed Research International*, 4239648. doi:10.1155/2017/4239648

Chuang YF, Tanaka T, Beason-Held LL et al. (2014) FTO genotype and aging: Pleiotropic longitudinal effects on adiposity, brain function, impulsivity and diet. *Molecular Psychiatry 20*, 1, 133–139. doi:10.1038%2Fmp.2014.49

Collet T-H, Dubern B, Mokrosinski J et al. (2017) Evaluation of a melanocortin-4 receptor (MC4R) agonist (Setmelanotide) in MC4R deficiency. *Molecular Metabolism 6*, 10, 1321–1329. doi:10.1016/j.molmet.2017.06.015

Contreras AV, Torres N, Tovar AR (2013) PPAR-α as a key nutritional and environmental sensor for metabolic adaptation. *Advances in Nutrition 4*, 4, 439–452. doi:10.3945/an.113.003798

Corella D, Peloso G, Arnett DK et al. (2009) APOA2, dietary fat, and body mass index: Replication of a gene-diet interaction in 3 independent populations. *Archives of Internal Medicine 169*, 20, 1897–1906. doi:10.1001/archinternmed.2009.343

de Luis DA, Aller R, Izaola O et al. (2015) Effects of a high-protein/low-carbohydrate diet versus a standard hypocaloric diet on weight and cardiovascular risk factors: Role of a genetic variation in the rs9939609 FTO gene variant. *Journal of Nutrigenetics and Nutrigenomics 8*, 128–136.

Delmonico MJ, Zmuda JM, Taylor BC et al. (2008) Association of the ACTN3 genotype and physical functioning with age in older adults. *Journals of Gerontology Series A: Biological Sciences and Medical Sciences 63*, 11, 1227–1234.

Diradourian C, Girard J, Pégorier JP (2005) Phosphorylation of PPARs: From molecular characterization to physiological relevance. *Biochimie 87*, 33–38.

Farooqi IS, Keogh J, Yeo G et al. (2003) Clinical spectrum of obesity and mutations in the melanocortin 4 receptor gene. *New England Journal of Medicine 348*, 12, 1085–1095.

Farooqi IS, Yeo G, Keogh JM et al. (2000) Dominant and recessive inheritance of morbid obesity associated with melanocortin 4 receptor deficiency. *Journal of Clinical Investigation 106*, 271–279.

Fawcett, KA & Barroso, I (2010). The genetics of obesity: FTO leads the way. *Trends in genetics: TIG 26*, 6, 266–274. doi:10.1016/j.tig.2010.02.006

Feige J, Gelman L, Michalik L et al. (2006) From molecular action to physiological outputs: Peroxisome proliferator-activated receptors are nuclear receptors at the crossroads of key cellular functions. *Progress in Lipid Research 45*, 120–159.

Figiel I (2008) Pro-inflammatory cytokine TNFα as a neuroprotective agent in the brain. *Acta Neurobiologiae Experimentalis 68*, 4, 526–534.

Gardner CD, Trepanowski JF, Del Gobbo LC et al. (2018) Effect of low-fat vs low-carbohydrate diet on 12-month weight loss in overweight adults and the association with genotype pattern or insulin secretion: The DIETFITS randomized clinical trial. *JAMA. 319*, 7, 667–679. doi:10.1001/jama.2018.0245

Gonzalez Y, Herrera MT, Soldevila G et al. (2012) High glucose concentrations induce TNF-α production through the down-regulation of CD33 in primary human monocytes. BMC Immunology 13, 19. doi:10.1186/1471-2172-13-19

Greenfield JR, Miller JW, Keogh JM et al. (2009) Modulation of blood pressure by central melanocortinergic pathways. New England Journal of Medicine 360, 1, 44–52.

Hatoum I, Stylopoulos N, Vanhoose A et al. (2012) Melanocortin-4 receptor signaling is required for weight loss after gastric bypass surgery. Journal of Clinical Endocrinology and Metabolism 97, 6, E1023–1031.

Houweling PJ, Berman YD, Turner N et al. (2017) Exploring the relationship between α-actinin-3 deficiency and obesity in mice and humans. International Journal of Obesity 41, 7, 1154–1157. doi:10.1038/ ijo.2017.72

Hu C, Jia W, Fang Q et al. (2006) Peroxisome proliferator-activated receptor (PPAR) delta genetic polymorphism and its association with insulin resistance index and fasting plasma glucose concentrations in Chinese subjects. Diabetic Medicine 23, 12, 1307–1312.

Kane E (2017) Life on a membrane. Paper presented during the Membrane Medicine Seminar on 18 November.

Konijeti GG, Kim N, Lewis JD et al. (2017) Efficacy of the autoimmune protocol diet for inflammatory bowel disease. Inflammatory Bowel Diseases 23, 11, 2054–2060. doi:10.1097/MIB.0000000000001221

Lai CQ, Smith CE, Parnell LD (2018) Epigenomics and metabolomics reveal the mechanism of the APOA2-saturated fat intake interaction affecting obesity. American Journal of Clinical Nutrition 108, 1, 188–200. doi:10.1093/ajcn/nqy081

Liu L, Li J, Yan M et al. (2017) TCF7L2 polymorphisms and the risk of schizophrenia in the Chinese Han population. Oncotarget 8, 17, 28614–28620.

Mattei J, Qi Q, Hu FB et al. (2012) TCF7L2 genetic variants modulate the effect of dietary fat intake on changes in body composition during a weight-loss intervention. American Journal of Clinical Nutrition 96, 5, 1129–1136. doi:10.3945/ajcn.112.038125

Mitra SR, Tan PY, Amini F (2019) Association of ADRB2 rs1042713 with obesity and obesity-related phenotypes and its interaction with dietary fat in modulating glycaemic indices in Malaysian adults. Journal of Nutrition and Metabolism 2019, 8718795. doi:10.1155/2019/8718795

Monaco C, Nanchahal J, Taylor P et al. (2014) Anti-TNF therapy: Past, present and future. International Immunology 27, 1, 55–62.

Motawi TK, Shaker OG, Ismail MF et al. (2017) peroxisome proliferator-activated receptor gamma in obesity and colorectal cancer: The role of epigenetics. Scientific Reports 7, 1, 10714. doi:10.1038/s41598-017-11180-6

Nielsen AO, Poulsen SS, Dahl M (2018) Role of β2-adrenergic receptor in cigarette smoke-induced COPD in mice. European Respiratory Journal 52, suppl 62, PA939. doi:10.1183/13993003.congress-2018.PA939

Nohara A, Kawashiri MA, Claudel T et al. (2007) High frequency of a retinoid X receptor γ gene variant in familial combined hyperlipidemia that associates with atherogenic dyslipidemia. Arteriosclerosis, Thrombosis, and Vascular Biology 27, 4, 923–928.

Panigrahy D, Singer S, Shen LQ et al. (2002) PPARγ ligands inhibit primary tumor growth and metastasis by inhibiting angiogenesis. Journal of Clinical Investigation 110, 923–932.

Sanders K (2016) Do genetics affect how the body uses fatty acids? Natural Medicine Journal 8, 9. www.naturalmedicinejournal.com/journal/2016-09/ genetics-and-effects-fatty-acids

Schwartzenberg-Bar-Yoseph F, Armoni M, Karnieli E (2004) The tumor suppressor p53 down-regulates glucose transporters GLUT1 and GLUT4 gene expression. Cancer Research 64, 2627–2633,

Shao W, Wang D, Chiang Y-T et al. (2013) The Wnt signaling pathway effector TCF7L2 controls gut and brain proglucagon gene expression and glucose homeostasis. Diabetes 62, 3, 789–800. doi:10.2337/ db12-0365

Smart NA, Larsen AI, Le Maitre JP et al. (2011) Effect of exercise training on interleukin-6, tumour necrosis factor alpha and functional capacity in heart failure. Cardiology Research and Practice 2011, 532620. doi:10.4061/2011/532620

Speakman JR (2015) The 'fat mass and obesity related' (FTO) gene: Mechanisms of impact on obesity and energy balance. *Current Obesity Reports 4*, 1, 73–91. doi:10.1007/s13679-015-0143-1.

Stutzmann F, Tan K, Vatin V *et al.* (2008) Prevalence of MC4R deficiency in Europeans and their age-dependant penetrance in multi-generational pedigrees. *Diabetes 2008*, 57, 2511-2518.

Tan PY, Mitra SR, Amini F (2019) Lifestyle Interventions for weight control modified by genetic variation: A review of the evidence. *Public Health Genomics 21*, 5–6, 169–175.

Tian Y, Zhang W, Zhao S *et al.* (2016) FADS1-FADS2 gene cluster confers risk to polycystic ovary syndrome. *Scientific Reports 6*, 21195. doi:10.1038/srep21195

Vaquero AR, Ferreira NE, Omae SV *et al.* (2012) Using gene-network landscape to dissect genotype effects of TCF7L2 genetic variant on diabetes and cardiovascular risk. *Physiological Genomics 44*, 19, 903–914. doi:10.1152/physiolgenomics.00030.2012

Wang L, Shao YY, Ballock RT (2006) Peroxisome Proliferator-Activated Receptor Promotes Adipogenic Changes in Growth Plate Chondrocytes In Vitro. *PPAR*, 2006, 67297. doi: 10.1155/PPAR/2006/67297

Wood AR, Tyrrell J, Beaumont R *et al.* (2016) Variants in the *FTO* and *CDKAL1* loci have recessive effects on risk of obesity and type 2 diabetes, respectively. *Diabetologia 59*, 6, 1214–1221. doi:10.1007/s00125-016-3908-5.

Yang J, Loos RJ, Powell JE *et al.* (2012) FTO genotype is associated with phenotypic variability of body mass index. *Nature 490*, 7419, 267–272. doi:10.1038/nature11401.

Yang N, MacArthur DG, Gulbin JP *et al.* (2003) ACTN3 genotype is associated with human elite athletic performance. *American Journal of Human Genetics 73*, 3, 627–631. doi:10.1086/377590

Zamani E, Sadrzadeh-Yeganeh H, Sotoudeh G *et al.* (2017) The interaction between ApoA2 -265T>C polymorphism and dietary fatty acids intake on oxidative stress in patients with type 2 diabetes mellitus. *European Journal of Nutrition 56*, 5, 1931–1938. doi:10.1007/s00394-016-1235-8

Zheng Y, Huang T, Zhang X *et al.* (2015) Dietary fat modifies the effects of FTO genotype on changes in insulin sensitivity. *Journal of Nutrition 145*, 5, 977–982. doi:10.3945/jn.115.210005

Zhou Y, Park SY, Su J *et al.* (2014) TCF7L2 is a master regulator of insulin production and processing. *Human Molecular Genetics 23*, 24, 6419–6431. doi:10.1093/hmg/ddu359

7

Genes Associated with Neurodegenerative Disease

Apolipoprotein E: ApoE genes

The ApoE gene is well known for its influence on the development of Alzheimer's disease. This gene instructs an enzyme to combine a protein with a lipid to create a lipoprotein. These lipoproteins are responsible for wrapping up cholesterol and other fats and distributing them throughout the body, via the bloodstream. Cholesterol homeostasis is vastly important for the prevention of heart disease, Alzheimer's and cardiovascular accident or stroke.

There are three major alleles of concern and these are e2, e3 and e4. The e3 allele is the most common, occurring in over 50% of the general population. The ApoE4 allele appears to be the one carrying the highest risk of Alzheimer's disease.

Alzheimer's disease occurs when the receptors for certain substrates are unable to uptake their respective molecules. Vitamin D, brain-derived neurotropic factor and synapse-specific molecules may be in short supply, so the amyloid precursor proteins instruct for the destruction of neurons and synaptic destruction. ApoE4 is key to management of the reduction of amyloid plaque peptides. However, it also enters the nucleus of the cell and binds efficiently to DNA (Bredesen 2017, p.94); in fact, ApoE4 can bind to promoters of any of 1700 genes, reducing associated protein production.

ApoE4 is a huge promoter of inflammation due to its ability to shut down the SirT1 gene and activate nuclear factor kappa B (NF-kB) (Cacabelos *et al.* 2019). SirT1 is the longevity molecule activated by resveratrol and NF-kB promotes inflammation.

There are three major subtypes of Alzheimer's: hot or inflammatory, cold or atrophic, and vile or toxic, according to Bredesen (2017).

Type 1 inflammatory (hot): Occurs more often in those who carry one of two alleles of the ApoE4 gene. It tends to run in families. Inflammation is, of course, a natural immune reaction to foreign stimuli that would have stopped us bleeding to death from punctured feet before the days of leather shoes. It would have saved us from pathogenic invasion from eating raw meat. In effect, inflammation is a lifesaver in certain situations. However, in today's lifestyle choices and as a factor of ageing, it can also promote conditions such as cardiovascular disease, arthritis and Alzheimer's. ApoE2 is associated with a lower risk of Alzheimer's disease. Of note with type 1 is that other genes if expressing can up-regulate the inflammatory response. These include tumour necrosis factor (TNF) and interferon-γ (IFN-gamma).

Table 7.1: APOE genes distribution and outcome

ApoE gene SNPs	Number of carriers of the gene	Number of copies	Risk of Alzheimer's	Age of onset	Best outcome approach
ApoE3	Most	2	low risk		
ApoE4	75 million (USA)	1	30%	Late 50s to 60s	Recode protocol
ApoE4	7 million	2	50%	Late 40s to 50s	Recode protocol
	Markers include: > C-reactive protein, > interleukin 6, > tumour necrosis factor, insulin resistance, high homocysteine				

Adapted from Bredesen (2017)
Recode protocol is the comprehensive personalized
programme designed by Bredesen.

Type 2 atrophic (cold): Occurs more frequently in those with two copies of the ApoE4 gene. Typically, signs and symptoms arise ten years later than with the inflammatory type and are marked by lower levels of hormones and vitamin D. Low levels of brain-derived neurotropic factor (BDNF) can impact negatively on neuronal and synaptic growth.

Markers for the type 2 atrophic Alzheimer's include: suboptimal levels of hormones (thyroid, adrenal, oestrogen, progesterone, testosterone and pregnenolone) and vitamin D. Insulin resistance or low insulin may be an issue as may high homocysteine. This type tends to be slower to respond to support.

Types 1 and 2 can occur together, resulting in chronically high glucose levels with glycation (alteration to various proteins) and inflammation.

Type 3 toxic (vile): This tends to occur in those who carry a homozygous presentation of the common ApoE3 gene and therefore doesn't run in families. Symptoms tend to commence between the ages of late 40s to early 60s. Stress tends to be a strong trigger and cognitive deficits, such as difficulties with executive functioning, speech or number application, appear prior to memory loss. This type could typically occur after the death of a spouse, for example.

While the first two types represent strategic downsizing of the hierarchy of brain structure, the third type is like tossing a hand grenade into a room. Old as well as recent memories are lost; episodic (discrete life event facts) and procedural (speaking, board game playing) memory are lost, leading to increased stress and confusion. The striking finding with these people is the incredibly low levels of serum zinc (Brewer 2014) and low levels of triglycerides (de Chaves & Narayanaswami 2008). These people are often classified as atypical Alzheimer's. Their MRI scans show brain atrophy and neuroinflammation, serum zinc in the low 50s and serum copper up to 170. Typically, they are also known to experience HPA axis hormone dysregulation (Peavy *et al.* 2007). This may manifest in biomarkers such as low cortisol, high reverse T3, low free T3, low pregnenolone, low estradiol, low testosterone or other abnormal hormones, high levels of mycotoxin and/or heavy metals such as mercury. Serum mercury would not represent evidence of mercury in the brain, so a urine mercury with a chelating challenge to pull mercury out of tissues may be the best choice of functional test. Mainstream medicine is still not accepting of heavy metals as a possible contributing factor due to the unavailability of constant qualitative evidence. However, there are studies consistent with high levels of aluminium (Tomljeno-vic 2011). Xu *et al.* (2014) have reviewed the incidence of metals in the pathogenesis of Alzheimer's and concluded that to date there is a lack of understanding of the mechanism associated in each of the three types.

Chronic inflammatory response syndrome (CIRS) may be relevant with this profile. CIRS is a reaction to mycotoxin in mould. For this reason, other genes may be relevant such as GSTM1, methylation genes and MTHFR. The genes of the glutathione-S-transferase family are vital for the conjugation of many metabolic toxins, carcinogens and environmental toxins, and are therefore relevant in this third type of Alzheimer's presentation. GSTM1 has been discussed in detail within the section on transsulphuration in Chapter 5. However, with regard to GSTM1 expression and type 3 Alzheimer's, practitioners need to be mindful of identifying and addressing the underlying causes of oxida-tive stress and inflammation, then supporting glutathione-producing enzymes with vitamins C (Waly *et al.* 2015) and E (Van Haaften *et al.* 2003). Also consider the recycling of glutathione via glutathione per-oxidase enzyme, which requires selenium as a cofactor (Nogales *et al.* 2013), and glutathione reductase enzyme, which requires riboflavin as a cofactor (Mulherin *et al.* 1996).

Methylation controls genetic expression. Recall that methylation adds a methyl group to genes, enzymes, hormones, neurotransmitters and vitamins within the body. If the system fails, genes are likely to be switched on when they should be off and vice versa. If methylation is switching genes on that promote the production of B-amyloid, then that may offer some protection, within reason, for type 1 and type 3. If methylation is down-regulating the genes of transsulphuration, then that could be detrimental for all types (Bredesen 2017).

MTHFR is the gene everyone has grown to know and love. It has been discussed in more depth in the methylation section. This is the gene that is effectively the starter motor for the methylation cycle. So in terms of type 3 Alzheimer's, synthesis of SAMe might be lowered, leading to fewer methyl donors and therefore undermethylation. The term 'undermethylation' is used rather loosely here as distinct over- and undermethylation are now outdated terms. When working effectively, the methylation system is a homeostatic mechanism.

These three types of Alzheimer's each require a different approach. If B-amyloid is removed from a person with the inflammatory subtype (type 1), this may be detrimental as there may be microbes left behind that are being fought by the inflammatory response. If beta amyloid is removed from a person with a toxic presentation (type 3), this too can present negatively, as part of the protection provided by the beta amyloid may be lost. Understanding the three subtypes has provided a more exclusive and personalized approach when supporting individuals with Alzheimer's. While the basics of these three approaches will be outlined below, readers are advised to consult the works of Dr Dale Bredesen (2017) when consulting with these patients.

Patients should be evaluated for the following:

- genetic ApoE and other genes that may raise the risk of Alzheimer's
- inflammation (C-reactive protein, albumin to globulin ratio, red cell membrane fatty acids, interleukin 6, TNFα)
- infections (herpes simplex 1, *Borrelia*, *P. gingivitis*, various fungi)
- homocysteine (usually high)
- B6, B12 and folate (usually low)
- vitamin D (aim for 50–80ng/ml 25-hydroxycholecalciferol)
- fasting insulin level (usually high levels of insulin and glucose)
- hormonal status (thyroid, oestrogen, progesterone, testosterone, cortisol, pregnenolone and DHEA)
- toxic exposure (heavy metals and minerals)
- red blood cell magnesium
- selenium and glutathione
- immune system (autoantibodies)
- microbiome
- gluten sensitivity
- mycotoxins
- blood–brain barrier function (herpes simplex 1, syphilis (*Treponema pallidum*) and Lyme (*Borrelia burgdorferi*) can all be culprits)

- body mass index
- pre-diabetes
- Volumetrics
- sleep, sleep and mouth breathing – sleep deprivation is associated with increased amyloid production (Shokri-Kokori *et al.* 2018).

Doctors who have trained in naturopathy or functional medicine generally undertake nutritional and lifestyle approaches towards the reversal of Alzheimer's disease because, if not caught early, medications may be a necessary part of treatment, even though they would not be regarded as first-line. Every abnormality needs to be identified and addressed by bringing the patient's markers to within 25% of the median value on each marker.

The anti-Alzheimer's diet

- Aiming for mild ketosis so the liver produces specific ketone bodies of acetoacetate, beta-hydroxybutyrate and acetone by breaking down fat. This appears optimal for the production of brain-derived neurotropic factor (BDNF), a synapse-supporting molecule. It switches metabolism from carbohydrate burning and insulin resistant to fat burning and sensitive.
- Following a low-carbohydrate diet; omitting simple carbs (sugars, confectionary, white bread, white rice, white potato, soft drinks, alcohol and processed foods), moving to a more ketogenic base (Rusek *et al.* 2019).
- Fasting for 12 hours overnight to promote ketosis and autophagy (a cell recycling and renewal process, from damaged proteins and mitochondria), although some would refute the necessity of fasting (Wirrell *et al.* 2002).
- Consuming fats such as MCT (medium-chain triglycerides) oil (Taylor *et al.* 2019), extra-virgin olive oil (Román *et al.* 2019), avocado or nuts.
- All foods should be below 35 on the glycemic index scale (Bredesen 2017).

- All foods should be organic or on the list of the clean fifteen (Bredesen 2017).
- Avoidance of fruit juices, switching these for low-sugar fruits with the fibre (Bredesen 2017), although Dai *et al.* (2006) found the antioxidants in fruit and vegetable juices were useful for prevention of Alzheimer's.
- Avoid gluten (Mohan *et al.* 2020) and dairy (Bredesen 2017). Dairy is a very interesting one because a meta-analysis by Wu and Sun (2016) found mixed results, with some studies pointing to a definite benefit to consuming dairy. However, the authors do point out that studies to date are very small, so no firm conclusions can be made.
- Reducing toxin load by eating specific plants know to support detoxification, such as cruciferous vegetables, avocado, beets, dandelions, garlic, ginger, lemon and seaweed (Hodges & Minich 2015).
- Fish is optional. Always eat wild-caught versions of salmon, mackerel, anchovies, sardines and herring, avoiding bigger fish that may contain higher levels of mercury (Ajith 2018).
- Meat, eaten as a condiment rather than a main course. Buy grass- and pasture-fed meat and poultry to preserve the fatty acid ratio and minimize toxins (Bredesen 2017).
- Protein can also be provided from pulses, eggs and nuts.
- Fermented foods provide natural probiotics, so encourage kimchi, sauerkraut, sour pickles, miso soups and kombucha to support gut microbiome (Jang 2021).
- Moderate exercise – at least 150 minutes of brisk walking per week (Meng 2020).

Inducers of ApoE

- Low levels of serum zinc (Brewer 2014).
- Low levels of triglycerides (de Chaves & Narayanaswami 2008).
- High serum copper or copper dysregulation (Morris *et al.* 2006).
- HPA axis hormone dysregulation (Peavy *et al.* 2007).
- Aluminium (Tomljenovic 2011).

- Heavy metals (Xu *et al.* 2014).
- Mycotoxins (Bredesen 2016).
- Standard American diet.
- Gluten (Mohan *et al.* 2020).
- Dairy (Bredesen 2017).

Inhibitors of APOe

- Plant-based foods to support detoxification (Hodges & Minich 2015).
- Fermented foods to support rebalancing of the gut microbiome (Jang *et al.* 2021).
- MCT oil (Taylor *et al.* 2019).
- Olive oil (Román *et al.* 2019).
- Fasting (Wirrell *et al.* 2002).
- Ketogenic/high-fat, low-carbohydrate diet (Włodarek 2019).

ELLA'S APOE GENES

All Ella's ApoE genes were identified as wild card or normal. However, her father had the common ApoE3 gene (vile version) and he developed Alzheimer's within two months of her mother's death. Recall that this was a concern of Ella's when her dopamine levels were low. As pyroluria has been supported for Ella, her predisposition to Alzheimer's type 3 may have been significantly reduced.

Tumour necrosis factor alpha: TNF

This gene encodes a multifunctional pro-inflammatory cytokine that belongs to the tumour necrosis factors super family. Cell proliferation, apoptosis, cell differentiation, lipid metabolism and coagulation are all biological processes that TNFα is involved in regulating. Elevations of TNFα, a major pro-inflammatory cytokine, have been implicated in a number of diseases such as rheumatoid and psoriatic arthritis, insulin resistance and cancer. This has led to the introduction of monoclonal antibodies or biologics therapies for the autoimmune conditions. Chang *et al.* (2017) have identified some interesting findings with regard to TNF and Alzheimer's. Their findings are most notably that raised TNF impacts negatively on a number of areas associated with the management of B-amyloid. In particular, they found increased levels of amyloid beta being produced via up-regulation of β-secretase expression and γ-secretase activity. This resulted in synaptic loss, neuronal loss and dysfunction, and neuronal cell death. However, anti-TNFα medications were not helpful in this scenario as the molecules from these are too large to cross the blood–brain barrier (Boado *et al.* 2010). TNFα also inhibits the glucocorticoid receptor genes, inducing glucocorticoid resistance or poor response to the anti-inflammatory aspects of glucocorticoids (Dendoncker *et al.* 2019). TNFα is expressed in fat cells, dendritic cells, fibroblasts, T cells and macrophages, and can become activated by a chronic infection. This can also cause lectin sensitivity.

Possible interventions based on TNF genetic expression
Helpful medicinal inhibitors of TNF enzyme activity
Biologics therapy or monoclonal antibodies (etanercept, infliximab, adalimumab, certolizumab pegol and golimumab) and antihistamine (fexofenadine) (Ciprandi *et al.* 2004).

Helpful nutrient inhibitors of TNF enzyme activity

- Glycine (Alarcon-Aguilar *et al.* 2008).
- Chromium (Jain *et al.* 2012).
- Bromelain (Huang *et al.* 2008).
- Berberine (Zhang *et al.* 2014).
- Apple polyphenols (Denis *et al.* 2013).
- Phytosterols (Valerio *et al.* 2011).
- Glucosamine (Ju *et al.* 2008).
- NAD (Van Gool *et al.* 2009).
- EGCGs (Niu *et al.* 2013).

Helpful foods to inhibit TNF enzyme activity

Nutritional yeast/beta-glucans in mushrooms (Zhu *et al.* 2013), stevia (Cho *et al.* 2013), garlic (Makris *et al.* 2005), berry anthocyanidins (Fu *et al.* 2014), brassicas/sulphoraphane (Kuntz & Kunz 2014), beets (Ahmadi *et al.* 2020), coriander (Park *et al.* 2014), slippery elm (Lee & Choi 2007) and dandelion (L Liu *et al.* 2010).

PRACTITIONER NOTES

TNF does increase C-reactive protein (CRP), a serum marker for inflammation. However, it may not be adequate to rely on CRP in chronic cases as the marker may normalize when the condition becomes chronic.

Interferon-gamma: IFN-/IFNG

The IFN-γ gene encodes for the enzyme interferon-gamma, which is produced by lymphocytes (white blood cells). Its role in the body is to prevent viruses from replicating. However, a further function is as a macrophage activator. Macrophages are required to become activated at the site of infection. IFN-γ can help other types of interferons to work while preventing cell replication when the cell danger response is active. Rs1861493 and rs1861494 appear to be the two most researched alleles, with the latter being more related to amygdala reactivity and emotional stimuli. This gene also appears to moderate early life stress on emotion processing (Redlich *et al.* 2015).

Monteiro *et al.* (2016) have demonstrated in knockout mice that absence of IFN-γ selectively enhances hippocampal-related cognitive tasks. In the dorsal part of the hippocampus, the absence of IFN-γ appears to lead to newly formed neurons in the dentate gyrus. This is known to support learning and memory. In addition, synaptic plasticity was also moderately increased. Interestingly, Cozachenco *et al.* (2019) have also identified IFN-γ as a potential gene connecting Alzheimer's and vascular dementia with diabetes.

Inhibitors and inducers for this enzyme have been excluded due to lack of updated evidence and lack of clarity from the original evidence of the 1990s.

Brain-derived neurotropic factor: BDNF

Brain-derived neurotropic factor is a neurotrophin, belonging to a family or proteins that promote survival functions and the development of neurons (Ng *et al.* 2019) – in other words, synaptic plasticity. BDNF is crucial for the development of entorhinal cortical neurons. When these begin to dysfunction, short-term memory begins to fail (Giuffrida *et al.* 2018), leading potentially to Alzheimer's disease. A number of rsids are relevant in the evidence base: rs6265, rs41282918, rs2049046, rs56164415 and rs2072446.

Lim *et al.* (2014) recruited 333 adults aged 70 with normal cognitive function, to assess whether ApoE4 and BDNF genes together would exacerbate cognitive deterioration. Their findings demonstrated that those who had both expressing genes deteriorated faster into cognitive decline. Those who only had the BDNF gene barely changed in 4.5 years, as did those who carried neither gene nor a negative amyloid scan. In their calculations, the authors predicted that those with ApoE only would take a further ten years to decline to the same degree. Those with amyloid only would reach the same degenerative point in 27 years.

Possible interventions based on BDNF genetic expression
Inducers and cofactors that may increase BDNF enzyme activity

- Exercise (De La Rosa *et al.* 2019; Loprinzi 2019; Liu & Nusslock 2018).
- Deep sleep (Mahboubi *et al.* 2019; Garner *et al.* 2018).
- Meditation (Cahn *et al.* 2017).
- Polyphenols (Sangiovanni *et al.* 2017; De Nicoló *et al.* 2013).
- Coffee (Lee *et al.* 2018; Lao-Peregrín *et al.* 2017).
- Bulletproof coffee.
- Hypoxia (Satriotomo *et al.* 2016).

- Sunlight (Molendijk *et al.* 2012).
- Nootropics (Sangiovanni *et al.* 2017).

Unhelpful inhibitors that reduce BDNF enzyme function

- Stress (Licznerski & Jonas 2018; Eckert *et al.* 2017).
- Sugar (Krabbe *et al.* 2007).
- Social isolation (Murínová *et al.* 2017; Zaletel *et al.* 2017).

Inflammation

Other genes have been identified as inflammation promoters in Alzheimer's disease. There are CLU, CR1, PICALM, BIN1, ABCA7, MS4A, CD33, EPHA1 and CD2AP. They have not all been included in the analysis for this section because although they are available in some DTC-GTs, the applications for interpretation of DTC-GTs do not always include them.

Interleukin 6: IL6

IL6 is a cell signalling protein that, when activated by various triggers, initiates an inflammatory response. It encodes a cytokine that functions in inflammation and in maturation of β-lymphocytes. The rs1800795 appears to be the most prominent allele. IL6 is a signalling protein that is secreted by T cells and macrophages. This is an acute response that is stimulated under conditions such as infection and trauma, so is produced at the sites of acute or chronic inflammation and then secreted into the serum. Burns notably stimulate it. A mutated gene that is expressing will induce a chronic inflammatory response. Mutated IL6 genes have been associated with type 2 diabetes mellitus (Akbari *et al.* 2018), type 1 diabetes (Purohit *et al.* 2018) and juvenile rheumatoid arthritis (Akioka 2019; Bielak *et al.* 2018).

Possible interventions based on IL6 genetic expression
Helpful medicinal inhibitors that reduce IL6 enzyme activity
Tociluzumab (a monoclonal antibody) (Atsushi *et al.* 2019).

Helpful natural inhibitors that reduce IL6 enzyme activity

- Curcumin (Ghandadi & Sahebkar 2017).
- Polyphenols such as curcumin and resveratrol (Kloesch *et al.* 2012).
- Omega 3 fatty acids (Allam-Ndoul *et al.* 2017).
- Regular exercise (Gómez-Rubio & Trapero 2019).

TNF receptor associated factor 1: TRAF1

The TRAF1 gene encodes the protein TNF receptor associated factor. This protein formation can be enhanced by the presence of the Epstein–Barr virus. TRAF1 and TRAF2 form a complex, which is needed to activate mitogen-activated protein kinases MAPK8/JNK and NF-kB enzymes by TNFα. The complex also interacts with a protein responsible for inhibiting apoptosis and controls signals from TNFα which helps prevent apoptosis or cell death. Rs3761847 appears to be the most researched TRAF1 gene. MAP kinases are activated by a number of stressors such as environmental, heat shock, pathogens, growth factors, ultraviolet radiation and osmotic shock (C Yang *et al.* 2014).

TRAF genes have been implicated in a whole host of inflammatory conditions. Being versatile and indispensable regulators of inflammation and inflammatory responses, where expression is seen in TRAFs, this is known to contribute to the pathogenesis of inflammatory disease (Lalani *et al.* 2018). Expression of TRAF1 is restricted to testis, spleen and lung under normal conditions (Lee & Chol 2007). It has been implicated in conditions such as atherosclerosis, liver and lung inflammation and rheumatoid arthritis in both animal and human studies (Lalani *et al.* 2018). Subsequent studies have identified TRAF1 as a predictor of therapeutic response to anti-TNF therapies in patients with rheumatoid arthritis (Canhão *et al.* 2015). TRAF1 may also express in non-alcoholic fatty liver disease (Xiang *et al.* 2016). Zhu *et al.* (2018) identified and reviewed the function of seven TRAF genes in relation to specific forms of pathogen-induced cancer. One example the authors cite is the belief that *Helicobacter pylori* is a major cause of gastric cancer. They also cite an indirect contribution by TRAF genes on the development of tumour genesis and metastasis via their effects on chronic inflammation, bone resorption, tumour immunity and the tumour microenvironment.

Possible interventions based on TRAF1 genetic expression
Helpful nutrient inhibitors to reduce TRAF enzyme function

- Curcumin (Hashem *et al.* 2016).
- Fish oil (Tan *et al.* 2018).
- Phosphatidylcholine (Treede *et al.* 2009).
- Polyphenols (Lacroix *et al.* 2018; Bhullar & Rupasinghe 2013).

> PRACTITIONER NOTES
>
> Please be aware that many studies are using serum-derived fatty acids as a biological marker for deranged fatty acid profiles. However, Sun *et al.* (2007) and Harris *et al.* (2013) would argue that red cell membrane fatty acids are the most accurate as a biomarker.

Sirtuins 1–7: SIRT1 (2, 3, 4, 5, 6, 7)

The silent information regulator 2 family of proteins or sirtuins use NAD to regulate a number of metabolic pathways including adipogenesis (the formation of fats cells from stem cells), mitochondrial biogenesis (the process used by cells to increase mitochondrial mass), glucose utilization, fat oxidation and insulin secretion. One of the central proteins that regulate inflammation is NF-kB. SIRT 1 is a NAD+-dependent protein deacetylase that has been shown to depress NF-kB signalling. This results in a reduction in inflammatory responses (Yang *et al.* 2012). Higher levels of SIRT1 are said to provide a protective mechanism by increasing antioxidant capacity and reducing oxidative stress (Elibol & Kilic 2018).

Overexpression of SIRT1 or activation of SIRT1 with the use of resveratrol is said to protect microglia against β-amyloid toxicity in neurons (Chen *et al.* 2005). SIRT1 is decreased in smokers and humans with chronic obstructive pulmonary disease (COPD) (Rajendrasozhan *et al.* 2008). SIRT1 is the most frequent family member to be reported on in the literature. Low levels of SIRT1 and SIRT6 have been shown to be responsible for destabilizing of telomeres and activating a DNA damage response (Sahin & DePinho 2012).

Although all SIRT genes are thought to be protein deacetylasers, only Sirt1, 2, and 3 have robust deacetylase activity. SIRT4, 5, 6 and 7 have very weak or no detectable activity (Carafa *et al.* 2019). Sirtuins are located in three specific areas: cytoplasm, nucleus and mitochondria. SIRT1, 6 and 7 are located in the nucleus, SIRT2 is located in the cytoplasm and SIRT3, 4 and 5 are in the mitochondria, according to Carafa *et al.* McGuinness *et al.* (2011) advocate that some sirtuins can and do relocate in certain circumstances. Cell cycle phase, tissue type, stress factors and metabolic status can all influence this. SIRT1, 2 and 7 are often found both in the nucleus and in the cytoplasm (Michishita *et al.* 2005).

The SIRT family of genes are known as oncogenes, meaning they are known to be able to transform normal cells into tumours via their direct roles on cell proliferation, cell division and cell apoptosis. They can also be tumour suppressors depending on the environment of the cell (Deng *et al.* 2014). They do this via their action on three important tumour processes – namely, epithelial to mesenchymal transition (EMT), invasion and metastasis. EMT is the process of changing a polarized epithelial cell to a mesenchymal cell. This cell is then able to migrate away from the epithelium of its origin due to its increased migratory and invasive capacities. This is, however, a reversible process caused by widespread epigenetic reprogramming of gene expression. Mesenchymal to epithelial conversion is, of course, its counterpart (Lamouille *et al.* 2014).

Many SIRTs are responsible for celluar metabolic reprogramming and drug resistance by inactivating cell death pathways and promoting uncontrolled proliferation. Wang *et al.* (2017) confirmed elevated levels of expressed SIRT1 in several cancer lines associated with poor prognosis. This is particularly noted in gastric tumours (Nie *et al.* 2009; Zhang *et al.* 2017).

Possible interventions based on SIRT1 genetic expression
Inhibitors of SIRT1 enzyme activity (may be helpful
or unhelpful dependent on the case)
Resveratrol inhibits EMT in renal injury and fibrosis both *in vitro* and *in vivo*. Many non-steroidal anti-inflammatories with the exception of ketoprofen (Dell'Omo 2019).

Inducers that increase or promote SIRT1 enzyme activity
Resveratrol and other small molecule polyphenols were the first activating compounds to be discovered (Howitz *et al.* 2003). Other polyphenols include butein, piceatannol, isoliquiritigenin, fisetin, and quercetin (Link *et al.* 2010). Sirtuin-activating compounds/medications (STACS).

Resveratrol-mediated SIRT1 upregulation attenuated renal injury and fibrosis by inhibiting TGF-β pathway (Xiao *et al.* 2016).

PRACTITIONER NOTES

As can be seen above, resveratrol as a SIRT1 inducer or inhibitor is at the very least controversial. While some studies have identified resveratrol as an inhibitor of neoplastic lesions, others have demonstrated a reduction in proliferation of some cancers. However, breast and multiple myeloma were not cancers seen to have this effect. This may have been due to a dose-dependent or bioavailability issue in different tissues according to Baur and Sinclair (2006). SIRT1 activity can be ascertained by testing via fluorometric assay (Hubbard & Sinclair 2013).

Nuclear factor kappa B: NF-kB

NF-kB is a transcription regulator – in other words, it controls the expression of other genes. The rs28362491 allele appears to be the most influential, although there are a number of alleles for this gene.

NF-kB can be activated by a variety of extracellular stimuli in line with Naviaux's cell danger response theory (2020, 2014). Cytokines, oxidative stress, ultraviolet irradiation and viral or bacterial insults are the usual culprits for determining expression. Activated NF-kB is known to migrate into the nucleus of the cell where it stimulates the expression of over 200 known genes. This is why it is implicated and found to be chronically active in so many inflammatory diseases. Examples of those diseases include inflammatory bowel disease, arthritis, sepsis, gastritis, asthma and atherosclerosis (Monaco *et al.* 2004). NF-kB has also been found to be extremely active in schizophrenia (Song *et al.* 2009).

According to Gilmore and Herscovitch (2006), there are more than 780 inhibitors for NF-kB. These range from natural products, chemicals, metabolites, synthetic compounds, peptides, proteins (cellular, bacterial, fungal) and physical conditions. The authors have classified the inhibitors into agents that act directly on NF-kB direct gene transactivation; these act more upstream (at receptor or adapter level) or at NF-kB phosphorylation, ubiquitination (inactivates a protein) or proteosomal degradation and at DNA binding sites. A few major inhibitors will be discussed but practitioners will need to consult the evidence base for those appropriate to their case.

Possible interventions based on NF-kB genetic expression
Helpful inhibitors that reduce NF-kB enzyme activation

- N-acetylcysteine (Zheng *et al.* 2019; Michailidis *et al.* 2013).
- Polyphenols such as curcumin (Olivera *et al.* 2012).
- Resveratrol (Ren *et al.* 2013).
- Quercetin (Chekalina *et al.* 2018).
- Silymarin (Surai 2015).
- Plant polyphenols (Karunaweera *et al.* 2015).

Unhelpful inducers that increase NF-kB enzyme activity

- High levels of reactive oxygen species (Chien *et al.* 2011).
- Loss of mitochondrial integrity (Dai *et al.* 2012).
- Deficiencies in celluar housekeeping (Salminen *et al.* 2012).
- Activation of innate immunity and subsequent release of pro-inflammatory cytokines (Gilmore & Wolenski 2012).
- Excessive stimulation of insulin/IGF (Salminen & Kaarniranta 2010).

Nutritional interventions that may be of benefit

Caloric restriction is a good approach according to Speakman & Mitchell (2011). Four pathways that have been implicated in meditating the effects of caloric restriction include the insulin/IGF1 signalling pathway, the adenosine monophosphate pathway, the sirtuin pathway, the activate protein kinase pathway and mTOR pathway. For practitioners who would like to delve deeper into this topic, Balistreri *et al.* (2013b) have provided a useful review of the biochemistry.

Physical activity is also recommended (Ambarish *et al.* 2012) and pre- and probiotics (Balistreri *et al.* 2013a).

Mechanistic target of rapamycin: mTOR

MTOR is a protein that in humans is encoded by the mTOR gene. MTOR forms two functional complexes known as C1 and C2. C1 is the complex that is more significant to health and disease. When activated, it allows us to increase muscle mass and fat (Laplante & Sabatini 2012). It regulates cell growth, cell proliferation, cell motility, cell survival, protein synthesis, autophagy and transcription. One of these roles is specifically to deal with autophagy – the process of removal of debris by the cell. The failure of autophagy has been one theory put forward to explain the accumulation of cell damage during the ageing process. This pathway has been implicated in a number of pathological conditions including cancer, specifically non-small-cell lung cancer (Besse *et al.* 2014), gastric cancer (Riquelme *et al.* 2016), colorectal cancer (Zhang *et al.* 2009), renal cell carcinoma (Grabiner *et al.* 2014), bladder cancer (Park *et al.* 2011), prostate cancer (Stelloo *et al.* 2017), breast cancers (Hare & Harvey 2017) and cancers of the head and neck (Freudlsperger *et al.* 2011). Other conditions include obesity (Ye *et al.* 2019), NIDDM (Tuo & Xiang 2019) and neurodegeneration (Francois *et al.* 2016). Blagosklonny (2010) suggests having a higher SIRT1 activation during early adulthood can escalate the ageing process.

The mTOR-signalling pathway is known to sense and integrate many environmental cues in order to regulate growth of the organism and promote homeostasis. One hypothesis that has been put forward is that caloric restriction, as mentioned above, may increase lifespan by reducing mTOR activity. Decreasing mTOR activity has been found to increase lifespan in animal studies. MTOR activation in the hypothalamus has been shown to increase satiety and reduce body weight. Leptin is known to regulate weight via this pathway by signalling within the hypothalamus (Cota *et al.* 2006).

MTOR is said to increase the production of mitochondria (Laplante & Sabatini 2012) and also to increase mitochondrial metabolism by activating PGC1a (Summer *et al.* 2019). Conversely, there is also a suggestion that mTOR, when activated, may be involved in synaptic plasticity, so it is important in the reconsolidation of fear memory. Increasing activation in the brain could therefore be useful in cases of posttraumatic stress disorder (PTSD) (Blundell *et al.* 2008).

Possible interventions based on mTOR genetic expression
Inhibitors that reduce mTOR activation (helpful
or unhelpful depending on the case)

- Calorie restriction (Dogan *et al.* 2011).
- Curcumin (Du *et al.* 2015).
- Protein restriction (Fontana *et al.* 2013).
- Exercise (Watson & Baar 2014). NB: Inhibits mTOR in the liver and fat cells but activates it in the brain, muscle and heart.
- Intermittent fasting (Dogan *et al.* 2011).
- Resveratrol (Liu *et al.* 2010).
- Quercetin (Bruning 2013).

- Pomegranate polyphenols (Banerjee *et al.* 2013).
- Reishi mushroom (Suarez-Arroyo *et al.* 2013).
- Silymarin (Gharagozloo *et al.* 2013).
- Aloe emodin (Liu *et al.* 2012).
- Omega 3 fatty acids (Deng *et al.* 2015; Chen *et al.* 2013).

Inducers that activate mTOR activity (helpful
or unhelpful depending on the case)

- Testosterone (Basualto-Alarcón *et al.* 2012).
- Insulin (Yoon 2017).
- Ghrelin in the hypothalamus (Martins *et al.* 2012).
- Leptin in the hypothalamus (Cota *et al.* 2006).
- Excess thyroid hormone/hyperthyroidism (Varela *et al.* 2012).

> PRACTITIONER NOTES
>
> For health and longevity, mTOR needs to be in low activation most
> of the time with occasional short bursts of activation. The evidence
> suggests that mTOR activity should occur in the brain and muscles
> rather than in fat cells and liver. Exercise provides the mechanism
> for this (Watson & Baar 2014).

Nuclear factor erythroid-derived 2: NRF2

Also known as NFE2L2, NRF2 is a protein transcription factor that
increases the expression of antioxidant proteins triggered in response to
injury and inflammation. NRF2 is found in the highest concentrations
in the kidney, muscle, heart, liver and brain (Gold *et al.* 2012). NRF2 is
known to stimulate NQO1, which in turn donates and detoxifies a number of chemicals and medications in phase two of the liver. It provides
one of the most important rate-limiting steps in glutathione production. Glutamate cysteine ligase (GCLC), catalytic GCLC and modifier
(GCLM) become bound to form glutathione. These are all produced

from NRF2 (Lu 2009). NRF2 is really important for the protection of mitochondria from oxidative stress (Strom *et al.* 2016). This is crucial for protection against cardiovascular disease (Dinkova-Costova & Abramov 2015). NRF2 is highly regulated, meaning either too much or too little can be detrimental to the cell (Satta *et al.* 2017).

Glutathione-S-transferase (GST) allows glutathione to bind to toxins, enabling safe elimination. GSTs are produced by NRF2 activation. NRF2 has also been found to induce UGT1A1 and UGT1A6 to enable conjugation of glucuronic acid to toxins and chemicals. Bilirubin and paracetamol require glucoronidation (Mehboob *et al.* 2017).

There can be a negative side to activation of NRF2 and this is that it may lead to higher levels of cholesterol and possible heart disease. It has also been found to promote the development of cancerous tumours. Low levels of cholesterol may therefore indicate the need to explore the possibility of NRF2 overactivation. This has led to the development of NRF2 inhibitors for NRF2-addicted cancers (Tsuchida *et al.* 2017).

There are a number of alleles that determine regulation of NRF2:

Rs10183914, rs16865105, rs1962142, rs2886161, rs35652124, rs6706649, rs6721961, rs6726395, rs7557529.

Possible interventions based on NRF2 genetic expression
Helpful inducers that help to increase NRF2

- Exercise (Pall & Levine 2015).
- Vitamin D (Jiménez-Osorio *et al.* 2015).
- Sulphorophane from broccoli sprouts (Kensler *et al.* 2013).
- Butyrate (Yaku *et al.* 2012).
- Garlic (Pall & Levine 2015).
- Curcumin (Macciò and Madeddu 2012).
- Luteolin (Zhang *et al.* 2013). This appears to be dose-dependent as too much can also inhibit NRF2 (Smith *et al.* 2016).

Less effective ways that still may be worth trying include:

- Pyrroloquinoline quinone (PQQ) (Zhang *et al.* 2012).

- Green tea catechins – EGCG (Ye *et al.* 2015): This appears to be dose-dependent as too much can also inhibit NRF2 (Smith *et al.* 2016).
- Astaxanthin (Saw *et al.* 2013).
- Resveratrol (Ungvari *et al.* 2010).
- Liquorice (Gong *et al.* 2015).
- Ginger (Peng *et al.* 2015).

Unhelpful inhibitors that reduce or inhibit NRF2 activity

- N-acetylcysteine (Lee *et al.* 2015). Note that although NAC is known to down-regulate NRF2, it is an antioxidant in its own right, thereby decreasing oxidative stress directly.
- Ochratoxin A (mould toxin) (Zeraik & Yariwake 2010).
- Ascorbic acid at high doses (Zeraik & Yariwake 2010).

Cyclooxygenase: COX OR prostaglandin-endoperoxide synthase 2: PTGS2

Practitioners may also know this gene and its respective enzyme as prostaglandin-endoperoxide synthase (PTGS). The PTGS2 gene provides the instructions for making the PTGS2/COX2 enzyme. Prostaglandins are fatty acids that act as hormones to stimulate inflammation and allergic response. COX2 is the main enzyme for making prostaglandins. Two forms of PTGS enzymes are known – a form that is permanently active (PTGS1) and an inducible form that can be switched on (PTGS2). They differ in the way they regulate cyclooxygenase and their location in the body. The PTGS2 gene encodes the inducible form and is regulated by specific events that stimulate its function. This suggests it is responsible for the prostanoid synthesis involved in the conversion of arachidonic acid to prostaglandin H_2, an important precursor of prostacyclin and thromboxane A2 among others.

COX2 has been researched for many years in relation to specific COX2 inhibitors because blocking or inhibiting COX2 reduces prostaglandins, thereby reducing inflammation (Bhardwaj *et al.* 2017).

Medications that are designed as COX2 inhibitors include non-steroidal anti-inflammatory (NSAIDs) agents such as amlodipine, celecoxib, valdecoxib and rofecoxib. These newer medications are specific for the COX2 enzyme, whereas the over-the-counter NSAIDs such as ibuprofen and aspirin also block COX1 (Bhardwaj *et al.* 2017). Due to COX1 having a protective effect on the stomach, long-term use of NSAIDs may increase the risk of stomach ulcers (Ballinger & Smith 2001).

COX2 overexpression has been linked to a number of diseases of inflammatory origin such as multiple sclerosis, amyotrophic lateral sclerosis, Parkinson's disease and Alzheimer's (Wu *et al.* 2011; Minghetti 2004).

Possible interventions based on PTGS2 genetic expression
Unhelpful inducers that increase COX2 activity

- Arachidonic acid is a precursor to inflammatory prostaglandins that COX2 produces (Hanna & Hafez 2018).
- Omega 6 fatty acids (Patterson *et al.* 2012).
- Stress (Attiq *et al.* 2018).

Helpful inhibitors that reduce COX2 enzyme activity

- Fish, seafood and omega 3 fatty acids (Chen 2010).
- Olive oil (Scoditti *et al.* 2012).
- Curcumin (Rao 2007).
- Ginger (van Breemen *et al.* 2011).
- Cinnamon (Rao & Gan 2014).
- Fennel (Hotta *et al.* 2010).
- Flaxseed oil (Nunes *et al.* 2014).
- Garlic (Colín-González *et al.* 2011).
- Ketogenic diet (Jeong *et al.* 2011).

Nutritional supplements that may also inhibit COX2

- Butyrate (Tong *et al.* 2004).
- PQQ (Yang *et al.* 2014).

- Quercetin (Attiq *et al.* 2018).
- Glucosamine (Song *et al.* 2014).
- Astaxanthin (Yasui *et al.* 2011).
- Sulphorophane (Shan *et al.* 2009).
- Bromelain (Huang *et al.* 2008).
- Rooibos (Chen *et al.* 2017).

PRACTITIONER NOTES

The Attiq paper (2018) provides a very comprehensive review of the inflammatory pathways pertaining to COX2, diseases associated and the natural therapies that may be of benefit.

Discussion and conclusion

Ella's complex nutrigenomic case has highlighted a number of important points for the practitioner to consider in order to be practising safely and ethically within this doctrine. First, there are many approaches that may persuade the practitioner to adopt a particular doctrine because many are advocating the benefits. The benefits of paleo, autoimmune paleo, high-fat/low-carbohydrate, ketogenic, neurolipid keto, raw vegan, FODMAP and many other nutritional approaches are purported everywhere. It is really easy to follow the doctrine, but in essence humans are individuals, and the more complex the client, the less likely they are to fit into a designated category.

In Ella's case, neurolipid keto, ketogenic or paleo should have been ideal for her. She is also a type O blood group, so technically this is said to support a more paleo-led nutritional approach that Butler (2017) has summarized from the work of D'Adamo. However, Ella's digestion from the outset was never going to be strong enough to support those approaches. Ella had to be taught, with the help of the NSA sessions, to listen to her own body, be mindful about what her body needed at specific times and use her own intuition to guide her eating patterns. Ella was given basic rules in a visual format such as the BANT Eatwell plates (https://bant.org.uk/bant-wellbeing-guidelines) to enable her to balance fats, proteins and carbohydrates in each meal and snack. Ella's experience led her finally to a diet of 70–80% plant. She therefore ate little animal protein. Ella was taught to read her symptoms so that she understood when she needed animal protein. It was found that the introduction of fish every 3–4 days for one meal was ample. Eggs were an excellent source of protein for Ella, especially when she had a mountain of mental work ahead. Egg yolk, of course, is a great source of phosphatidylcholine (Smolders *et al.* 2019).

It may seem to practitioners reading this case study that the individual pathways were addressed in linear fashion. It may therefore be difficult for inexperienced practitioners to grasp the interconnectedness of them all. It is important to note that Ella's case took three years to solve and remediate, so all these approaches had their own place and time in Ella's timeline and sometimes a particular pathway had to be revisited. The reason for their inclusion was to make this accessible for practitioners who may wish to help their clients more but don't have the knowledge and experience to do so.

There is no one diet/biomedical approach that suits all and no one diet/biomedical approach that suits an individual for life. Learning to listening to the body's innate wisdom is the cornerstone to good health.

For those practitioners who may be excited by the idea of expanding their knowledge beyond what has been presented to date or excited to acquaint themselves with the models used to guide this case, please continue to Chapter 8 for further exploration. Klinghardt's 5 levels of healing and Epstein's reorganizational healing models will be discussed in depth.

For those practitioners who are just starting out on the journey into nutrigenomics or find the subject overwhelming, start small with the companies who gene-test mostly for diet and nutrition purposes. These are usually the ones aimed at serious athletes. Start by running your own genetic profile and appropriate functional tests. A list of competencies can be found in Chapter 9.

References

Ahmadi H, Nayeri Z, Minuchehr Z *et al.* (2020) Betanin purification from red beetroots and evaluation of its anti-oxidant and anti-inflammatory activity on LPS-activated microglial cells. *PLoS ONE 15*, 5. doi: 10.1371/journal.pone.0233088

Ajith TA (2018) A recent update on the effects of omega-3 fatty acids in Alzheimer's disease. *Current Clinical Pharmacology 13*, 4, 252–260. doi:10.2174/1574884713666180807145648

Akbari M, Hassan-Zadeh V (2018) IL-6 signalling pathways and the development of type 2 diabetes. *Inflammopharmacology 26*, 3, 685–698. doi:10.1007/s10787-018-0458-0

Akioka S (2019) Interleukin-6 in juvenile idiopathic arthritis. *Modern Rheumatology 29*, 2, 275–286. doi:10.1080/14397595.2019.1574697

Alarcon-Aguilar FJ, Almanza-Perez J, Blancas G *et al.* (2008) Glycine regulates the production of pro-inflammatory cytokines in lean and monosodium glutamate-obese mice. *European Journal of Pharmacology 599*, 1–3, 152–158. doi:10.1016/j.ejphar..09.047

Allam-Ndoul B, Guénard F, Barbier O *et al.* (2017) Effect of different concentrations of omega-3 fatty acids on stimulated THP-1 macrophages. *Genes and Nutrition 12*, 7. doi:10.1186/s12263-017-0554-6

Ambarish V, Chandrashekara S, Suresh KP (2012) Moderate regular exercises reduce inflammatory response for physical stress. *Indian Journal of Physiology and Pharmacology 56*, 1, 7–14.

Atsushi O, Yasuhiro K, Shinji H *et al.* (2019) IL-6 inhibitor for the treatment of rheumatoid arthritis: A comprehensive review. *Modern Rheumatology 29*, 2, 258–267. doi:10.1080/14397595.2018.1546357

Attiq A, Jalil J, Husain K *et al.* (2018) Raging the war against inflammation with natural products. *Frontiers in Pharmacology 9*, 976. doi:0.3389/fphar.2018.00976

Balistreri CR, Accardi G, Candore G (2013a) Probiotics and prebiotics: Health promotion by immune modulation in the elderly. In RR Watson, VR Preedy (eds) *Bioactive Food as Dietary Interventions for Arthritis and Related Inflammatory Diseases*. San Diego, CA: Academic Press.

Balistreri CR, Candore G, Accardi G *et al.* (2013b) NF-κB pathway activators as potential ageing biomarkers: Targets for new therapeutic strategies. *Immunity and Ageing 10*, 24. doi:10.1186/1742-4933-10-24

Ballinger A, Smith G (2001) COX-2 inhibitors vs. NSAIDs in gastrointestinal damage and prevention. *Expert Opinion on Pharmacotherapy 2*, 1, 31–40. doi:10.1517/14656566.2.1.31

Banerjee N, Kim H, Talcott S *et al.* (2013) Pomegranate polyphenolics suppressed azoxymethane-induced colorectal aberrant crypt foci and inflammation: Possible role of miR-126/VCAM-1 and miR-126/PI3K/AKT/mTOR. *Carcinogenesis 34*, 12, 2814–2822. doi:10.1093/carcin/bgt295

Basualto-Alarcón C, Jorquera G, Altamirano F *et al.* (2013) Testosterone signals through mTOR and androgen receptor to induce muscle hypertrophy. *Medicine and Science in Sports and Exercise 45*, 9, 1712–1720. doi:10.1249/MSS.0b013e31828cf5f3

Baur JA and Sinclair DA (2006) Therapeutic potential of resveratrol: The in vivo evidence. *Nature Reviews Drug Discovery 5*, 493–506. doi:10.1038/nrd2060

Besse B, Leighl N, Bennouna J *et al.* (2014) Phase II study of everolimus-erlotinib in previously treated patients with advanced non-small-cell lung cancer. *Annals of Oncology 25*, 409–415. doi:10.1093/annonc/mdt536

Bhardwaj A, Kaur J, Wuest M *et al.* (2017) In situ click chemistry generation of cyclooxygenase-2 inhibitors. *Nature Communications 8*, 1, 1. doi:10.1038/s41467-016-0009-6

Bhullar KS, Rupasinghe HPV (2013) Polyphenols: Multipotent therapeutic agents in neurodegenerative diseases. *Oxidative Medicine and Cell Longevity*, 891748. doi:10.1155/2013/891748

Bielak M, Husmann E, Weyandt N *et al.* (2018) IL-6 blockade in systemic juvenile idiopathic arthritis – achievement of inactive disease and remission (data from the German AID-registry). *Pediatratric Rheumatology 16*, 1, 22. doi:10.1186/s12969-018-0236-y

Blagosklonny MV (2010) Why men age faster but reproduce longer than women: mTOR and evolutionary perspectives. *Aging 2*, 5, 265–273. doi:10.18632/aging.100149

Blundell J, Kouser M, Powell CM (2008) Systemic inhibition of mammalian target of rapamycin inhibits fear memory reconsolidation. *Neurobiol Learn Mem 90*, 1, 28–35. doi: 10.1016/j.nlm.2007.12.004.

Boado RJ, Hui EK, Lu JZ et al. (2010) Selective targeting of a TNFR decoy receptor pharmaceutical to the primate brain as a receptor-specific IgG fusion protein. *Journal of Biotechnology 146*, 1–2, 84–91. doi:10.1016/j.jbiotec.2010.01.011

Bredesen D (2017) *The End of Alzheimer's: The First Programme to Prevent and Reverse the Cognitive Decline of Dementia*. London: Vermillion.

Bredesen DE (2016) Inhalational Alzheimer's disease: An unrecognized – and treatable – epidemic. *Aging 8,* 2, 304–313. doi:10.18632/aging.100896

Brewer GJ (2014) Alzheimer's disease causation by copper toxicity and treatment with zinc *Frontiers in Aging Neuroscience*. doi:10.3389/fnagi.2014.00092

Bruning A (2013) Inhibition of mTOR signaling by quercetin in cancer treatment and prevention. *Anti-Cancer Agents in Medicinal Chemistry 13*, 7, 1025–1031. doi:10.2174/18715206113139990114

Butler N (2017) Does the O blood type diet work? *Medical News Today*. www.medicalnewstoday.com/articles/319303.php

Cacabelos R, Carril JC, Cacabelos N et al. (2019) Sirtuins in Alzheimer's disease: SIRT2-related genophenotypes and implications for pharmacoepigenetics. *International Journal of Molecular Sciences 20*, 5, 1249. doi:10.3390%2Fijms20051249

Cahn BR, Goodman MS, Peterson CT et al. (2017) Yoga, meditation and mind-body health: Increased bdnf, cortisol awakening response, and altered inflammatory marker expression after a 3-month yoga and meditation retreat. *Frontiers in Human Neuroscience 11*, 315. doi:10.3389/fnhum.2017.00315

Canhão H, Rodrigues AM, Santos MJ et al. (2015) TRAF1/C5 but not PTPRC variants are potential predictors of rheumatoid arthritis response to anti-tumor necrosis factor therapy. *Biomed Research International 2015*, 490295. doi:10.1155/2015/490295

Carafa V, Altucci L, Nebbioso A (2019) Dual tumor suppressor and tumor promoter action of sirtuins in determining malignant phenotype. *Frontiers in Pharmacology 10*. doi:10.3389/fphar.2019.00038

Chang R, Yee KL, Sumbria RK (2017) Tumor necrosis factor α inhibition for Alzheimer's disease. *Journal of Central Nervous System Disease 9*, 1179573517709278. doi:10.1177%2F1179573517709278

Chekalina N, Burmak Y, Petrov Y et al. (2018) Quercetin reduces the transcriptional activity of NF-kB in stable coronary artery disease. *Indian Heart Journal 70*, 5, 593–597. doi:10.1016/j.ihj.2018.04.006

Chen C (2010) COX-2's new role in inflammation. *Nature Chemical Biology 6*, 401–402. doi:10.1038/nchembio.375

Chen D, Steele AD, Lindquist S et al. (2005) Increase in activity during calorie restriction requires Sirt1. *Science 310*, 5754, 1641. doi:10.1126/science.1118357.

Chen X-M, Kitts DD, Ma Z (2017) Demonstrating the relationship between the phytochemical profile of different teas with relative antioxidant and anti-inflammatory capacities. *Functional Foods in Health and Disease 7*, 6, 375–395. doi:10.31989/ffhd.v7i6.342

Chen Z, Zhang Y, Jia C et al. (2013) mTORC1/2 targeted by n-3 polyunsaturated fatty acids in the prevention of mammary tumorigenesis and tumor progression. *Oncogene 33*, 37, 4548–4557. doi:10.1038/onc.2013.402

Chien Y, Scuoppo C, Wang X et al. (2011) Control of the senescence-associated secretory phenotype by NF-κB promotes senescence and enhances chemosensitivity. *Genes and Development 25*, 2125–2136. doi:10.1101/gad.17276711

Cho BO, Ryu HW, So Y et al. (2013) Anti-inflammatory effect of austroinulin and 6-O-acetyl-austroinulin from Stevia rebaudiana in lipopolysaccharide-stimulated RAW264.7 macrophages. *Food and Chemical Toxicology 62*, 638-44. doi:10.1016/j.fct.2013.09.011

Ciprandi G, Cirillo I, Vizzaccaro A (2004) Mizolastine and fexofenadine modulate cytokine pattern after nasal allergen challenge. *European Annals of Allergy and Clinical Immunology 36*, 4, 146–150.

Colín-González AL, Ortiz-Plata A, Villeda-Hernández J *et al.* (2011) Aged garlic extract attenuates cerebral damage and cyclooxygenase-2 induction after ischemia and reperfusion in rats. *Plant Foods for Human Nutrition 66*, 4, 348–354. doi:10.1007/s11130-011-0251-3

Cota D, Proulx K, Smith KA *et al.* (2006) Hypothalamic mTOR signaling regulates food intake. *Science 312*, 5775, 927–930. doi:10.1126/science.1124147

Cozachenco D, Selles MC, Ribeiro FC (2019) Interferon-γ as a potential link between diabetes mellitus and dementia. *Journal of Neuroscience 39*, 24, 4632–4635. doi:10.1523/JNEUROSCI.3046-18.2019

Dai DF, Rabinovitch PS, Ungvari Z (2012) Mitochondria and cardiovascular aging. *Circulation Research 110*, 1109–1124. doi:10.1161/CIRCRESAHA.111.246140

Dai Q, Borenstein AR, Wu Y *et al.* (2006) Fruit and vegetable juices and Alzheimer's disease: The Kame Project. *American Journal of Medicine 119*, 9, 751–759. doi:10.1016/j.amjmed.2006.03.045

de Chaves EP, Narayanaswami V (2008) Apolipoprotein E and cholesterol in aging and disease in the brain. *Future Lipidology 3*, 5, 505–530. doi:10.2217/17460875.3.5.505

De la Rosa A, Solana E, Corpas R *et al.* (2019) Long-term exercise training improves memory in middle-aged men and modulates peripheral levels of BDNF and Cathepsin B. *Scientific Reports 9*, 3337. doi:10.1038/s41598-019-40040-8

Dell'Omo G, Crescenti D, Vantaggiato C *et al.* (2019) Inhibition of SIRT1 deacetylase and p53 activation uncouples the anti-inflammatory and chemopreventive actions of NSAIDs. *Br J Cancer 120*, 537–546. doi:10.1038/s41416-018-0372-7

De Nicoló S, Tarani L, Ceccanti M *et al.* (2013) Effects of olive polyphenols administration on nerve growth factor and brain-derived neurotrophic factor in the mouse brain. *Nutrition 29*, 4, 681–687. doi:10.1016/j.nut.2012.11.007

Dendoncker K, Timmermans S, Vandewalle J *et al.* (2019) TNF-α inhibits glucocorticoid receptor-induced gene expression by reshaping the GR nuclear cofactor profile. *PNAS 116*, 26, 12942–12951. doi:10.1073/pnas.1821565116

Deng S, Zhu S, Wang B *et al.* (2014) Chronic pancreatitis and pancreatic cancer demonstrate active epithelial-mesenchymal transition profile, regulated by miR-217-SIRT1 pathway. *Cancer Letters 355*, 184–191. doi:10.1016/j.canlet.2014.08.007

Deng X, Dong Q, Bridges D *et al.* (2015) Docosahexaenoic acid inhibits proteolytic processing of sterol regulatory element-binding protein-1c (SREBP-1c) via activation of AMP-activated kinase. *Biochimica et Biophysica Acta 1851*, 12, 1521–1529.

Denis MC, Furtos A, Dudonné S *et al.* (2013) Apple peel polyphenols and their beneficial actions on oxidative stress and inflammation. *PLOS ONE 8*, 1, e53725. doi:10.1371/journal.pone.0053725

Dinkova-Kostova AT, Abramov AY (2015) The emerging role of Nrf2 in mitochondrial function. *Free Radical Biology and Medicine 88*, B, 179–188.

Dogan S, Johannsen AC, Grande JP *et al.* (2011) Effects of intermittent and chronic calorie restriction on mammalian target of rapamycin (mTOR) and IGF-1 signaling pathways in mammary fat pad tissues and mammary tumors. *Nutrition and Cancer 63*, 3, 389–401. doi:10.1080/01635581.2011.535968

Du Y, Long Q, Zhang L *et al.* (2015) Curcumin inhibits cancer-associated fibroblast-driven prostate cancer invasion through MAOA/mTOR/HIF-1α signaling. *International Journal of Oncology 47*, 6, 2064–2072.

Eckert A, Karen S, Beck J *et al.* (2017) The link between sleep, stress and BDNF. *European Psychiatry 41*, S282. doi:10.1016/j.eurpsy.2017.02.132

Elibol B, Kilic U (2018) High levels of SIRT1 expression as a protective mechanism against Disease-Related Conditions. *Frontiers in Endocrinology 9*, 614. doi:10.3389/fendo.2018.00614

Fontana L, Adelaiye RM, Rastelli AL *et al.* (2013) Dietary protein restriction inhibits tumor growth in human xenograft models. *Oncotarget 4*, 12, 2451–2461. doi:10.18632/oncotarget.1586

Francois A, Verite J, Bilan AR *et al.* (2016) The mTOR signaling pathway in neurodegenerative diseases. *Molecules to Medicine with mTOR 2016*, 85–104. doi:10.1016/B978-0-12-802733-2.00011-6

Freudlsperger C, Burnett JR, Friedman JA *et al.* (2011) EGFR-PI3K-AKT-mTOR signaling in head and neck squamous cell carcinomas: Attractive targets for molecular-oriented therapy. *Expert Opinion on Therapeutic Targets 15*, 63–74. doi:10.1517/14728222.2011.541440

Fu Y, Zhou E, Wei Z *et al.* (2014) Cyanidin-3-O-β-glucoside ameliorates lipopolysaccharide-induced acute lung injury by reducing TLR4 recruitment into lipid rafts. *Biochemical Pharmacology 90*, 2, 126–134. doi:10.1016/j.bcp.2014.05.004

Garner JM, Chambers J, Barnes AK *et al.* (2018) Changes in brain-derived neurotrophic factor expression influence sleep–wake activity and homeostatic regulation of rapid eye movement sleep. *Sleep 41*, 2, zsx194. doi:10.1093/sleep/zsx194

Ghandadi M, Sahebkar A (2017) Curcumin: An effective inhibitor of interleukin-6. *Current Pharmaceutical Design 23*, 6, 921–931. doi:10.2174/1381612822666161006151605

Gharagozloo M, Javid EN, Rezaei A *et al.* (2013) Silymarin inhibits cell cycle progression and mTOR activity in activated human T cells: Therapeutic implications for autoimmune diseases. *Basic and Clinical Pharmacology and Toxicology 112*, 4, 251–256. doi:10.1111/bcpt.12032

Gilmore T, Herscovitch M (2006) Inhibitors of NF-κB signaling: 785 and counting. *Oncogene 25*, 6887–6899. doi:10.1038/sj.onc.1209982

Gilmore TD, Wolenski FS (2012) NF-κB: Where did it come from and why? *Immunological Reviews 246*, 14–35. doi:10.1111/j.1600-065X.2012.01096.x

Giuffrida ML, Copani A, Rizzarelli E (2018) A promising connection between BDNF and Alzheimer's disease. *Aging 10*, 8, 1791–1792. doi:10.18632/aging.101518

Gold R, Kappos L, Arnold DL *et al.* (2012) Placebo-controlled phase 3 study of oral BG-12 for relapsing multiple sclerosis. *New England Journal of Medicine 367*, 12, 1098–1107.

Gómez-Rubio P, Trapero I (2019)The effects of exercise on IL-6 levels and cognitive performance in patients with schizophrenia. *Diseases 7*, 1, 11. doi:10.3390/diseases7010011

Gong H, Zhang BK, Yan M *et al.* (2015) A protective mechanism of licorice (Glycyrrhiza uralensis): Isoliquiritigenin stimulates detoxification system via Nrf2 activation. *Journal of Ethnopharmacology 162*, 134–139. doi:10.1016/j.jep.2014.12.043

Grabiner BC, Nardi V, Birsoy K *et al.* (2014) A diverse array of cancer-associated MTOR mutations are hyperactivating and can predict rapamycin sensitivity. *Cancer Discovery 4*, 554–563. doi: 10.1158/2159-8290.CD-13-0929

Hanna VS, Hafez EAA (2018) Synopsis of arachidonic acid metabolism: A review. *Journal of Advanced Research 11*, 23–32. doi:10.1016/j.jare.2018.03.005

Hare SH, Harvey AJ (2017) mTOR function and therapeutic targeting in breast cancer. *American Journal of Cancer Research 7*, 383–404.

Harris WS, Varvel SA, Pottala JV *et al.* (2013) Comparative effects of an acute dose of fish oil on omega-3 fatty acid levels in red blood cells versus plasma: Implications for clinical utility. *Journal of Clinical Lipidology 7*, 5, 433–440. doi:10.1016/j.jacl.2013.05.001

Hashem RM, Mohamed RH, Abo-El-matty DM (2016) Effect of curcumin on TNFR2 and TRAF2 in unilateral ureteral obstruction in rats. *Nutrition 32*, 4, 478–485. doi:10.1016/j.nut.2015.10.005

Hodges RE, Minich DM (2015) Modulation of metabolic detoxification pathways using foods and food-derived components: A scientific review with clinical application. *Journal of Nutrition and Metabolism 2015*, 760689. doi:10.1155/2015/760689

Hotta M, Nakata R, Katsukawa M *et al.* (2010) Carvacrol, a component of thyme oil, activates PPARalpha and gamma and suppresses COX-2 expression. *Journal of Lipid Research 51*, 1, 132–139. doi:10.1194/jlr.M900255-JLR200

Howitz KT, Bitterman KJ, Cohen HY *et al.* (2003) Small molecule activators of sirtuins extend *Saccharomyces cerevisiae* lifespan. *Nature 425*, 191–196. doi:10.1038/nature01960

Huang JR, Wu CC, Hou RC *et al.* (2008) Bromelain inhibits lipopolysaccharide-induced cytokine production in human THP-1 monocytes via the removal of CD14. *Immunological Investigations 37*, 4, 263–277. doi:10.1080/08820130802083622

Hubbard BP, Sinclair DA (2013) Measurement of sirtuin enzyme activity using a substrate-agnostic fluorometric nicotinamide assay. *Methods in Molecular Biology 1077*, 167–177. doi:10.1007/978-1-62703-637-5_11

Jain SK, Kahlon G, Morehead L *et al.* (2012) Effect of chromium dinicocysteinate supplementation on circulating levels of insulin, TNF-α, oxidative stress, and insulin resistance in type 2 diabetic subjects: Randomized, double-blind, placebo-controlled study. *Molecular Nutrition and Food Research 56*, 8, 1333–1341. doi:10.1002/mnfr.201100719

Jang CH, Oh J, Lim JS *et al.* (2021) Fermented soy products: Beneficial potential in neurodegenerative diseases. *Foods 10*, 3, 636. doi:10.3390/foods10030636

Jeong EA, Jeon BT, Shin HJ *et al.* (2011) Ketogenic diet-induced peroxisome proliferator-activated receptor-γ activation decreases neuroinflammation in the mouse hippocampus after kainic acid-induced seizures. *Experimental Neurology 232*, 2, 195–202. doi:10.1016/j.expneurol.2011.09.001

Jiménez-Osorio AS, González-Reyes S, Pedraza-Chaverri J (2015) Natural Nrf2 activators in diabetes. *Clinica Chimica Acta 448*, 182–192. doi:10.1016/j.cca.2015.07.009

Ju Y, Hua J, Sakamoto K *et al.* (2008) Modulation of TNF-alpha-induced endothelial cell activation by glucosamine, a naturally occurring amino monosaccharide. *International Journal of Molecular Medicine 22*, 6, 809–815.

Karunaweera N, Raju R, Gyengesi E *et al.* (2015) Plant polyphenols as inhibitors of NF-κB induced cytokine production-a potential anti-inflammatory treatment for Alzheimer's disease? *Frontiers in Molecular Neuroscience 8*, 24. doi:10.3389/fnmol.2015.00024

Kensler TW, Egner PA, Agyeman AS *et al.* (2013) Keap1-nrf2 signaling: A target for cancer prevention by sulforaphane. *Natural Products in Cancer Prevention and Therapy 329*, 163–177. doi:10.1007/128_2012_339

Kloesch B, Dietersdorfer E, Broell J *et al.* (2012) The polyphenols curcumin and resveratrol effectively block IL-1β and PMA-induced IL-6, IL-8 and VEGF-A expression in human rheumatoid synovial fibroblasts. *Annals of the Rheumatic Diseases 71*, S1, A90–A91.

Krabbe KS, Nielsen AR, Krogh-Madsen R *et al.* (2007) Brain-derived neurotrophic factor (BDNF) and type 2 diabetes. *Diabetologia 50*, 2, 431–438. doi:10.1007/s00125-006-0537-4

Kuntz S, Kunz C (2014) Extracts from *Brassica oleracea* L. convar. acephala var. sabellica inhibit TNF-α stimulated neutrophil adhesion *in vitro* under flow conditions. *Food and Function 5*, 6, 1082–1090. doi:10.1039/c3fo60562k

Lacroix S, Klicic Badoux J, Scott-Boyer MP *et al.* (2018) A computationally driven analysis of the polyphenol-protein interactome. *Scientific Reports 8*, 1, 2232. doi:10.1038/s41598-018-20625-5

Lalani AI, Zhu S, Gokhale S *et al.* (2018) TRAF molecules in inflammation and inflammatory diseases. *Current Pharmacology Reports 4*, 1, 64–90. doi:10.1007/s40495-017-0117-y

Lamouille S, Xu J, Derynck R (2014) Molecular mechanisms of epithelial-mesenchymal transition. *Nature Reviews Molecular Cell Biology 15*, 178–196. doi:10.1038/nrm3758

Lao-Peregrín C, Ballesteros JJ, Fernández M *et al.* (2017) Caffeine-mediated BDNF release regulates long-term synaptic plasticity through activation of IRS2 signaling. *Addiction Biology 22*, 6, 1706–1718. doi:10.1111/adb.12433

Laplante M, Sabatini DM (2012) MTOR signaling in growth control and disease. *Cell 149*, 2, 274–293.

Lee D, Kook SH, Ji H *et al.* (2015) N-acetyl cysteine inhibits H2O2-mediated reduction in the mineralization of MC3T3-E1 cells by down-regulating Nrf2/HO-1 pathway. *BMB Reports 48*, 11, 636–641. doi:10.5483/bmbrep.2015.48.11.112

Lee IT, Sheu WH, Lee WJ *et al.* (2018) Serum brain-derived neurotrophic factor predicting reduction in pulse pressure after a one-hour rest in nurses working night shifts. *Scientific Reports 8*, 1, 5485. doi:10.1038/s41598-018-23791-8

Lee SY, Choi Y (2007) TRAF1 and its biological functions. *Advances in Experimental Medicine and Biology 597*, 25–31. doi:10.1007/978-0-387-70630-6_2

Licznerski P, Jonas EA (2018) BDNF signaling: Harnessing stress to battle mood disorder. *PNAS 115*, 15, 3742–3744. doi:10.1073/pnas.1803645115

Lim YY, Villemagne VL, Laws SM *et al.* (2014) APOE and BDNF polymorphisms moderate amyloid β-related cognitive decline in preclinical Alzheimer's disease. *Molecular Psychiatry 20*, 11, 1322–1328. doi:10.1038/mp.2014.123

Link A, Balaguer F, Goel A (2010) Cancer chemoprevention by dietary polyphenols: Promising role for epigenetics. *Biochemical Pharmacology 80*, 12, 1771–1792. doi:10.1016/j.bcp.2010.06.036

Liu L, Xiong H, Ping J *et al.* (2010) Taraxacum officinale protects against lipopolysaccharide-induced acute lung injury in mice. *Journal of Ethnopharmacology 130*, 2, 392–397. doi:10.1016/j.jep.2010.05.029

Liu M, Wilk SA, Wang A *et al.* (2010) Resveratrol inhibits mTOR signaling by promoting the interaction between mTOR and DEPTOR. *Journal of Biological Chemistry 285*, 47, 36387–36394. doi:10.1074/jbc.M110.169284

Liu PZ, Nusslock R (2018) Exercise-mediated neurogenesis in the hippocampus via BDNF. *Frontiers in Neuroscience 12*. doi:10.3389/fnins.2018.00052

Loprinzi PD (2019) Does brain-derived neurotrophic factor mediate the effects of exercise on memory? *The Physician and Sportsmedicine 47*, 4, 395–405. doi:10.1080/00913847.2019.1610255

Lu SC (2009) Regulation of glutathione synthesis. *Molecular Aspects of Medicine 30*, 1–2, 42–59. doi:10.1016/j.mam.2008.05.005

Macciò A, Madeddu C (2012) Management of anemia of inflammation in the elderly. *Anemia 2012*, 563251. doi:10.1155/2012/563251

Mahboubi S, Nasehi M, Imani A *et al.* (2019) Benefit effect of REM-sleep deprivation on memory impairment induced by intensive exercise in male wistar rats: With respect to hippocampal BDNF and TrkB. *Nature and Science of Sleep 11*, 179–188. doi:10.2147/NSS.S207339

Makris A, Thornton CE, Xu B *et al.* (2005) Garlic increases IL-10 and inhibits TNFalpha and IL-6 production in endotoxin-stimulated human placental explants. *Placenta 26*, 10, 828–834. doi:10.1016/j.placenta.2004.10.019

Martins L, Fernández-Mallo D, Novelle MG *et al.* (2012) Hypothalamic mTOR signaling mediates the orexigenic action of ghrelin. *PLOS ONE 7*, 10, e46923. doi:10.1371/journal.pone.0046923

McGuinness D, McGuinness DH, McCaul JA *et al.* (2011) Sirtuins, bioageing, and cancer. *Journal of Aging Research 2011*, 235754. doi:10.4061/2011/235754

Mehboob H, Tahir IM, Iqbal T *et al.* (2017) Effect of UDP-glucuronosyltransferase (UGT) 1A polymorphism (rs8330 and rs10929303) on glucuronidation status of acetaminophen. *Dose Response 15*, 3, 1559325817723731. doi:10.1177/1559325817723731

Meng Q, Lin MS, Tzeng IS (2020) Relationship between exercise and Alzheimer's disease: A narrative literature review. *Frontiers in Neuroscience 14*, 131. doi:10.3389/fnins.2020.00131

Michailidis Y, Karagounis LG, Terzis G *et al.* (2013) Thiol-based antioxidant supplementation alters human skeletal muscle signaling and attenuates its inflammatory response and recovery after intense eccentric exercise. *American Journal of Clinical Nutrition 98*, 1, 233–245.

Michishita E, Park JY, Burneskis J *et al.* (2005) Evolutionarily conserved and nonconserved cellular localizations and functions of human SIRT proteins. *Molecular Biology of the Cell 16*, 4623–4635. doi:10.1091/mbc.e05-01-0033

Minghetti L (2004) Cyclooxygenase-2 (COX-2) in inflammatory and degenerative brain diseases. *Journal of Neuropathology and Experimental Neurology 63*, 9, 901–910. doi:10.1093/jnen/63.9.901

Mohan M, Okeoma CM, Sestak K (2020) Dietary gluten and neurodegeneration: A case for preclinical studies. *International Journal of Molecular Sciences 21*, 15, 5407. doi:10.3390/ijms21155407

Molendijk ML, Haffmans JP, Bus BA *et al.* (2012) Serum BDNF concentrations show strong seasonal variation and correlations with the amount of ambient sunlight. *PLOS ONE 7*, 11, e48046. doi:10.1371/journal.pone.0048046

Monaco C, Andreakos E, Kiriakidis S *et al.* (2004) Canonical pathway of nuclear factor κB activation selectively regulates proinflammatory and prothrombotic responses in human atherosclerosis. *PNAS 101*, 15, 5634– 5639. doi:10.1073/pnas.0401060101

Monteiro S, Ferreira F, Pinto V *et al.* (2016) Absence of IFNγ promotes hippocampal plasticity and enhances cognitive performance. *Translational Psychiatry 6*, e707. doi:10.1038/tp.2015.194

Morris MC, Evans DA, Tangney CC *et al.* (2006) Dietary copper and high saturated and trans fat intakes associated with cognitive decline. *Archives of Neurology 63*, 8, 1085–1088. doi:10.1001/archneur.63.8.1085

Mulherin DM, Thurnham DI, Situnayake RD (1996) Glutathione reductase activity, riboflavin status, and disease activity in rheumatoid arthritis. *Annals of the Rheumatic Diseases 55*, 11, 837–840. doi:10.1136/ard.55.11.837

Murínová J, Hlaváčová N, Chmelová M *et al.* (2017) The evidence for altered BDNF expression in the brain of rats reared or housed in social isolation: A systematic review. *Frontiers in Behavioral Neuroscience 11*, 101. doi:10.3389/fnbeh.2017.00101

Naviaux RK (2014) Metabolic features of the cell danger response. *Mitochondrion 16*, 7–17. doi:10.1016/j.mito.2013.08.006

Naviaux RK (2020) Perspective: Cell danger response biology – the new science that connects environmental health with mitochondria and the rising tide of chronic illness. *Mitochondrion 51*, 40–45. doi:10.1016/j.mito.2019.12.005

Ng TKS, Ho CSH, Tam WWS *et al.* (2019) Decreased serum brain-derived neurotrophic factor (BDNF) levels in patients with Alzheimer's disease (AD): A systematic review and meta-analysis. *International Journal of Molecular Sciences 20*, 2, 257. doi:10.3390/ijms20020257

Nie Y, Erion DM, Yuan Z *et al.* (2009) STAT3 inhibition of gluconeogenesis is down-regulated by SirT1. *Nature Cell Biology 11*, 492–500. doi:10.1038/ncb1857

Niu Y, Na L, Feng R *et al.* (2013) The phytochemical, EGCG, extends lifespan by reducing liver and kidney function damage and improving age-associated inflammation and oxidative stress in healthy rats. *Aging Cell 12*, 6, 1041–1049. doi:10.1111/acel.12133

Nogales F, Ojeda ML, Fenutría M *et al.* (2013) Role of selenium and glutathione peroxidase on development, growth, and oxidative balance in rat offspring. *Reproduction 146*, 6, 659–667. doi:10.1530/REP-13-0267

Nunes DO, Almenara CC, Broseghini-Filho GB *et al.* (2014) Flaxseed oil increases aortic reactivity to phenylephrine through reactive oxygen species and the cyclooxygenase-2 pathway in rats. *Lipids in Health and Disease 13*, 107. doi:10.1186/1476-511X-13-107

Olivera A, Moore TW, Hu F *et al.* (2012) Inhibition of the NF-κB signaling pathway by the curcumin analog, 3,5-Bis(2-pyridinylmethylidene)-4-piperidone (EF31): Anti-inflammatory and anti-cancer properties. *International Immunopharmacology 12*, 2, 368–377. doi:10.1016/j.intimp.2011.12.009

Pall ML, Levine S (2015) Nrf2, a master regulator of detoxification and also antioxidant, anti-inflammatory and other cytoprotective mechanisms, is raised by health promoting factors. *Sheng Li Xue Bao 67*, 1, 1–18.

Park G, Kim HG, Lim S *et al.* (2014) Coriander alleviates 2,4-dinitrochlorobenzene-induced contact dermatitis-like skin lesions in mice. *Journal of Medicinal Food 17*, 8, 862–868. doi:10.1089/jmf.2013.2910

Park SJ, Lee TJ, Chang IH (2011) Role of the mTOR pathway in the progression and recurrence of bladder cancer: An immunohistochemical tissue microarray study. *Korean Journal of Urology 52*, 466–473. doi:10.4111/kju.2011.52.7.466

Patterson E, Wall R, Fitzgerald GF (2012) Health implications of high dietary omega-6 polyunsaturated fatty acids. *Journal of Nutrition and Metabolism 2012*, 539426. doi:10.1155/2012/539426

Peavy GM, Lange KL, Salmon DP *et al.* (2007) The effects of prolonged stress and APOE genotype on memory and cortisol in older adults. *Biological Psychiatry 62*, 5, 472–478. doi:10.1016/j.biopsych.2007.03.013

Peng S, Yao J, Liu Y *et al.* (2015) Activation of Nrf2 target enzymes conferring protection against oxidative stress in PC12 cells by ginger principal constituent 6-shogaol. *Food and Function 6*, 8, 2813–2823. doi:10.1039/c5fo00214a

Purohit S, Sharma A, Zhi W *et al.* (2018) Proteins of TNF-α and IL6 pathways are elevated in serum of type-1 diabetes patients with microalbuminuria. *Frontiers in Immunology 9*, 154. doi:10.3389/fimmu.2018.00154

Rajendrasozhan S, Yang SR, Kinnula VL *et al.* (2008) SIRT1, an antiinflammatory and antiaging protein, is decreased in lungs of patients with chronic obstructive pulmonary disease. *American Journal of Respiratory and Critical Care Medicine 177*, 861–870.

Rao CV (2007) Regulation of COX and LOX by curcumin. *Advances in Experimental Medicine and Biology 595*, 213–226. doi:10.1007/978-0-387-46401-5_9

Rao PV, Gan SH (2014) Cinnamon: A multi-faceted medicinal plant. *Evidence-Based Complementary and Alternative Medicine 2014*, 642942. doi:10.1155/2014/642942

Redlich R, Stacey D, Opel N *et al.* (2015) Evidence of an IFN-γ by early life stress interaction in the regulation of amygdala reactivity to emotional stimuli. *Psychoneuroendocrinology 62*, 166–173. doi:10.1016/j.psyneuen.2015.08.008

Ren Z, Wang L, Cui J *et al.* (2013) Resveratrol inhibits NF-KB signaling through suppression of p65 and IkappaB kinase activities. *Pharmazie 68*, 8, 689–694.

Riquelme I, Tapia O, Espinoza JA *et al.* (2016) The gene expression status of the PI3K/AKT/mTOR pathway in gastric cancer tissues and cell lines. *Pathology Oncology Research 22*, 4, 797–805. doi:10.1007/s12253-016-0066-5

Román GC, Jackson RE, Reis J *et al.* (2019) Extra-virgin olive oil for potential prevention of Alzheimer disease. *Revue Neurologique 175*, 10, 705–723. doi:10.1016/j.neurol.2019.07.017

Rusek M, Pluta R, Ułamek-Kozioł M *et al.* (2019) Ketogenic diet in Alzheimer's disease. *International Journal of Molecular Sciences 20*, 16, 3892. doi:10.3390/ijms20163892

Sahin E, DePinho RA (2012) Axis of ageing: Telomeres, p53 and mitochondria. *Nature Reviews Molecular Cell Biology 13*, 6, 397–404. doi:10.1038/nrm3352

Salminen A, Kaarniranta K (2010) Genetics vs. entropy: Longevity factors suppress the NF-kappaB-driven entropic aging process. *Ageing Research Reviews 9*, 3, 298–314. doi:10.1016/j.arr.2009.11.001

Salminen A, Kaarniranta K, Kauppinen A (2012) Inflammaging: Disturbed interplay between autophagy and inflammasomes. *Aging 4*, 3, 166–175.

Sangiovanni E, Brivio P, Dell'Agli M *et al.* (2017) Botanicals as modulators of neuroplasticity: Focus on BDNF. *Neural Plasticity 2017*, 5965371. doi:10.1155/2017/5965371

Satriotomo I, Nichols NL, Dale EA *et al.* (2016) Repetitive acute intermittent hypoxia increases growth/neurotrophic factor expression in non-respiratory motor neurons. *Neuroscience 322*, 479–488. doi:10.1016/j.neuroscience.2016.02.060

Satta S, Mahmoud AM, Wilkinson FL *et al.* (2017) The role of Nrf2 in cardiovascular function and disease. *Oxidative Medicine and Cellular Longevity 2017*, 9237263. doi:10.1155/2017/9237263

Saw CL, Yang AY, Guo Y *et al.* (2013) Astaxanthin and omega-3 fatty acids individually and in combination protect against oxidative stress via the Nrf2-ARE pathway. *Food and Chemical Toxicology 62*, 869–875. doi:10.1016/j.fct.2013.10.023

Scoditti E, Calabriso N, Massaro M *et al.* (2012) Mediterranean diet polyphenols reduce inflammatory angiogenesis through MMP-9 and COX-2 inhibition in human vascular endothelial cells: A potentially protective mechanism in atherosclerotic vascular disease and cancer. *Archives of Biochemistry and Biophysics 527*, 2, 81–89. doi:10.1016/j.abb.2012.05.003

Shan Y, Wu K, Wang W *et al.* (2009) Sulforaphane down-regulates COX-2 expression
by activating p38 and inhibiting NF-kap-
paB-DNA-binding activity in human
bladder T24 cells. *International Journal of
Oncology 34*, 4, 1129–1134. doi:10.3892/
ijo_00000240

Shokri-Kojori E *et al.* (2018) β-Amyloid
accumulation in the human brain after one
night of sleep deprivation. *PNAS 115, 17*,
4483–4488. doi:10.1073/pnas.1721694115

Smith RE, Tran K, Smith CC *et al.* (2016) The
role of the Nrf2/ARE antioxidant system in
preventing cardiovascular diseases. *Diseases
4*, 4, 34. doi:10.3390/diseases4040034

Smolders L, de Wit NJW, Balvers MGJ *et al.*
(2019) Natural choline from egg yolk
phospholipids is more efficiently absorbed
compared with choline bitartrate:
Outcomes of a randomized trial in healthy
adults. *Nutrients 11*, 11, 2758. doi:10.3390/
nu11112758

Song KH, Kang JH, Woo JK *et al.* (2014) The
novel IGF-IR/Akt-dependent anticancer
activities of glucosamine. *BMC Cancer 14*,
31. doi:10.1186/1471-2407-14-31

Song XQ, Lv LX, Li WQ *et al.* (2009) The interaction of nuclear factor-κB and cytokines
is associated with schizophrenia. *Biological
Psychiatry 65*, 6, 481–488. doi:10.1016/j.
biopsych.2008.10.018

Speakman JR, Mitchell SE (2011) Caloric
restriction. *Molecular Aspects of Medicine 32*,
159–221. doi:10.1016/j.mam.2011.07.001

Stelloo S, Sanders J, Nevedomskaya E *et al.*
(2016) mTOR pathway activation is a
favorable prognostic factor in human
prostate adenocarcinoma. *Oncotarget 7*, 22,
32916–32924. doi:10.18632/oncotarget.8767

Strom J, Xu B, Tian X *et al.* (2016) Nrf2 protects
mitochondrial decay by oxidative stress.
FASEB Journal 30, 1, 66–80.

Suarez-Arroyo IJ, Rosario-Acevedo R,
Aguilar-Perez A *et al.* (2013) Anti-tumor
effects of *Ganoderma lucidum* (reishi) in
inflammatory breast cancer in in vivo and
in vitro models. *PLOS ONE 8*, 2, e57431.
doi:10.1371/journal.pone.0057431

Summer R, Shaghaghi H, Schriner D *et al.*
(2019) Activation of the mTORC1/PGC-1
axis promotes mitochondrial biogenesis
and induces cellular senescence in the
lung epithelium. *American Journal of
Physiology – Lung Cellular and Molecular
Physiology 316*, 6, L1049–L1060. doi:10.1152/
ajplung.00244.2018

Sun Q, Ma J, Campos H *et al.* (2007) Comparison between plasma and erythrocyte fatty
acid content as biomarkers of fatty acid
intake in US women. *American Journal of
Clinical Nutrition 86*, 1, 74–81. doi:10.1093/
ajcn/86.1.74

Surai PF (2015) Silymarin as a natural
antioxidant: An overview of the current
evidence and perspectives. *Antioxidants 4*, 1,
204–247. doi:10.3390/antiox4010204

Tan A, Sullenbarger B, Prakash R *et al.* (2018)
Supplementation with eicosapentaenoic
acid and docosahexaenoic acid reduces
high levels of circulating proinflammatory
cytokines in aging adults: A randomized,
controlled study. *Prostaglandins, Leukotrienes, and Essential Fatty Acids 132*, 23–29.
doi:10.1016/j.plefa.2018.03.010

Taylor MK, Swerdlow RH, Sullivan DK
(2019) Dietary neuroketotherapeutics
for Alzheimer's disease: An evidence
update and the potential role for diet
quality. *Nutrients 11*, 8, 1910. doi:10.3390/
nu11081910

Tomljenovic L (2011) Aluminum and Alzheimer's disease: After a century of controversy,
is there a plausible link? *Journal of Alzheimer's Disease 23*, 4, 567–598. doi:10.3233/
JAD-2010-101494

Tong X, Yin L, Giardina C (2004) Butyrate
suppresses Cox-2 activation in colon
cancer cells through HDAC inhibition.
*Biochemical and Biophysical Research Com-
munications 317*, 2, 463–471. doi:10.1016/j.
bbrc.2004.03.066

Treede I, Braun A, Jeliaskova P *et al.* (2009)
TNF-α-induced up-regulation of
pro-inflammatory cytokines is reduced
by phosphatidylcholine in intestinal
epithelial cells. *BMC Gastroenterology 9*, 1,
53. doi:10.1186/1471-230X-9-53

Tsuchida K, Tsujita T, Hayashi M *et al.* (2017) Halofuginone enhances the chemo-sensitivity of cancer cells by suppressing NRF2 accumulation. *Free Radical Biology and Medicine 103*, 236–247. doi:10.1016/j.freeradbiomed.2016.12.041

Tuo Y, Xiang M (2019) mTOR: A double-edged sword for diabetes. *Journal of Leukocyte Biology 106*, 2, 385–395. doi:10.1002/JLB.3MR0317-095RR

Ungvari Z, Bagi Z, Feher A *et al.* (2010) Resveratrol confers endothelial protection via activation of the antioxidant transcription factor Nrf2. *American Journal of Physiology – Heart and Circulatory Physiology 299*, 1, H18–H24. doi:10.1152/ajpheart.00260.2010

Valerio M, Liu HB, Heffner R *et al.* (2011) Phytosterols ameliorate clinical manifestations and inflammation in experimental autoimmune encephalomyelitis. *Inflammation Research 60*, 5, 457–465. doi:10.1007/s00011-010-0288-z

van Breemen RB, Tao Y, Li W (2011) Cyclooxygenase-2 inhibitors in ginger (Zingiber officinale). *Fitoterapia 82*, 1, 38–43. doi:10.1016/j.fitote.2010.09.004

Van Gool F, Gallí M, Gueydan C *et al.* (2009) Intracellular NAD levels regulate tumor necrosis factor protein synthesis in a sirtuin-dependent manner. *Nature Medicine 15*, 2, 206–210. doi:10.1038/nm.1906

Van Haaften RM, Evelo C, Penders J *et al.* (2001) Inhibition of human glutathione S-transferase P1-1 by tocopherols and α-tocopherol derivatives. *Biochimica et Biophysica Acta – Protein Structure and Molecular Enzymology 1548*, 1, 23–28 doi:10.1016/S0167-4838(01)00211-4

Varela L, Martínez-Sánchez N, Gallego R *et al.* (2012) Hypothalamic mTOR pathway mediates thyroid hormone-induced hyperphagia in hyperthyroidism. *Journal of Pathology 227*, 2, 209–222. doi:10.1002/path.3984

Waly MI, Al-Attabi Z, Guizani N (2015) Low Nourishment of vitamin C induces glutathione depletion and oxidative stress in healthy young adults. *Preventive Nutrition and Food Science 20*, 3, 198–203. doi:10.3746/pnf.2015.20.3.198

Wang C, Yang W, Dong F *et al.* (2017) The prognostic role of Sirt1 expression in solid malignancies: A meta-analysis. *Oncotarget 8*, 66343–66351. doi:10.18632/oncotarget.18494

Watson K, Baar K (2014) mTOR and the health benefits of exercise. *Seminars in Cell and Developmental Biology 36*, 130–139. doi:10.1016/j.semcdb.2014.08.013

Wirrell EC, Darwish HZ, Williams-Dyjur C *et al.* (2002) Is a fast necessary when initiating the ketogenic diet? *Journal of Child Neurology 17*, 3, 179–182. doi:10.1177/088307380201700305

Włodarek D (2019) Role of ketogenic diets in neurodegenerative diseases (Alzheimer's disease and Parkinson's disease). *Nutrients 11*, 1, 169. doi:10.3390/nu11010169

Wu L, Sun D (2016) Meta-analysis of milk consumption and the risk of cognitive disorders. *Nutrients 8*, 12, 824. doi:10.3390/nu8120824

Wu T, Wu H, Wang J *et al.* (2011) Expression and cellular localization of cyclooxygenases and prostaglandin E synthases in the hemorrhagic brain. *Journal of Neuroinflammation 8*, 22. doi:10.1186/1742-2094-8-22

Xiang M, Wang PX, Wang AB *et al.* (2016) Targeting hepatic TRAF1-ASK1 signaling to improve inflammation, insulin resistance, and hepatic steatosis. *Journal of Hepatology 64*, 6, 1365–1377.

Xiao Z, Chen C, Meng T *et al.* (2016) Resveratrol attenuates renal injury and fibrosis by inhibiting transforming growth factor-β pathway on matrix metalloproteinase 7. *Experimental Biology and Medicine 241*, 2, 140–146. doi:10.1177/1535370215598401

Xu H, Finkelstein DI, Adlard PA (2014) Interactions of metals and Apolipoprotein E in Alzheimer's disease. *Frontiers in Aging Neuroscience 6*, 121. doi:10.3389/fnagi.2014.00121

Yaku K, Enami Y, Kurajyo C *et al.* (2012) The enhancement of phase 2 enzyme activities by sodium butyrate in normal intestinal epithelial cells is associated with Nrf2 and p53. *Molecular and Cellular Biochemistry 370*, 1–2, 7–14. doi:10.1007/s11010-012-1392-x

Yang C, Yu L, Kong L *et al.* (2014) Pyrroloquinoline quinone (PQQ) inhibits lipopolysaccharide induced inflammation in part via downregulated NF-κB and p38/JNK activation in microglial and attenuates microglia activation in lipopolysaccharide treatment mice. *PLOS ONE 9*, 10, e109502. doi:10.1371/journal.pone.0109502

Yang H, Zhang W, Pan H *et al.* (2012) SIRT1 activators suppress inflammatory responses through promotion of p65 deacetylation and inhibition of NF-κB activity. *PLOS ONE 7*, 9, e46364. doi:10.1371/journal. pone.0046364

Yang Y, Kim SC, Yu T *et al.* (2014) Functional roles of p38 mitogen-activated protein kinase in macrophage-mediated inflammatory responses. *Mediators of Inflammation 2014*, 352371. doi:10.1155/2014/352371

Yasui Y, Hosokawa M, Mikami N *et al.* (2011) Dietary astaxanthin inhibits colitis and colitis-associated colon carcinogenesis in mice via modulation of the inflammatory cytokines. *Chemico-Biological Interactions 193*, 1, 79–87. doi:10.1016/j.cbi.2011.05.006

Ye T, Zhen J, Du Y *et al.* (2015) Green tea polyphenol (–)-epigallocatechin-3-gallate restores Nrf2 activity and ameliorates crescentic glomerulonephritis. *PLOS ONE 10*, 3, e0119543. doi:10.1371/journal. pone.0119543

Ye Y, Liu H, Zhang F *et al.* (2019) mTOR signaling in brown and beige adipocytes: Implications for thermogenesis and obesity. *Nutrition and Metabolism 16*, 74. doi:10.1186/s12986-019-0404-1

Yoon MS (2017) The role of mammalian target of rapamycin (mTOR) in insulin signaling. *Nutrients 9*, 11, 1176. doi:10.3390/nu9111176

Zaletel I, Filipović D, Puškaš N (2017) Hippocampal BDNF in physiological conditions and social isolation. *Reviews in the Neurosciences 28*, 6, 675–692. doi:10.1515/ revneuro-2016-0072

Zeraik ML, Yariwake JH (2010) Quantification of isoorientin and total flavonoids in *Passiflora edulis* fruit pulp by HPLC-UV/ DAD. *Microchemical Journal 96*, 86–91. doi:10.1016/j.microc.2010.02.003

Zhang S, Huang S, Deng C *et al.* (2017) Co-ordinated overexpression of SIRT1 and STAT3 is associated with poor survival outcome in gastric cancer patients. *Oncotarget 8*, 18848–18860. doi:10.18632/ oncotarget.14473

Zhang Y, Li X, Zhang Q *et al.* (2014) Berberine hydrochloride prevents postsurgery intestinal adhesion and inflammation in rats. *Journal of Pharmacology and Experimental Therapeutics 349*, 3, 417–426. doi:10.1124/ jpet.114.212795

Zhang Y-C, Gan F-F, Shelar SB *et al.* (2013) Antioxidant and Nrf2 inducing activities of luteolin, a flavonoid constituent in *Ixeris sonchifolia* Hance, provide neuroprotective effects against ischemia-induced cellular injury. *Food and Chemical Toxicology 59*, 272–280. doi:10.1016/j.fct.2013.05.058

Zhang YJ, Dai Q, Sun DF *et al.* (2009) mTOR signaling pathway is a target for the treatment of colorectal cancer. *Annals of Surgical Oncology 16*, 2617–2628. doi:10.1245/ s10434-009-0555-9

Zheng R, Tan Y, Gu M *et al.* (2019) N-acetyl cysteine inhibits lipopolysaccharide-mediated synthesis of interleukin-1β and tumor necrosis factor-α in human periodontal ligament fibroblast cells through nuclear factor-kappa B signaling. *Medicine 98*, 40, e17126. doi:10.1097/ MD.0000000000017126

Zhu S, Jin J, Gokhale S *et al.* (2018) Genetic alterations of TRAF proteins in human cancers. *Frontiers in Immunology*. doi:10.3389/ fimmu.2018.02111

Zhang Q, Ding M, Gao XR *et al.* (2012) Pyrroloquinoline quinone rescues hippocampal neurons from glutamate-induced cell death through activation of Nrf2 and up-regulation of antioxidant genes. *Genet Mol Res 11*, 3, 2652–64. doi: 10.4238/2012.June.27.3.

Zhu W, Ma H, Miao J *et al.* (2013) β-Glucan modulates the lipopolysaccharide-induced innate immune response in rat mammary epithelial cells. *International Immunopharmacology 15*, 2, 457–465. doi:10.1016/j. intimp. 12.007

8
Insightful Models for Further Exploration

Klinghardt's 5 levels of healing

Klinghardt's theory has not yet reached the domains of peer-reviewed journals; equally, he isn't the only person to discuss aspects of health from the perspective of physics as well as biochemistry. Klinghardt's theory stems from his work as a medical doctor in India where he studied the ancient medicines of Tibetan, Ayurveda and Traditional Chinese (TCM) in the Himalayan mountains. It also stems from his knowledge and interpretation of the Yoga sutras of Patanjali. The teachings of these doctrines have largely been lost in Western culture; however, there is much evidence behind the four thousand years of TCM.

Klinghardt's (2005) model is unique and may in fact lead the way in how practitioners address health in the future. The information and evidence is there but has not been entered into a model in this way prior to Klinghardt's publication of his work over the preceding 20 years. His rationale for the development of his model stems from his observations that many patients are not getting well from basic biological treatments comprising diet and nutritional supplements, medications and exercise. Practitioners who see a variety of complex, chronic and disabling conditions would no doubt agree at least in part. Klinghardt states very clearly that patients need assistance on all five levels to effect a full recovery. So what are these five levels?

The five bodies	Level body/sphere	Our experience at this level	Anatomical and conceptual designation	Related science	'Diagnostic' method	Related medical treatment and healing techniques
	5th Level Spirit Body	Bliss Oneness with God Satori	Spirit Higher consciousness Connection to God Faith – belief	Religion	Knowing and awareness Witness – experience Divine Virtues – life changing Grace – humility – love – Fruits of the Spirit Supernatural endurance	Love yourself – self-healing Love God – serve others Prayer, praise, worship God True meditation, gratitude, chanting, Holy Eucharist, adoration, laying on of hands
	4th Level Intuitive Body	Intuition, gifts of knowledge, Prophecy, symbols, trance meditative states, dreams, magic, curses, spirit possession, out-of-body and near-death experiences, archetypes	Collective unconscious 'No mind' The fourth level Tunya	Mathematics and quantum physics	APN II, Jungian approach, systemic family constellation, Radiesthesia, Dream analysis, psycho-kinesiology, sound and voice analysis, syntonic optometry, art therapy, shamanistic approaches, discernment of spirits – light or dark	Hypnotherapy, Jungian psychotherapy, music/singing, systemic family constellation, forgiveness – gratitude – love, colour and sound therapies, radionics, rituals, shamanism, induced drug states with psychotropics

5SB
4IB
3MB
2EB
1PB

Spheres Model

cont.

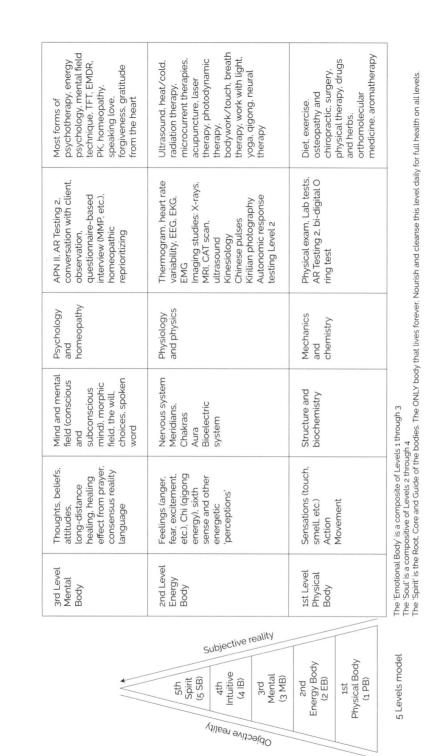

3rd Level Mental Body	Thoughts, beliefs, attitudes, long-distance healing, healing effect from prayer, consensus reality language	Mind and mental field (conscious and subconscious mind), morphic field, the will, choices, spoken word	Psychology and homeopathy	APN II, AR Testing 2, conversation with client, observation, questionnaire-based interview (MMP, etc.), homeopathic reprioritizing	Most forms of psychotherapy, energy psychology, mental field technique, TFT, EMDR, PK, homeopathy, speaking love, forgiveness, gratitude from the heart
2nd Level Energy Body	Feelings (anger, fear, excitement, etc.), Chi (qigong energy), sixth sense and other energetic 'perceptions'	Nervous system Meridians, Chakras Aura Bioelectric system	Physiology and physics	Thermogram, heart rate variability, EEG, EKG, EMG Imaging studies: X-rays, MRI, CAT scan, ultrasound Kinesiology Chinese pulses Kirlian photography Autonomic response testing Level 2	Ultrasound, heat/cold, radiation therapy, microcurrent therapies, acupuncture, laser therapy, photodynamic therapy, bodywork/touch, breath therapy, work with light, yoga, qigong, neural therapy
1st Level Physical Body	Sensations (touch, smell, etc.) Action Movement	Structure and biochemistry	Mechanics and chemistry	Physical exam, Lab tests, AR Testing 2, bi-digital O ring test	Diet, exercise, osteopathy and chiropractic, surgery, physical therapy, drugs and herbs, orthomolecular medicine, aromatherapy

The 'Emotional Body' is a composite of Levels 1 through 3
The 'Soul' is a compositive of Levels 2 through 4
The 'Spirit' is the Root, Core and Guide of the bodies. The ONLY body that lives forever. Nourish and cleanse this level daily for full health on all levels.

5 Levels model

Figure 8.1: The 5 levels of healing (Klinghardt 2005)

With grateful thanks to Dr Dietrich Klinghardt for his 5 levels of healing model. © Klinghardt, D (2005) The 5 levels of healing. Explore 14, 4, 1–7

Level 1: Physical body

If Klinghardt's model is considered in the same way one would consider Abraham Maslow's (1968) 'hierarchy of need' model, it can be seen that the physical body is the foundation on which everything else is built. The physical body is what can be perceived through our five senses. Doctrines such as nutrition, nutrigenomics, exercise, physical therapies, medications, herbs and nutritional supplements are all level 1 interventions. While these are absolutely necessary, they only address the biochemistry of the body. Many complex patients are known to react negatively to interventions at this level, so practitioners who work solely at level 1 may be left wondering why.

Level 2: Energy body

The energy body is very much based in physiology and physics-related sciences. It is not only due to neuronal activity within the body, although all practitioners are familiar with this concept. Somatic and autonomic nerve signals travel up and down the body longitudinally, and the nerve currents they produce create a magnetic field in and around the body that is said to extend theoretically into infinity. The earth's gravitational field also exists in this plane.

The energy body encompasses the meridians, chakras, aura, nervous system, glycosaminoglycans, biophoton field, nadis and bioelectric system. It houses feelings such as happiness, sadness, anger and excitement. What might be termed the sixth sense would be assigned to the energy body.

For those practitioners who would like to explore this further, Lynn McTaggart has written extensively in her book *The Field*, although most of the credit is assigned to Fritz-Albert Popp. The biophoton field, according to Popp (2003), is created by light emissions around the body. Every cell in the body is said to emit biophotons, which are squeezed and polarized, highly coherent forms of light. These light emissions are said to regulate most enzymes in the body. Individuals are beginning to understand how important sunlight is for so many processes such as vitamin D assimilation and sulphation, and PubMed houses 3000 papers on light therapy, so none of this is new.

Energy medicine has been available in the forms of qigong, acupuncture, yoga, breath therapy, pulse electromagnetic frequency therapies (PEMF), bioresonance, bodywork and basic meditation practices for many years and is now receiving a surge of interest. There are 5000 papers on PubMed about PEMF, 3000 papers on red light therapy. All practitioners should be familiar with the use of a light box for seasonal affective disorder and the evidence pointing to the negative effects of blue light on human physiology. Some would say energy medicine is the medicine of the future.

Western medicine uses energy to measure heart and brain traces in the form of electrocardiograph and electroencephalograph in addition to computerized tomography, X-rays and magnetic resonance, so again this is not a new science.

Interestingly, the best energetic daily routine according to Klinghardt is qigong, and Wang *et al.* (2019) highlight the benefits to those with chronic pain and depression. Cleaning up electro-smog in the home is a must and spending time in nature, such as forest bathing, may restore energetic balance (Antonelli *et al.* 2019).

Therapies that may be useful at this level include neural therapy, microcurrent therapies, acupuncture, bodywork, touch tui na, breath therapy, yoga qigong, relaxation and meditation, radiation therapy, ultrasound and laser detox.

Level 3: Mental body

Level 3 considers both the conscious and subconscious mind, becoming more esoteric. It governs thoughts, attitudes and beliefs, and extends into infinity. Rupert Sheldrake has called this level the morphic field which is discussed in his 2009 book *A New Science of Life* and includes the concept that humans are all interconnected. An example of extrasensory perception might explain this easily. Why is it when one human thinks about another close family member or friend, the telephone rings and that person is on the other end? How is it that when a person has had an accident or is in some other form of trouble, their mother, spouse or sibling knows something bad has happened to them? There is also that sense of being stared at. Morphic fields are said to underpin our perceptions and mental activity. For those practitioners interested in further reading, Rupert Sheldrake has some interesting papers on his site at www.sheldrake.org/research/morphic-resonance.

Klinghardt discusses the recoding of life events in this section, being clear that the brain has no circuitry for the establishment of long-term memory. Resulting from this is that hypnosis can and has been used to reduce the symptoms of Alzheimer's disease and dementia (Duff 2008). Under hypnosis, patients with 40% loss of brain capacity have been able to access previously lost memory.

While psychology still debates this concept, it is understood from works such as Lipton (2015), Dispenza, McTaggart and others that a perception and a thought or a chain of thoughts precedes every emotion. When this event occurs, there is a trigger of change in the physical body as seen also in the work of Bessel van der Kolk (2015). These types of illness require a far more holistic approach than those available at level 1 and 2.

Psychology, homeopathy, Popp's biophoton physics, global scaling (Müller 2018) are the related sciences of the mental body. Appropriate therapies and healing techniques include the following: applied psycho-neurobiology (APN1), personal and transpersonal psychotherapy, mental field therapy, psychokinesiology, thought field therapy (TFT), emotion freedom techniques (EFT), eye movement desensitization reprogramming (EMDR), be set free fast (BSSF), brain working recursive therapy (BWRT), body talk, network spinal analysis, homeopathy.

The purpose of these therapies is threefold:

1. to bring suppressed events from the past into consciousness
2. to uncouple the illness-making effects of the traumatic events from the autonomic nervous system
3. to replace limiting beliefs around the trauma with liberating beliefs. Limiting beliefs are an ineffective way to deal with trauma.

Level 4: Intuitive body

This fourth level is more esoteric, within the realm of dreams and intuition. Klinghardt states that this is the level of near-death experiences, past lives, archetypes and ecstatic states. Trans-generational family issues that remain unresolved are said to express at this level. It is also the highest level a practitioner can interact with a client. Conceptually, at this stage is what is termed collective mind or universal connection; the Network Spinal advocates would call this awakening. This level is measurable mathematically so the evidence that exists is purely within the domains of mathematics and physics.

Klinghardt uses autonomic response testing (ART) and family constellations as diagnostic tools for this level. Other tools include sound and voice analysis, dream analysis, syntonic optometry and radiesthesia (dowsing). When APN II therapy is initiated at this level, healing is said to occur when the client is connected with his or her core feelings in relation to the trauma/family conflict. APN is the work of John Bradshaw and is clearly outlined as a procedure in his book *Family Secrets*. In a light trance state, the client can have a healing dialogue with the other person that comes from an attitude of deep respect. Analyzing and interpreting of this type of session at level 3 is necessary. However, at level 4 the soul is said to complete the process in the unconscious state.

Healing dialogue has a number of components that must be addressed during the session as follows:

1. Acknowledge the event in full and frank truth, using words that expose the truth.
2. See your own responsibility. Acting out the event the client needs to take full responsibility for their part or healing will not occur.
3. Seeing the dynamic at play.
4. Feeling the feelings – these may be primary (deep/strong), secondary (superficial) or feelings carried for someone else. The deeper feelings are short-lasting but intense and they always move the client forward in a profound way with incredible insights and lasting changes. This in turn promotes healing.

Although this is so difficult to measure and therefore quantify in a scientific sense, what Klinghardt has stated from Bradshaw's original work also happens in network spinal analysis.

Appropriate healing techniques include APN II, family constellations, shamanism, hypnotherapy, network spinal analysis, Jungian psychotherapy, radionics or colour and sound therapies. The Klinghardt academy trains practitioners to use autonomic response therapy as a diagnostic tool for all levels 1 to 4.

Level 5: Spirit body

This is a very interesting level, aptly described as the level of self-healing that is outside the understanding of many. Satori (awakening), bliss, at one, connected to spirit/the universe and at one with God are terms that might be experienced at this level. This is conceptualized as spiritual or higher consciousness with its foundations in the science of religion and spirituality.

This level cannot be enhanced with practitioner input and practitioners shouldn't interfere or overstep the boundary at this level. While NSA and APN II can take the client to the gateway, hypothetically speaking, only self-healing, true meditation, chanting and prayer are said to be the healer. Louise Hay, Joe Dispenza, Greg Braden, Bruce Lipton and many other well-respected researchers have all made their life's work out of these phenomena. There are many life stories of those who healed following near-death experiences such as Anita Moorjani in her book *Dying to Be Me.* The case presented in this book is not quite so profound but is strikingly similar.

What rules govern the 5 levels of healing?

From Klinghardt's observations, each level is its own entity with its own rules. If a person gains a trauma at a higher level, this can migrate into the lower levels, and also a trauma at a lower level can migrate upwards. Each trauma may therefore impact more than one level. A healing intervention must be initiated on the level of the trauma or above because healing impulses created at a lower level are unable to penetrate upwards. An example might be a client who has a diagnosis of PTSD, which is a level 3 disorder. Supplying him with B vitamins or supporting his methylation at level 1 is not going to penetrate upwards, reversing his PTSD. The practitioner therefore needs a referral network in order to access tools at all levels. He or she also needs the knowledge or intuition to know which tool is appropriate at which point in time.

Practitioners familiar with energy healing modalities, such as acupuncturists, will understand fully that where a symptom or an illness is visible physically, it can also be detected on different levels. Pulse and tongue diagnosis, for example, can highlight early warning signs before symptoms occur. Bioresonance can identify bacteria, parasites and viruses that may not be identified on blood testing as the pathogens may be residing deep in tissue behind biofilms created for their survival. As Klinghardt clearly points out, the lower levels provide the foundation and boundaries for the client to exist in and energy or nourishment to the higher levels. The higher levels provide an organizing influence on the level(s) below. In effect, this is true integrative or holistic medicine.

Klinghardt (2005) provides a beautiful case example of a client with an eating disorder to demonstrate how all the 5 levels of healing manifest. He advocates supporting all the lower three levels with as much energy as can be mustered in order to support healing at the top two levels. This is where the magic of healing is said to occur.

Network spinal analysis (NSA) based on the 12 stages of healing (Epstein 1994)

With grateful thanks to Dr Donald Epstein for kindly editing this section.

Network chiropractic or network spinal analysis (NSA) was chosen for Ella as it covers levels 2–4 of Klinghardt's 5 levels of healing and this would negate the need for multiple therapies or a repeat of therapies Ella had previously found limited in effect. Ella had mentioned that she had encountered counselling/psychotherapy sessions in earlier times, but they caused her to ruminate on her bad memories. NSA, as mentioned earlier, is said to tap into the body's own innate wisdom, allowing healing. NSA has been evolved based on academic research and practitioner assessments into Network Spinal. NSA and the newer Network Spinal seek to enhance and grow levels of spinal and neural (nervous system) integrity while producing and refining the Network Wave. Instead of looking to correct anything, the body is able to better self-regulate and heal. It does this with the unique Network Wave that creates reorganization as an expression of a person's healing signature.

NSA isn't a talking therapy; in fact, practitioners are encouraged to talk only when necessary and not to discuss the experience of the client. This slots NSA very firmly between levels 3 and 4 of Klinghardt's model. Ella felt NSA would be really beneficial. She did volunteer that she had previously and without realizing manipulated other practitioners, who were practicing well known talking therapies. Ella admitted to a distinct lack of trust in most practitioners.

Three decades of research and clinical findings related to NSA suggest an important role for the spine in how an individual maintains stability amid change (McEwen *et al.* 2015), more readily deals with stress, stays well (Antonovsky 1979) and achieves higher levels of living and wellness characterized as reorganizational healing (Epstein *et al.* 2009; Senzon *et al.* 2011) These findings include the dynamics of the spinal wave as a central pattern generator (Jonkheere *et al.* 2010), the development of a respiratory wave visibly rocking every vertebra of the spine (Blanks *et al.* 2001), the stress-busting effect of NSA care (Miller & Redmond 1998; Senzon 2003; Kidoo 2001) and the emergence of increased patient self-reported quality of life with statistically significant impacts on wellness lifestyles. Case studies include conditions such as inattention (Pauli 2007), psoriasis (Behrendt 1998) and in vitro fertilization (Senzon 2003), although addressing rebalancing of the central nervous system may have an impact on so many conditions. One self-reporting study (Blanks *et al.* 2001) found on measures of physical symptoms, mental/emotional symptoms, stress indictor scale and enjoyment scale that individuals reported improvements in wellness scores.

NSA really comes under the umbrella term reorganizational healing (ROH) (Epstein *et al.* 2014; Epstein *et al.* 2009). ROH as an academic concept has evolved into EpiHealing, beyond ordinary healing with an expanded model and experience of the forces that self-organize the body and life.

ROH effectively provides a map for the individual to assess their strengths to create sustainable change. The works of theorists such Grof, Maslow, Wilber and Washburn have influenced the evolution of ROH. It uses tools under three central elements. These include the four seasons of wellbeing, the triad of change and the five energetic intelligences. The model is an emerging wellness growth and behavioural change paradigm, growing from empirical evidence on the discovery of reproducible and measurable neurophysiological spinal wave phenomena (Epstein *et al.* 2009; Senzon 2011) and a healing process that Epstein has structured into 12 stages of somatic and respiratory integration (Epstein 1994).

This is a very interesting model as it considers disease as being attributed to and arising from the individual's or society perspectives, worldviews and overall life stressors. Diseases of meaning in this respect are viewed as a call to know the self and the body–mind connection more intimately. In doing this, the individual can link their perception of self to their health to effect change. The tool allows the individual to use the meanings of their symptoms or problems and life stressors as a catalyst to taking action to improve resilience and a more fulfilling life. With that comes improved health outcomes. Bessel van der Kolk, Gabor Mate and Candace Pert are all pioneers of this work.

The reader is advised to read Epstein *et al.* (2009) and Epstein *et al.* (2014) for a full discussion of the model below as a broad range of methodologies and applications can use this model to further inform. Epstein's latest development, EpiHealing, links cutting-edge science, body–mind–spirit understandings and applications with centuries-old spiritual wisdom. EpiHealing considers the bio, emotional, mental and spiritual organizing intelligences and integrates the person's individual healing strategies consistent with their own unique way of using energy to fuel their organizing wisdom, health and life. EpiHealing is an expression of EpiEnergetics, the conscious and ecological use of energy and information to create the extraordinary. Epstein *et al.* point out clearly the contrast between this and restorative therapeutics used in allopathic medicine. Here is a brief synopsis.

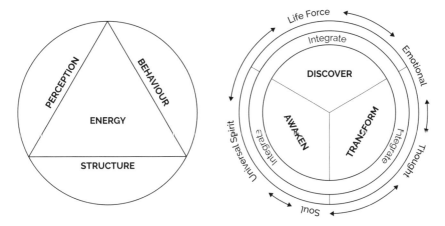

Figure 8.2: Elements of reorganizational healing (Epstein 2009)
*Source: Reproduced from Epstein et al. (2009), with
grateful thanks to Dr Donald Epstein*

Energy (on the left) is seen as fuel for growth so where the body holds/
traps the energy as a result of being in defence model, this is felt as pain,
tension or stiffness. The pain/tension/stiffness results from a lack of
body awareness so the therapy uses breath, energy and movement to
redirect the energy. This encourages a heightened level of awareness
in the individual that goes beyond the cognitive. It is hypothesized that
the frontal lobes of the cerebral cortex and the vagal centres become
more available to assess perception, structure and behaviour when the
physiology is less in defence (Epstein 2005).

The four seasons of wellbeing (right) – discover, transform, awaken
and integrate– refer to distinct rhythms or periods in an individual's life
journey. An individual may need to live in one season at a certain point
in time and for a specific reason but may not necessarily progress in a
linear or sequential fashion.

In *discover*, the focus is on the physical: How has one caused pain for
oneself or others in an attempt to disconnect or avoid pain? Discover
uses the breath, energy and movement to facilitate the transition from
fear, blame and reaction (behaviour), pain, stiffness, feeling stuck (structural), victim, disassociated, nothing works (perception) to security and
safety. If the individual seeks CAM therapies in this season, they seek
out of fear, reaction, frustration or hopes of a magical cure.

Transform is really about attention and action to transform relationships. Blame no longer exists and problems are replaced by opportunities, goals and deliberate action. The individual becomes more flexible, growth oriented, adaptable, optimistic (structure), decisive, deliberate, seeking opportunity (behaviour) and focused on goals, excited, courageous (perception).

Awaken is what could also be called conscious or collective consciousness as in Klinghardt's level 4. This is about the experience of effortless being and knowing (intuition). In awaken, gratitude, awe, amazement, love and benevolence develop. The body becomes more expansive/spacious. The individual uses the new expanded consciousness to formulate new actions. This season relates more to the need to give love and contribute to the world. It is also the time of spiritual growth and inner work. Individuals are more likely to seek CAM therapies for the advancement of their own evolution. They are more able to connect into subtle energies and achieve optimal health.

The season of *integrate* is when the individual revisits a previous season while maintaining the learning from previous seasons. Integrate is the season where the individual is able to make conscious life choices and be resourceful.

An example of this might be:

The individual is being triggered into patterns of negative behaviours that have been programmed from subconscious memories, by the behaviours of someone close without realizing. This often brings confusion and physical defence, maybe even anger. The individual would then need to live in 'discover' for a while in order to work out what is happening. They may be 'awakened' by the insight and use that to 'transform' the old behaviours into ones that are more conducive to the relationship.

The seasons of wellbeing are ever changing throughout the lifetime of the individual. The evolution from discover to awaken, while available to most, is not guaranteed. Low-functioning individuals may only ever experience the season of discover. Over-achievers may only ever experience the season of transform. Self-actualizers, after Maslow (1968), may continually experience the season of awaken and new age circles are able to conceptualize and explain the season well. The key to working with an individual is to work at the season congruent with where the individual is at the point of the session.

The triad of change (perception, behaviour and structure) is the central focus and the power of the therapy arises from the synergy of two sides of the model (i.e. perception and behaviour) entraining the third (structure). The key to successful and sustainable change is congruence.

What is interesting in Epstein's work is that working purely with the restorative therapeutics can be a huge challenge as this is where the individual tends to feel inadequate, useless and never good enough. The greatest psychological wounds are located here, giving rise to resistance and defensiveness. By only supporting one aspect of the triad, there is the tendency for the other two sides to bring the challenged side to its previous state, enhancing the 'nothing ever works' perception.

In conclusion, Ella is one case of many seen in clinical practice on a weekly basis. The use of nutrigenomics tools was instrumental in solving the underlying features of this case. However, respect and gratitude have to be given for the healing modalities that allowed greater expansion of practitioner knowledge and the tools to identify and remediate the true root cause. Nutrigenomic competencies produced as a result of this and other cases follow this section. Further tools to reduce anxiety can be found in the Appendix.

> We cannot solve our problems with the same thinking we used when we created them.
>
> *Albert Einstein*

References

Antonelli M, Barbieri G, Donelli D (2019) Effects of forest bathing (shinrin-yoku) on levels of cortisol as a stress biomarker: A systematic review and meta-analysis. *International Journal of Biometeorology 63*, 1117–1134. doi:10.1007/s00484-019-01717-x

Antonovsky A (1979) *Health, Stress and Coping.* San Francisco, London: Jossey-Bass.

Behrendt M (1998) Reduction of psoriasis in a patient under network spinal analysis care: A case report. *Journal of Vertebral Subluxation Research 2*, 4, 1–5.

Blanks RH, Schuster TL, Dobson M *et al.* (2001) Assessment of Network Spinal Analysis in retrospective and prospective research design formats using a survey of Self-Reported Health and Wellness. https://static1.squarespace.com/static/5b15520e1137a6d3c0a46f5f/t/5b-1de9a36d2a73d2cc21c0f8/1528687011638/uc-irvine+nsa+study.pdf

Bradshaw J (1996) *Family Secrets: The Path to Self-Acceptance and Reunion*. New York, NY: Bantam Books.

Duff S (2008) Hypnosis shown to reduce symptoms of dementia. *ScienceDaily*, 29 July. www.sciencedaily.com/releases/2008/07/080728111402.htm

Epstein D (1994) *The Twelve Stages of Healing: A Network Approach to Wholeness*. San Rafael, CA: Amber Allen

Epstein D (2005) *Theoretical Basis and Clinical Application of Network Spinal Anaylsis (NSA) and Evidence-based Document*. Longmont, CO: Innate Intelligence.

Epstein DM, Senzon SA, Lemberger DC (2009) Reorganizational healing: A paradigm for the advancement of wellness, behaviour change, holistic practice and healing. *Journal of Alternative and Complimentary Medicine 15*, 5, 475–487.

Epstein DM, Senzon SA, Lemberger DC (2014) The Seasons of Wellbeing as an evolutionary map for transpersonal medicine. *International Journal of Transpersonal Studies 33*, 1, 102–130.

Jonkheere E, Lohsoonthorne P, Musuvarthy S *et al.* (2010) On a standing wave central pattern generator and the coherence problem. *Biomedical Signal Processing and Control 5*, 4, 336-347. doi:10.1016/j.bspc.2010.04.002

Kidoo K (2001) The role of network spinal analysis in augmenting psychotherapy. Paper presented at the Association for Network Care, Scientific Research Conference, Como, Italy.

Klinghardt D (2005) The 5 levels of healing. *Explore 14*, 1–7.

Klinghardt D (2018) Autism solutions seminar: The biological treatment of children and adults with an autism spectrum disorder. Klinghardt Institute. www.klinghardtinstitute.com

Lipton BH (2015) *The Biology of Belief: Unleashing the Power of Consciousness, Matter, and Miracles*. Carlsbad, CA: Hay House.

Maslow AH (1968) *Toward a Psychology of Being*, 2nd edn. New York, NY: D. Van Nostrand.

McEwen BS, Gray JD, Nasca C (2015) 60 years of neuroendocrinology: Redefining neuroendocrinology: Stress, sex and cognitive and emotional regulation. *Journal of Endocrinology 226*, T67–T83. doi:10.1530/joe-15-0121

McTaggart L (2003) *The Field: The Quest for the Secret Force of the Universe*. London: Element.

Miller E, Redmond P (1998) Changes in digital skin temperature, surface electromyography and electrodermal activity in subjects receiving network spinal analysis care. *Journal of Vertebral Subluxation Research 2*, 2, 1–9.

Moorjani A (2012) *Dying to Be Me: My Journey from Cancer to Near Death to True Healing*. Carlsbad, CA: Hay House.

Müller H (2018) *Global Scaling: The Fundamentals of Interscalar Cosmology*. Brooklyn, NY: New Heritage Publishers. www.ptep-online.com/books/muller2018.pdf

Pauli Y (2007) Improvement in attention in patients undergoing network spinal analysis: A case series using objective measures of attention. *Journal of Vertebral Subluxation Research*, 1–9.

Popp FA (2003) Properties of biophotons and their theoretical implications. *Indian Journal of Experimental Biology 41*, 5, 391–402.

Sheldrake R (2009) *A New Science of Life*. London: Icon Books. First published 1981.

Senzon SA (2011) Constructing a philosophy of chiropractic: Evolving worldviews and postmodern core. *Journal of Chiropractic Humanities 18*, 1, 39–63. doi:10.1016/j.echu.2011.10.001

Senzon S (2003) Successful in vitro fertilization in a poor responder while under network spinal analysis care: A case report. *Journal of Vertebral Subluxation Research*, 14, 1–6.

Senzon S, Epstein D, Lemberger D (2011) Reorganizational healing as an integrally informed framework for integral medicine. *Journal of Integral Theory and Practice 6*, 4, 113–130.

Van Der Kolk B (2015) *The Body Keeps the Score: Mind, Brain and Body in the Transformation of Trauma*. New York, NY: Penguin.

Wang CC, Li K, Choudhury A, Gaylord S (2019) Trends in yoga, tai chi, and qigong use among us adults, 2002–2017. *American Journal of Public Health 109*, 5, 755–761. doi:10.2105/AJPH.2019.304998

9

Nutrigenomic Competencies

The book would not be complete without providing a set of competencies that should underpin work with nutrigenomics. Given the nature of the work and the current zeitgeist, it is imperative that practitioners understand and have the support to work with nutrigenomic testing should they wish. To this end I have written a set of competencies for the profession that are aligned with national occupational standards (Skills for Health n.d.). That document is reproduced in full below.

Nutrigenomics competencies for integrative medicine practitioners

Introduction

This document contains nutrigenomics competencies for nutrigenomic (NG) training and is applicable to all education and training providers offering study of NG.

This nutrigenomics competency document forms the skeleton around which the delivery of a course or programme leading to the practice of nutrigenomics in integrative medicine should take place. As such, it sets out the minimum standard required for independent, safe and effective practice in addition to everything in the Core Curriculum (CC) and the National Occupational Standards (NOS) document developed in terms of learning outcomes of increasing complexity. Training should encourage the development of a reflective, research-minded practitioner with qualities of integrity, humanity, caring, trust, responsibility, respect and confidentiality.

This document should be read in conjunction with the NOS and CC but the following information is provided to assist your understanding and use of the nutrigenomics competencies.

Knowledge and understanding required of nutritional therapists

Nutrigenomics clinical practice

The overall aim of clinical practice must be to prepare a lawful, safe and effective nutritional therapy practitioner who is able to practise nutrigenomics with autonomy. This requires competence at level 6 and all practitioners must be in receipt of a certificate of successful completion of their respective profession. Training providers (TPs) will need to demonstrate that their graduates feel confident to practise safely and effectively.

Assessment

Assessment methods must demonstrate an evolving process of complexity and preparation to practise in a professional capacity and relate to the learning outcomes. Professional competence to practise as a nutrigenomics practitioner requires an effective synthesis of a wide range of knowledge and skills, and graduates must demonstrate intellectual flexibility within a realistic clinical practice on completion. This is a HE Level 6 skill. Assessment methods are to be decided by the TPs and should support the development of practice but must include case studies containing both genetic interpretive reports and appropriate functional tests.

Academic assessment methods

Aside from the obvious short-answer assignments, essays, various tests including multiple choice and examinations, some of which may be conducted as open book, it is also helpful to include a wide variety of other assessment methods, some of which will be formative and others summative. These may include oral presentations and discussions, poster presentations and production of leaflets, information sheets, a specific literature review, evaluation of treatment for a named disease, critique of a scientific paper. Assessments should include an element of reflective practice. Clinical practice assessment will be unnecessary as these are considered as postgraduate qualifications.

SEEC/HE LEVEL6: relates to application of knowledge in a complex autonomous environment where the process needs to be critically evaluated (relates to former HE Level 3).

Core elements

1: Client care

Aims

- To ensure client is fully informed and supported and that the practitioner has fully prepared the client before recommending nutrigenomic testing.
- To ensure that the practitioner has recommended the best type of nutrigenomics analysis for the client, given their health concerns, risk factors and goals for achievement.

Learning outcomes

LO1: The practitioner fully understands the variety of nutrigenomics testing and interpretations within and outside the profession.

LO2: The practitioner can fully explain the risk and benefit of nutrigenomics testing to the client when undertaking nutrigenomics testing.

LO3: The practitioner can explain and provide a comprehensive overview and plan to the client to ensure patient safety, comfort and compliance.

1:1 Appropriateness of nutrigenomics testing

1:1:1 Explain the limitations of nutrigenomics information to the client – nutrigenomics testing should not be used in isolation to provide nutritional recommendations.

1:1:2 Explain the need for functional testing in addition to nutrigenomics interpretation.

1:1:3 Undertake nutrigenomics counselling to address client concerns such as data protection, use of genetic data by the health industry.

1:1:4 Undertake an assessment to ascertain whether foundational work has been completed prior to nutrigenomics assessment.

1:1:5 Provide an in-depth explanation of the process and cost of nutrigenomics testing and interpretation.

1:1:6 Explain the difference between single-gene disorders and nutrigenomics.

1:1:7 Explain the difference between epigenetic and nutrigenomics factors.

1:2 Benefits to the client

1:2:1 Explain benefits to the client including the potential for improved health and/or fitness.

1:2:2 Note and explain to the clients that the providers of genetics raw data are unable to provide health risk from the epidemiological data collected.

1:2:3 Explain how nutrigenomics may be used in order to assist the client to achieve optimal health.

1:2:4 Explain how the use of nutrigenomics may help reduce disease risk or the risk of family health-related conditions.

1:2:5 Explain that although nutrigenomics testing provides information on inherited disease, this is not a guarantee of contracting the disease.

1:3 Interpretation and reporting

1:3:1 Prioritize the approach based on client main aims, symptomology and those single nucleotide polymorphism (SNP) combinations that are expressing according to functional testing.

1:3:2 Production of a report comprising nutrigenomics, relevant functional tests and history.

1:3:3 Provide nutrition and lifestyle management programme based on the FM approach and encompassing the results from nutrigenomics testing, functional testing and a full case history.

1:3:4 Fully explain the difference between null, homozygous and heterozygous SNPs and their significance to the case/client.

2: Professional and ethical practice

Aims

- To ensure the practitioner can work ethically, safely and effectively with nutrigenomics.
- To ensure the practitioner understands their own limits to competence and applies that successfully in the best interests of the client.

Learning outcomes

LO1: To ensure that the practitioner is fully aware of his or her limits of competence and can refer as appropriate.

LO2: To ensure the practitioner complies with all professional boundaries and professional competencies.

LO3: To ensure the practitioner is knowledgeable in the field of nutrigenomics and demonstrates a sensitivity and willingness to work to the client needs.

2:1 Limits to competence

2:1:1 The practitioner demonstrates the recognition of their own limits to competence and can refer appropriately as necessary.

2:1:2 The practitioner demonstrates sensitivity to client needs and requirements and can meet the client at their level of understanding, accounting for possible developmental age and use of appropriate language.

2:2 Ethical considerations

2:2:3 The practitioner can delivery appropriate care without coercion or bias.

2:2:4 The practitioner is fully aware of confidentiality and data protection and can discuss client concerns regarding sharing of genetic data.

2:2:5 The practitioner must disclose the acceptance of commissions from tests and supplements.

2:2:7 Dealing with client concerns regarding personal data and adapt for differences in ethnicity, cultural and ethical beliefs and intellect.

3: Personal and professional development

Aims

- To ensure adequate training and development in the field of nutrigenomics, appreciating this as an evolving science.

Learning outcomes

LO1: To understand SNPs and their potential expression from a functional medicine perspective.

LO2: To develop an understanding of how foods, nutrients and environmental exposures affect SNPs.

LO3: To understand how to interpret patterns of heterozygous and homozygous SNPs and apply that knowledge to simple and complex cases.

LO4: To gain a thorough understanding of the strengths and weaknesses of different methods of DNA testing and the adjunctive functional testing.

LO5: To understand the benefits and limitations of the various available genetic interpretive applications.

LO6: To appreciate the need for appropriate and additional functional testing.

LO7: To develop an awareness of limits to competence and the importance of appropriate counselling when necessary for the client.

LO8: To ensure professional boundaries by compliance with BANT and CNHC codes of professional conduct.

3:1 Appreciate the importance of working in a holistic and/or collaborative way

3:1:1 Understand the concept of nutrigenomics, epigenetics and SNPs as an evolving science so there is a need to be connected to a practitioner forum.

3:1:2 Understand when there is a need to refer and who would be the most appropriate person to refer to.

3:1:3 Understand the need for collaboration with other HCPs in order to share best practice and experience.

3:1:4 Understand and recognize the need for further CPD training and ensure this personal need is met.

3:1:5 The practitioner must demonstrate an understanding of the importance of the family history and predisposition for disease.

3:2 Understanding biochemical pathways

3:2:1 Demonstrate understanding of specific biochemical pathways associated with nutrigenomics support.

3:2:2 Demonstrate understanding of how the specific biochemical pathways interrelate.

3:2:3 Demonstrate which pathways to support and in which order according to history, genomics interpretation and functional test results.

3:2:4 Demonstrate a good underpinning knowledge of cofactors, inhibitors, promoters and reactive oxygen species in relation to gene expression.

3:3 Evaluate interpretive applications

3:3:1 Demonstrate an awareness of a number of interpretive applications and their individual limitations.

3:3:2 Understand the basic concepts of nutrigenomics and genetics and the differences between them.

3:2:3 Appreciate the importance of being a good generalist.

3:2:4 Demonstrate the ability to choose appropriate functional tests, given the client's history and genetic data.

3:2:5 Knowing and understanding the interrelationships between groups of SNPs and between pathways.

3:2:6 Demonstrate application of knowledge and understanding within the functional medicine (FM) framework.

Reference

Skills for Health (n.d.) National Occupational Standards Overview. Accessed on 30/03/2021 at www.skillsforhealth.org.uk/info-hub/national-occupational-standards-overview

Appendix

HeartMath – what is it?

HeartMath is a set of tools to help the individual convert stress into resilience. It is an excellent tool for the technically savvy individual because it combines a sensor to measure heart rate variability (HRV) with an application to teach the user how to breathe mindfully. The sensor can be attached to the ear or finger and to the application on any mobile phone, iPad or laptop. There are versions for practitioners and for the general public. The application contains a number of meditations, games, a diary and, most importantly, feedback for the user in the form of a line graph while using the device. There are also various forms of presenting graphical data so the user can measure their own progress. For those who love to compete, not only can they compete with the software but they can also compete with others in the world via the cloud. Once the techniques have been learned, HeartMath can be used anywhere without the user feeling self-conscious. The latest innovative addition to the HeartMath portfolio is the opportunity to join regular online meditations with nations. They also support the moments of mass mindfulness (MOMM) group, who are working towards collective consciousness – or collective coherence, as HeartMath prefer. Biofeedback offers real-time insight into the individual's emotions, thoughts and behaviours, allowing the development of self-regulation.

HRV has been used as a measure of physiological coherence, stretching back 25 years. It is used extensively in sports. Coherence is an altered state of the autonomic nervous system towards increased parasympathetic activity. A reduction in autonomic outflow results in a lowered HRV. When an individual is coherent, there is an increased synchronicity between the heart and the brain. As the body becomes more into parasympathetic dominance, positive emotional shifts are said to trigger the release of DHEA and oxytocin, rather than the cortisol release from sympathetic dominance. Physicians and researchers consider HRV to be a marker of health and fitness.

When the individual practises HeartMath techniques, the state of coherence can be measured as represented in the graph below.

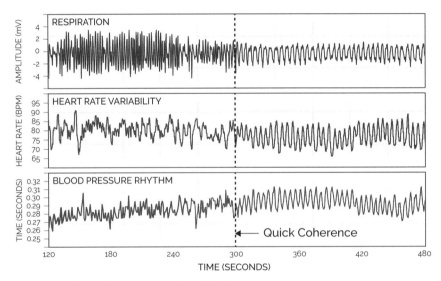

Figure A.1: The coherent state (HeartMath)
Image courtesy of the HeartMath® Institute – www.heartmath.org

This is a characteristic pattern of an individual who is clearly sympathetic dominant at commencement of HeartMath practice. The sine-wave-like pattern in the HRV trace can clearly be seen on the left (at the beginning) and on the right (at the end) of a session. There is an overall shift from sympathetic to parasympathetic dominance, indicating physiological entrainment or synchronicity of various body systems.

HRV research

Field *et al.* (2018) found HeartMath to be effective in improving HRV, coherence, mindfulness and relaxation in their mixed-methods study of individual with pharmaco-resistant focal epilepsy. Other studies have found a correlation between HeartMath practice and positive emotional states (Edwards 2015; McCraty & Schaffer 2015; Reiner *et al.* 2008). However, it would seem that consistent support with more guided training might be more effective than short training (Van der Zwan *et al.* 2015). Interestingly, Herrero *et al.* (2018), using intracranial electroencephalogram measurements, correlated limbic neuronal activity with the breath cycle. Breathing has always been thought to be an automatic process. They identified respiration-locked oscillation in the cortical and limbic areas of the brain. They also found stronger oscillations in the amygdala during voluntary rapid breathing. Hyperventilation is known to accompany high anxiety states (Homma & Masaoka 2008); behavioural performance may also be dependent on the breathing cycle, and fear recognition was faster when stimuli was presented on the inhalation peak (Zelano *et al.* 2016). Field *et al.* propose the use of breathing techniques to organize the cortical oscillations in the brain. Larger studies are needed to enhance this work.

ELLA'S CASE: LIFESTYLE APPROACHES TO REDUCE ANXIETY

The two initial HeartMath techniques taught to Ella were heart lock-in and quick coherence. For all HeartMath techniques, the grounding principle is to focus on the heart. Emotions such as love, compassion and gratitude are those to connect to for the session. As the client and practitioner identify the length and depth of breath that is appropriate, the client is also helped to find aspects of their life that they are grateful for. Gratitude is said to raise the individual's vibrational energy. Dr David Hawkins, an eminent psychiatrist and researcher, in his book *Power vs. Force* (1995), explains vibrational states in relation to human suffering, in his model 'Vibrational states of its corresponding emotion'. He is one of many researchers who suggest that to live in love and peace, humans need to raise their vibration to match that which they wish to attract. A lot of current life coaching, meditative practices and psycho-spiritual approaches are based on this foundation. Some would expand on this, stating that the word 'love' is not the individual romantic love one might assume, but an unconditional love created by collective consciousness.

Heart lock-in

After an initial coaching session using the emotional landscape template Ella was instructed on the heart lock-in exercise. It was recommended that Ella practise for five minutes twice daily, on waking and before retiring. This was to be gradually increased to 20 minutes per session. Ella felt she would find compliance easier with this timing than physically making time during the day. She did need something to help her during the day, in the event of her becoming overwhelmed by specific events or incidents.

Quick coherence

This was the second technique taught to Ella. This technique is a shortened version to be used in those 'curveball' moments that life can throw in to encourage personal growth. It takes 60–90 seconds to reset the stress response. If the individual is aware such an event is likely to happen (e.g. public speaking), the technique can be used immediately before and after the event. The first episode reduces the fear and the second rebalances the cortisol and adrenaline afterwards.

Meditation

Meditation was suggested to Ella at the first nutrigenomics appointment, but she had so much resistance to it at that point that the chances of being successful may have been severely limited, thereby feeding her lack of self-esteem at the time. This was a chance to explore the concept further. Ella had completed and enjoyed an eight-week course with the Brahma Kumaris group a few years earlier, but had not continued due to many life commitments that took her away from self-care. She was keen to revisit but explore the specific types of meditation to see how they resonated.

There are a number of types of meditation practice, the most common are listed below:

Loving kindness meditation

While breathing deeply, practitioners open their minds to loving kindness, then send messages of loving kindness to their loved ones, specific people or to the world. It is designed to promote feelings of compassion and love for oneself and others. Anger, frustration, resentment and interpersonal conflict are the types of emotions that may be helped by loving kindness. Lang *et al.* (2019), Kearney *et al.* (2014) and others found loving kindness meditation to be of benefit to those diagnosed with PTSD.

Body scan or progressive relaxation/somatic yoga

While breathing deeply, the practitioner scans their body, noticing tension and breathing into that or tightening the muscle, then letting go. This brings the body into a state or relaxation and encourages emotion/body awareness.

Mindfulness meditation

Mindfulness is about being present in the moment. Rather than dwelling on the past or fearing the future, mindfulness makes the individual aware of their current surroundings. Being in the moment means the individual ceases to judge. Mindfulness can be practised anywhere from the beach to the half-mile-long queue at the supermarket checkout. The checkout line is the best place to practise mindfulness, as the individual will note the wait without the judgement. Mindfulness has been shown to improve memory (Sevinc & Lazar 2019), improve focus (Vago & Zeiden 2016), reduce fixation on negative emotions (Wu *et al.* 2019), reduce impulsivity (Pozuelos *et al.* 2019), reduce emotional eating (Lattimore 2020) and improve relationship satisfaction (Campos *et al.* 2019), chronic kidney disease and hypertension (Thomas *et al.* 2017).

Breath awareness meditation
This meditation is about breathing deeply and slowly, focusing on the breath and no other thoughts. This offers the same benefits as mindfulness.

Kundalini yoga
Kundalini blends physical movement with deep breathing, awareness and mantras. Individuals need to learn from an experienced instructor before practising at home. Mental health such as depression and anxiety may be reduced, and physical strength is also improved. A chronic low-back pain study found that Kundalini reduced pain, increased energy and improved overall performance (Shannahoff-Khalsa 2005).

Zen meditation
Usually part of Buddhist practice, Zen may also be called Zazen. The practice requires more discipline than mindfulness due to the number of specific steps and postures required. Finding a comfortable position, focusing on the breath and mindfully observing thoughts without judgement makes this the type of meditation for those seeking a new spiritual path.

Transcendental meditation™
Transcendental meditation™ is a spiritual form of meditation. Remaining seated and breathing very slowly allows the individual to transcend above their current state of being. The focus is on a set of words or mantra that is repeated during the meditation. The teacher, based on a number of complex factors, chooses the mantra. The more contemporary version of TM allows individuals to choose their own mantra based on their own needs (e.g. 'I am not afraid of public speaking') while meditating. Those who practise transcendental meditation report a heightened state of awareness and spiritual experiences.

Meditation practices are sold to the general public with the best of intentions but this gives the individual the subliminal message that meditation is something very special that they need to buy into. William Bloom (2020) however, states that meditation is the human default mechanism. Humans use meditation to go inside themselves for healing. If Bloom's belief is taken into everyday life, meditation does not need to be sitting on a pranayama cushion cross-legged reciting OM. How many times do you drive for five miles and either miss a motorway exit or wonder how you got to this point? How many times do runners zone out while running? How many times do you zone out in front of the TV? Do you ever recall times when you have been driving on a long road and suddenly you gain insights? These are all reminders that humans are natural meditators. All humans require is to find the type that suits the individual at that point in time and appreciate this may change over time.

Specific recommended guided meditations that Ella found useful in the beginning when her focus on the mediation was poor included:

- Deepak Chopra free 21-day mediations – https://chopracenter-meditation.com
- Dr Joe Dispenza open heart meditation – www.youtube.com/watch?v=cVedMX8Qfww
- Kelly Howell binaural beats with guided meditations
  - Healing – https://youtu.be/QS7XowzEW0k
  - Inner peace – https://youtu.be/EVLVC7jlB5M
  - The secret universal mind – https://youtu.be/6tF14GnCJqk
- The Sensate pebble is a medical device designed by Dr Stefan Chmelik (www.getsensate.com). It is a Bluetooth device to help support vagal tone. It is a fairly new device that has been trialled with serious meditators and been found to enhance meditation practice. The device vibrates on the chest while medical resonance music or the sounds of nature are heard on headphones in the background. The music can be switched off so the listener can listen to other meditative sounds if needed and this was how Ella used the device for the most part.
- HeartMath Inner balance sensor and meditation app – www.heartmath.co.uk/shop.

References

Bloom W (2020) How meditation was invented (first published in *Cygnus Review* 2019). https://williambloom.com/2020/02/19/how-meditation-was-invented

Campos D, Modrego-Alarcón M, López-Del-Hoyo Y *et al.* (2019) Exploring the role of meditation and dispositional mindfulness on social cognition domains: A controlled study. *Frontiers in Psychology*. doi:10.3389/fpsyg.2019.00809

Edwards SD (2015) HeartMath: A positive psychology paradigm for promoting psychophysiological and global coherence. *Journal of Psychology in Africa 25*, 4, 367–374.

Field LH, Edwards SD, Edwards DJ *et al.* (2018) Influence of HeartMath training programme on physiological and psychological variables. *Global Journal of Health Science 10*. doi:10.5539/gjhs.v10n2p126

Hawkins DR (1995) *Power vs. Force: The Hidden Determinants of Human Behavior.* Carlsbad, CA: Hay House.

Herrero JL, Khuvis S, Yeagle E *et al.* (2018) Breathing above the brain stem: Volitional control and attentional modulation in humans. *Journal of Neurophysiology 119*, 1, 145–159. doi:10.1152/jn.00551.2017

Homma I, Masaoka Y (2008) Breathing rhythms and emotions. *Experimental Physiology 93*, 1011–1021. doi:10.1113/expphysiol.2008.042424

Kearney DJ, McManus C, Malte CA *et al.* (2014) Loving-kindness meditation and the broaden-and-build theory of positive emotions among veterans with posttraumatic stress disorder. *Medical Care 52*, 12 Suppl 5, S32–S38. doi:10.1097/MLR.0000000000000221

Lang AJ, Malaktaris AL, Casmar P *et al.* (2019) Compassion meditation for posttraumatic stress disorder in veterans: A randomized proof of concept study. *Journal of Traumatic Stress 32*, 2, 299–309. doi:10.1002/jts.22397

Lattimore P (2020) Mindfulness-based emotional eating awareness training: Taking the emotional out of eating. *Eating and Weight Disorders 25*, 3, 649–657. doi:10.1007/s40519-019-00667-y

McCraty R, Shaffer F (2015) Heart rate variability: New perspectives on physiological mechanisms, assessment of self-regulatory capacity, and health risk. *Global Advances in Health and Medicine 4*, 1, 46–61. doi:10.7453/gahmj.2014.073

Pozuelos JP, Mead BR, Rueda MR *et al.* (2019) Short-term mindful breath awareness training improves inhibitory control and response monitoring. *Progress in Brain Research 244*, 137–163. doi:10.1016/bs.pbr.2018.10.019

Reiner G, Atkinson M, McCraty R (2008) The physiological and psychological effects of compassion and anger. *Journal of Advancement in Medicine 8*, 2, 87–105.

Sevinc G, Lazar SW (2019) How does mindfulness training improve moral cognition: A theoretical and experimental framework for the study of embodied ethics. *Current Opinion in Psychology 28*, 268–272. https://doi.org/10.1016/j.copsyc.2019.02.006

Shannahoff-Khalsa DS (2005) Patient perspectives: Kundalini yoga meditation techniques for psycho-oncology and as potential therapies for cancer. *Integrative Cancer Therapies 4*, 1, 87–100. doi:10.1177/1534735404273841

Thomas Z, Novak M, Platas S *et al.* (2017) Brief mindfulness meditation for depression and anxiety symptoms in patients undergoing hemodialysis: A pilot feasibility study. *Clinical Journal of the American Society of Nephrology 12*, 12, 2008–2015. doi:10.2215/CJN.03900417

Vago DR, Zeidan F (2016) The brain on silent: mind wandering, mindful awareness, and states of mental tranquility. *Annals of the New York Academy of Sciences 1373*, 1, 96–113. doi:10.1111/nyas.13171

van der Zwan JE, de Vente W, Huizink AC *et al.* (2015) Physical activity, mindfulness meditation, or heart rate variability biofeedback for stress reduction: A randomized controlled trial. *Applied Psychophysiology and Biofeedback 40*, 4, 257–268. doi:10.1007/s10484-015-9293-x

Wu R, Liu L-L, Zhu H *et al.* (2019) Brief
mindfulness meditation improves emotion
processing. *Frontiers in Neuroscience 13*,
1074. doi:10.3389/fnins.2019.01074

Zelano C, Jiang H, Zhou G *et al.* (2016) Nasal
respiration entrains human limbic oscillations and modulates cognitive function.
Journal of Neuroscience 36, 49, 12448–12467.
doi:10.1323/JNEUROSCI.2586 16.2016

Subject Index

Author Index